State-of-the-Art Imaging of Head and Neck Tumors

Editor

GIRISH M. FATTERPEKAR

MAGNETIC RESONANCE IMAGING CLINICS OF NORTH AMERICA

www.mri.theclinics.com

Consulting Editors
SURESH K. MUKHERJI
LYNNE S. STEINBACH

February 2018 • Volume 26 • Number 1

ELSEVIER

1600 John F. Kennedy Boulevard • Suite 1800 • Philadelphia, Pennsylvania, 19103-2899

http://www.mri.theclinics.com

MRI CLINICS OF NORTH AMERICA Volume 26, Number 1
February 2018 ISSN 1064-9689, ISBN 13: 978-0-323-56988-0

Editor: John Vassallo (j.vassallo@elsevier.com)
Developmental Editor: Meredith Madeira

Magnetic Resonance Imaging Clinics of North America (ISSN 1064-9689) is published quarterly by Elsevier Inc., 360 Park Avenue South, New York, NY 10010-1710. Months of issue are February, May, August, and November. Business and Editorial Offices: 1600 John F. Kennedy Blvd., Ste. 1800, Philadelphia, PA 19103-2899. Customer Service Office: 3251 Riverport Lane, Maryland Heights, MO 63043. Periodicals postage paid at New York, NY and additional mailing offices. Subscription prices are $395.00 per year (domestic individuals), $701.00 per year (domestic institutions), $100.00 per year (domestic students/residents), $437.00 per year (Canadian individuals), $913.00 per year (Canadian institutions), $545.00 per year (international individuals), $913.00 per year (international institutions), and $275.00 per year (international and Canadian students/residents). International air speed delivery is included in all *Clinics* subscription prices. All prices are subject to change without notice. **POSTMASTER:** Send address changes to *Magnetic Resonance Imaging Clinics*, Elsevier Health Sciences Division, Subscription Customer Service, 3251 Riverport Lane, Maryland Heights, MO 63043. Customer Service (orders, claims, online, change of address): Elsevier Health Sciences Division, Subscription **Customer Service, 3251 Riverport Lane, Maryland Heights, MO 63043. Tel:1-800-654-2452 (U.S. and Canada); 314-447-8871 (outside U.S. and Canada). Fax: 314-447-8029. E-mail: journalscustomer service-usa@elsevier.com (for print support); journalsonlinesupport-usa@elsevier.com (for online support).**

Reprints. For copies of 100 or more of articles in this publication, please contact the Commercial Reprints Department, Elsevier Inc., 360 Park Avenue South, New York, NY 10010-1710. Tel.: 212-633-3874; Fax: 212-633-3820; E-mail: reprints@elsevier.com.

Magnetic Resonance Imaging Clinics of North America is covered in the *RSNA Index of Imaging Literature, MEDLINE/PubMed (Index Medicus),* and *EMBASE/Excerpta Medica.*

Contributors

CONSULTING EDITORS

SURESH K. MUKHERJI, MD, MBA, FACR
Professor and Chairman, Walter F. Patenge
Endowed Chair, Department of Radiology,
Michigan State University, Chief Medical
Officer and Director of Health Care Delivery,
Michigan State University Health Team, East
Lansing, Michigan, USA

LYNNE S. STEINBACH, MD, FACR
Professor of Radiology and Orthopaedic
Surgery, Department of Radiology and
Biomedical Imaging, University of California
San Francisco, San Francisco, California, USA

EDITOR

GIRISH M. FATTERPEKAR, MBBS, DNB, MD
Associate Professor, Department of Radiology,
NYU Langone Medical Center, NYU Radiology
Associates, Associate Section Chief, Division
of Neuroradiology, NYU School of Medicine,
New York, New York, USA

AUTHORS

ASHLEY H. AIKEN, MD
Associate Professor, Department of Radiology
and Imaging Sciences, Emory University
School of Medicine, Emory University Hospital,
Atlanta, Georgia, USA

YOSHIMI ANZAI, MD, MPH
Professor of Radiology, Associate Chief
Medical Quality Officer, Adjunct Professor of
Population Health Sciences, University of Utah
Health, Salt Lake City, Utah, USA

NAFI AYGUN, MD
Division of Neuroradiology, The Russell H.
Morgan Department of Radiology and
Radiologic Science, The Johns Hopkins
Hospital, Baltimore, Maryland, USA

PRADEEP BHAMBHVANI, MD
Department of Radiology, The University of
Alabama at Birmingham, Birmingham,
Alabama, USA

ARI BLITZ, MD
Division of Neuroradiology, The Russell H.
Morgan Department of Radiology and
Radiologic Science, The Johns Hopkins
Hospital, Baltimore, Maryland, USA

YIN JIE CHEN, MD
Department of Radiology, Perelman School of
Medicine University of Pennsylvania, Hospital
of the University of Pennsylvania, Philadelphia,
Pennsylvania, USA

MICHAEL CONNOLLY, MD
Department of Radiology, University of
Michigan, Ann Arbor, Michigan, USA

ADAM J. DAVIS, MD
Director of Research and Collaboration, Image
Processing Lab, Department of Radiology,
Clinical Associate Professor, NYU School of
Medicine, NYU Langone Medical Center,
New York, New York, USA

NAMAN S. DESAI, MD
Division of Neuroradiology, The Russell H.
Morgan Department of Radiology and
Radiologic Science, The Johns Hopkins
Hospital, Baltimore, Maryland, USA

GIRISH M. FATTERPEKAR, MBBS, DNB, MD
Associate Professor, Department of Radiology,
NYU Langone Medical Center, NYU Radiology
Associates, Associate Section Chief, Division
of Neuroradiology, NYU School of Medicine,
New York, New York, USA

REZA FORGHANI, MD, PhD
Assistant Professor, Department of Radiology,
Clinical Investigator, Segal Cancer Centre and
Lady Davis Institute for Medical Research,
Jewish General Hospital, McGill University,
Montreal, Quebec, Canada

SAMUEL J. GALGANO, MD
Department of Radiology, The University of
Alabama at Birmingham, Birmingham,
Alabama, USA

MARI HAGIWARA, MD
Assistant Professor, Department of Radiology,
NYU Langone Medical Center, NYU Radiology
Associates, New York, New York, USA

JENNY K. HOANG, MD
Department of Radiology, Duke University,
Duke University Medical Center, Durham,
North Carolina, USA

PATRICIA A. HUDGINS, MD
Professor, Department of Radiology and
Imaging Sciences, Emory University School of
Medicine, Emory University Hospital, Atlanta,
Georgia, USA

DEAN JEFFERY, MD
Division of Neuroradiology, The Russell H.
Morgan Department of Radiology and
Radiologic Science, The Johns Hopkins
Hospital, Baltimore, Maryland, USA

AMY JULIANO, MD
Staff Radiologist, Massachusetts Eye and Ear
Infirmary, Assistant Professor, Department of
Radiology, Harvard Medical School, Boston,
Massachusetts, USA

SURAJ J. KABADI, MD
Resident, Diagnostic Radiology, University of
Virginia Health System, Charlottesville,
Virginia, USA

CLAUDIA F.E. KIRSCH, MD
Professor of Neuroradiology and
Otolaryngology, Chief, Division of
Neuroradiology, Department of Radiology,
Northwell Health, Donald and Barbara Zucker
School of Medicine at Hofstra/Northwell,
Manhasset, New York, USA

SAMUEL J. KUZMINSKI, MD
Department of Radiological Sciences, The
University of Oklahoma Health Sciences
Center, College of Medicine, Oklahoma City,
Oklahoma, USA

RYAN V. MARSHALL, MD
Department of Otolaryngology, The University
of Alabama at Birmingham, Birmingham,
Alabama, USA

JONATHAN E. McCONATHY, MD, PhD
Department of Radiology, The University of
Alabama at Birmingham, Birmingham,
Alabama, USA

ERIK H. MIDDLEBROOKS, MD
Department of Radiology, The University of
Alabama at Birmingham, Birmingham,
Alabama, USA

JONATHAN MOGEN, MD
Fellow, Neuroradiology, NYU Langone Medical
Center, NYU Radiology Associates, New York,
New York, USA

SUYASH MOHAN, MD, PDCC
Assistant Professor of Radiology and
Neurosurgery, Department of Radiology,
Perelman School of Medicine University of
Pennsylvania, Hospital of the University of
Pennsylvania, Philadelphia, Pennsylvania, USA

GUL MOONIS, MD
Associate Professor, Department of Radiology,
Columbia University Medical Center, New
York, New York, USA

SOHIL H. PATEL, MD
Assistant Professor, Department of Radiology
and Medical Imaging, University of Virginia
Health System, Charlottesville, Virginia, USA

ALMUDENA PÉREZ-LARA, MD, PhD
Department of Radiology, Jewish General
Hospital, McGill University, Montreal, Quebec,
Canada

TANYA RATH, MD
Associate Professor, Departments of
Radiology and Otolaryngology, University of
Pittsburgh School of Medicine, Pittsburgh,
Pennsylvania, USA

RAZIA REHMANI, MD
Assistant Professor, Director of
Neuroradiology, St Barnabas Healthcare
System, Albert Einstein College of Medicine,
Bronx, New York, USA

ILONA M. SCHMALFUSS, MD
Department of Radiology, University of Florida,
Veterans Administration Medical Center,
Gainesville, Florida, USA

JULIE A. SOSA, MD
Department of Surgery, Duke University, Duke
University Medical Center, Durham, North
Carolina, USA

ASHOK SRINIVASAN, MD
Professor, Division of Neuroradiology,
Department of Radiology, University of
Michigan, Ann Arbor, Michigan, USA

JESSICA WEN, MD
The Russell H. Morgan Department of
Radiology and Radiologic Science, The
Johns Hopkins Hospital, Baltimore, Maryland,
USA

Contents

> Spectral computed tomography (CT) or dual-energy CT (DECT) is an advanced form of CT with increasing applications in head and neck radiology. This article provides an overview of the DECT technique and reviews current applications for the evaluation of neck pathology, focusing on oncologic applications. Included are an overview of the basic underlying principles and approaches for DECT scan acquisition and material characterization; a discussion of various DECT reconstructions and a brief overview of practical issues pertaining to DECT implementation, including those related to workflow impact of DECT; and a discussion of various applications of DECT for the evaluation of the neck, especially in oncology.

> Perfusion and permeability computed tomography and MR imaging applied to head and neck cancer provide powerful diagnostic and prognostic tools for clinicians. Understanding the basics of these techniques allows the radiologist to make informed decisions regarding the use of modeling algorithms, acquisition parameters, and postprocessing techniques. This helps to ensure that studies are acquired, analyzed, and reported appropriately and erroneous results are avoided. These techniques are highly automated, widely available, and can be easily and safely incorporated into daily imaging workflow.

> Head and neck cancers are among the most common cancers worldwide. More than 90% to 95% are squamous cell carcinomas (SCCs). Accurate staging at diagnosis optimizes treatment planning with improved outcomes. 18F-fluorodeoxyglucose (FDG) PET–computed tomography (CT) has shown tremendous value at diagnosis for accurate staging, treatment planning, and prognostication and after definitive therapy for assessing response and long-term surveillance. Novel non-FDG PET tracers are under investigation, which have great potential for improving patient care in this era of personalized medicine.

Pretreatment apparent diffusion coefficient (ADC) values can suggest the likelihood of response to treatment. DWI-obtained ADC values are able to look beyond the anatomy in posttreatment tumor beds and metastatic lymph nodes to evaluate for tumor recurrence. Further research should include large-scale, multiinstitutional studies to provide standardized ADC cutoff values for more widespread use.

Dynamic contrast-enhanced (DCE) MR imaging uses rapid sequential MR image acquisition before, during, and after intravenous contrast administration to elucidate information on the microvascular biologic function of tissues. The derived pharmacokinetic parameters provide useful information on tissue perfusion and permeability that may help to evaluate entities that otherwise appear similar by conventional imaging. When specifically applied to the evaluation of head and neck cancer, DCE-MR imaging may provide valuable information to help predict treatment response, discriminate between posttreatment changes and residual tumor, and discriminate between various head and neck neoplasms.

Primary hyperparathyroidism (PHPT) is characterized by excessive, dysregulated production of parathyroid hormone (PTH) by one or more abnormal parathyroid glands. Minimally invasive surgical techniques have created a need for more precise localization of the parathyroid lesion by imaging. A variety of imaging protocols and techniques have been used for this purpose, but no one modality is clearly superior. Nuclear medicine scintigraphy and ultrasound imaging are established modalities, although multiphase or 4-dimensional computed tomography is an emerging modality with several advantages. This article provides a background regarding PHPT and key anatomy and discusses these alternative parathyroid imaging modalities with updates.

Clinical PET/MR imaging is being implemented at institutions worldwide as part of the standard-of-care imaging for select oncology patients. This article focuses on oncologic applications of PET/MR imaging in cancers of the head and neck. Although the current published literature is relatively sparse, the potential benefits of a hybrid modality of PET/MR imaging are discussed along with several possible areas of research. With the increasing number of PET/MR imaging scanners in clinical use and ongoing research, the role of PET/MR imaging in the management of head and neck cancer is likely to become more evident in the near future.

MAGNETIC RESONANCE IMAGING CLINICS OF NORTH AMERICA

FORTHCOMING ISSUES

May 2018
Current MR Imaging of Breast Cancer
Jessica W. T. Leung, *Editor*

August 2018
MR Imaging of the Pancreas
Kumar Sandrasegaran and Dushyant V. Sahani,
Editors

November 2018
Advanced MSK Imaging
Roberto Domingues and Flavia Costa, *Editors*

RECENT ISSUES

November 2017
Update on Imaging Contrast Agents
Carlos A. Zamora and Mauricio Castillo, *Editors*

August 2017
Gynecologic Imaging
Katherine E. Maturen, *Editor*

May 2017
Hybrid PET/MR Imaging
Weili Lin, Sheng-Che Hung, Yueh Z. Lee, and
Terence Z. Wong, *Editors*

ISSUE OF RELATED INTEREST

Radiologic Clinics, November 2017 (Vol. 55, No. 6)
Cancer Screening
Dushyant V. Sahani, *Editor*
Available at: www.radiologic.theclinics.com

VISIT THE CLINICS ONLINE!
Access your subscription at:
www.theclinics.com

PROGRAM OBJECTIVE
The goal of *Magnetic Resonance Imaging Clinics of North America* is to keep practicing physicians up to date with current clinical practice by providing timely articles reviewing the state of the art in patient care.

TARGET AUDIENCE
All practicing physicians and healthcare professionals who provide patient care utilizing findings from Magnetic Resonance Imaging.

LEARNING OBJECTIVES
Upon completion of this activity, participants will be able to:
1. Review current evidence for PET-CT in head and neck cancer.
2. Discuss tips and strategies for the use of PET-MRI in imaging of head and neck cancer.
3. Recognize future directions for the use of PET-CT and PET-MRI in head and neck cancer.

ACCREDITATION
The Elsevier Office of Continuing Medical Education (EOCME) is accredited by the Accreditation Council for Continuing Medical Education (ACCME) to provide continuing medical education for physicians.

The EOCME designates this enduring material for a maximum of 15 *AMA PRA Category 1 Credit*(s)™. Physicians should claim only the credit commensurate with the extent of their participation in the activity.

All other healthcare professionals requesting continuing education credit for this enduring material will be issued a certificate of participation.

DISCLOSURE OF CONFLICTS OF INTEREST
The EOCME assesses conflict of interest with its instructors, faculty, planners, and other individuals who are in a position to control the content of CME activities. All relevant conflicts of interest that are identified are thoroughly vetted by EOCME for fair balance, scientific objectivity, and patient care recommendations. EOCME is committed to providing its learners with CME activities that promote improvements or quality in healthcare and not a specific proprietary business or a commercial interest.

The planning committee, staff, authors and editors listed below have identified no financial relationships or relationships to products or devices they or their spouse/life partner have with commercial interest related to the content of this CME activity:
Ashley H. Aiken, MD; Yoshimi Anzai, MD, MPH; Nafi Aygun, MD; Pradeep Bhambhvani, MD; Ari Blitz, MD; Yin Jie Chen, MD; Michael Connolly, MD; Naman S. Desai, MD; Girish M. Fatterpekar, MBBS, DNB, MD; Anjali Fortna; Samuel J. Galgano, MD; Mari Hagiwara, MD; Jenny K. Hoang, MD; Dean Jeffery, MD; Amy Juliano, MD; Suraj J. Kabadi, MD; Claudia F.E. Kirsch, MD; Samuel J. Kuzminski, MD; Leah Logan; Ryan V. Marshall, MD; Erik H. Middlebrooks, MD; Jonathan Mogen, MD; Gul Moonis, MD; Suresh K. Mukherji, MD, MBA, FACR; Sohil H. Patel, MD; Almudena Pérez-Lara, MD, PhD; Tanya Rath, MD; Razia Rehmani, MD; Ilona M. Schmalfuss, MD; Ashok Srinivasan, MD; Karthik Subramaniam; John Vassallo; Jessica Wen, MD.

The planning committee, staff, authors and editors listed below have identified financial relationships or relationships to products or devices they or their spouse/life partner have with commercial interest related to the content of this CME activity:
Adam J. Davis, MD is on the speakers' bureau for and a consultant/advisor for Siemens USA, and is a consultant/advisor for Olea Medical.
Reza Forghani, MD, PhD is a consultant/advisor for General Electric Company and Real Time Medical, and has stock ownership in Real Time Medical.
Patricia A. Hudgins, MD receives royalties/patents from Elsevier.
Jonathan E. McConathy, MD, PhD is a consultant/advisor for Blue Earth Diagnostics Limited; General Electric Company; and Eli Lilly and Company, is a consultant/advisor for AlphaSource, Inc, has research support from Blue Earth Diagnostics Limited and Eli Lilly and Company, and his spouse/partner has research support from AbbVie Inc. and Navidea Biopharmaceuticals, Inc.
Suyash Mohan, MD, PDCC has research support from Radiological Society of North America; Novocure; and Galileo CDS, Inc.
Julie A. Sosa, MD is a consultant/advisor for Novo Nordisk A/S; GlaxoSmithKline plc; AstraZeneca; and Eli Lilly and Company.

UNAPPROVED/OFF-LABEL USE DISCLOSURE
The EOCME requires CME faculty to disclose to the participants:
1. When products or procedures being discussed are off-label, unlabelled, experimental, and/or investigational (not US Food and Drug Administration [FDA] approved); and
2. Any limitations on the information presented, such as data that are preliminary or that represent ongoing research, interim analyses, and/or unsupported opinions. Faculty may discuss information about pharmaceutical agents that is outside of FDA-approved labelling. This information is intended solely for CME and is not intended to promote off-label use of these

medications. If you have any questions, contact the medical affairs department of the manufacturer for the most recent pre-scribing information.

TO ENROLL
To enroll in the *Magnetic Resonance Imaging Clinics of North America* Continuing Medical Education program, call customer service at 1-800-654-2452 or sign up online at http://www.theclinics.com/home/cme. The CME program is available to sub-scribers for an additional annual fee of USD 250.

METHOD OF PARTICIPATION
In order to claim credit, participants must complete the following:
1. Complete enrolment as indicated above.
2. Read the activity.
3. Complete the CME Test and Evaluation. Participants must achieve a score of 70% on the test. All CME Tests and Evalua-tions must be completed online.

CME INQUIRIES/SPECIAL NEEDS
For all CME inquiries or special needs, please contact elsevierCME@elsevier.com.

Foreword

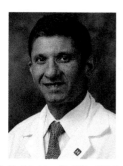

Suresh K. Mukherji, MD, MBA, FACR
Consulting Editor

Coincidentally, I received the request to write the Foreword to this issue on *Magnetic Resonance Imaging Clinics of North America* dedicated to Head and Neck Radiology as I was returning from the 2017 annual meeting of the American Society of Head and Neck Radiology. This issue, expertly edited by Dr Girish Fatterpekar, covers the most important topics discussed at this year's meeting! Therefore, I can undoubtedly say this issue of *Magnetic Resonance Imaging Clinics of North America* covers the most important and timely topics in Head and Neck Radiology. Dr Fatterpekar has done an outstanding job of inviting supremely talented article authors who are leaders in their field of expertise. I sincerely thank the authors for their wonderful contributions.

On a personnel note, Girish was my first international research fellow that I recruited as a junior faculty at UNC–Chapel Hill. He made the difficult decision to leave his family and travel halfway around the world to work with someone he had never met. The good Lord did not bestow many "gifts" upon me, but he did give me the ability to identify "talent" and "character" and I quickly realized Girish had both. Girish was an exemplary fellow, and I have been both happy and proud to watch him rapidly ascend the academic ranks. Girish....Congratulations on all you have accomplished and are destined to achieve....You truly deserve it, my friend!!

Suresh K. Mukherji, MD, MBA, FACR
Department of Radiology
Michigan State University
Michigan State University Health Team
846 Service Road
East Lansing, MI 48824, USA

E-mail address:
mukherji@rad.msu.edu

https://doi.org/10.1016/j.mric.2017.10.002
1064-9689/18/© 2017 Published by Elsevier Inc.

mri.theclinics.com

Preface

Advanced Imaging in Head and Neck Tumors

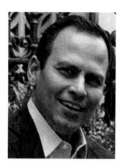

Girish M. Fatterpekar, MBBS, DNB, MD
Editor

The last few years of *Magnetic Resonance Imaging Clinics of North America* have not seen any focused Head and Neck issue. In fact, the last such publication that did concentrate on Head and Neck was in 2013. I would therefore like to thank Suresh Mukherji, MD (Consulting Editor) for providing me this opportunity, and truly consider it to be an honor to be the Guest Editor on this subject.

Head and Neck by itself can be pretty broad. To keep it focused, I considered tumors to be a good central theme. At the same time, I wanted to provide the readers with an issue that was cutting edge, "clinically relevant," and with the right technical support easy to implement. This current issue therefore concentrates on state-of-the-art computed tomography (CT) and MR imaging in head and neck tumors. Toward this, I would like to thank Dr Mukherji for allowing me to include some CT topics as well.

This particular issue has been largely organized such that the CT advances are discussed first, followed by MR applications, and finally, ending with PET-MR, which promises to play a significant role, albeit slowly, in our understanding and management of head and neck tumors. In addition, I have purposefully included a couple of articles that provide radiology pearls in terms of routine day-to-day imaging, including the imaging modality/sequences to use depending on the underlying clinical history, image acquisition strategies, and what to look for when evaluating different types of head and neck tumors. An article dedicated to generating a standardized report when evaluating head and neck tumors is also included.

I would like to take this opportunity to thank all the authors for their contributions. As the demand for RVUs (relative value units) keeps increasing with numerous other clinical and administrative responsibilities, I truly appreciate your efforts. Most of the authors are authoritative figures on the topic, and I think the readers stand to benefit from getting a wonderful, and, I dare say, much needed "update" on "Advanced Imaging in Head and Neck Tumors" from this single issue.

Finally, I would like to extend my gratitude to John Vassallo, Nicole Congleton, Meredith Madeira, and the staff at Elsevier for their patience and support.

It is my genuine hope that this issue will prove useful to the readers. Feedback is important and will be much appreciated. I can be reached at Girish.Fatterpekar@nyumc.org.

Girish M. Fatterpekar, MBBS, DNB, MD
Department of Radiology
NYU School of Medicine
660 1st Avenue, 2nd Floor, Room 224
New York, NY 10016, USA

E-mail address:
Girish.Fatterpekar@nyumc.org

Magn Reson Imaging Clin N Am 26 (2018) xv
https://doi.org/10.1016/j.mric.2017.10.001
1064-9689/18/© 2017 Published by Elsevier Inc.

Spectral Computed Tomography
Technique and Applications for Head and Neck Cancer

Almudena Pérez-Lara, MD, PhD[a], Reza Forghani, MD, PhD[b],*

KEYWORDS

- Dual-energy CT • Virtual monochromatic images • Spectral Hounsfield unit attenuation curves
- Iodine map • Squamous cell carcinoma • Cartilage invasion • Artifact reduction • Workflow

KEY POINTS

- There are increasing applications of spectral or dual-energy CT (DECT) for the evaluation of the neck, particularly head and neck squamous cell carcinoma (HNSCC).
- Low-energy DECT virtual monochromatic images can improve tumor visibility and soft tissue boundary delineation.
- High-energy DECT virtual monochromatic images and iodine maps can improve diagnostic evaluation of thyroid cartilage invasion; high-energy reconstructions can also be used to reduce dental artifact.
- Several other applications under investigation are likely to further increase the use and impact of DECT for diagnostic evaluation of the neck in the future.

INTRODUCTION

There is increasing use of spectral or dual-energy CT (DECT) in routine clinical practice. In the neck, multiple innovative applications of this technique have been shown to improve detection, characterization, and delineation of the extent of head and neck cancer, improving overall diagnostic evaluation.[1–4] This article provides an overview of the DECT technique and its applications in the neck, focusing on head and neck oncology. The review begins with an overview of the basic underlying principles and approaches for DECT scan acquisition and material characterization, which form the basis for different clinical applications of DECT and its optimal use. This is followed by a discussion of basic and essential information for the use of this technology in the clinical setting. The common types of DECT reconstructions that are generated are reviewed, followed by a brief overview of practical issues pertaining to DECT implementation, including those related to radiation dose and workflow impact of DECT. A detailed discussion of oncologic applications of DECT,

Disclosures: R. Forghani has acted as a consultant for GE Healthcare and has served as a speaker at lunch and learn sessions titled "Dual-Energy CT Applications in Neuroradiology and Head and Neck Imaging" sponsored by GE Healthcare at the 27th and 28th Annual Meetings of the Eastern Neuroradiological Society in 2015 and 2016 (no personal compensation or travel support for these sessions). A. Pérez-Lara declares no relevant conflict of interest.
[a] Department of Radiology, Jewish General Hospital, McGill University, Room C-212.1, 3755 Cote Ste-Catherine Road, Montreal, Quebec H3T 1E2, Canada; [b] Department of Radiology, Segal Cancer Centre and Lady Davis Institute for Medical Research, Jewish General Hospital, McGill University, Room C-212.1, 3755 Cote Ste-Catherine Road, Montreal, Quebec H3T 1E2, Canada
* Corresponding author.
E-mail address: rforghani@jgh.mcgill.ca

Magn Reson Imaging Clin N Am 26 (2018) 1–17
http://dx.doi.org/10.1016/j.mric.2017.08.001
1064-9689/18/© 2017 Elsevier Inc. All rights reserved.

mri.theclinics.com

focusing on head and neck squamous cell carcinoma (HNSCC), then follows. This includes a discussion of the use of specialized DECT reconstructions for improving tumor visualization and soft tissue boundary delineation, evaluation of thyroid cartilage invasion, and reduction of dental artifact for improving assessment of oral cavity and the oropharynx. A multiparametric approach using different DECT reconstructions is discussed, summarizing key reconstructions and their application. The article concludes with a brief discussion of applications under investigations and other exciting emerging applications of this technology in the head and neck.

OVERVIEW OF DUAL-ENERGY COMPUTED TOMOGRAPHY TECHNIQUE

A detailed discussion of the physics underlying DECT and different DECT systems is beyond the scope of this article and is found elsewhere.[5–9] However, familiarity with the basic principles underlying DECT scan acquisition, image processing, and analysis is essential for successful implementation and optimal use of this technique and is reviewed here. DECT consists of obtaining projecting data at two different peak energies. The raw data obtained from each of the two acquisitions are then processed and blended to generate different types of image reconstructions or to perform advanced quantitative analysis, such as generation of spectral Hounsfield unit attenuations curves (SHUACs) demonstrating the energy-dependent attenuation changes of a tissue of interest, as discussed in the subsequent sections. Although the terms DECT and spectral CT are sometimes used interchangeably, spectral CT could also encompass more advanced CT systems capable of discrimination between more than two spectra, such as the photon counting scanners currently under development experimentally.

The two different energy acquisitions in DECT are commonly at 80 to 100 kVp (lower energy acquisition) and 140 to 150 kVp (higher energy acquisition).[5,8] The reason behind this is that at energy peaks significantly lower than 80 kVp, a high proportion of the photons are absorbed by the tissues with little clinically useful information generated. At energy peaks significantly higher than 140/150 kVp, the dose may become prohibitively high and there is little soft tissue contrast, limiting usefulness in most clinical scenarios. These settings can vary depending on the scanner type, generation/model, other factors (eg, use of filters with dual source scanners), and for highly specialized applications. The basic requirements for DECT scan acquisition are summarized in Box 1.

DUAL-ENERGY COMPUTED TOMOGRAPHY SCANNING SYSTEMS: A REVIEW OF CURRENT AND EMERGING TECHNOLOGY

Since the first DECT scanner was approved for clinical use in 2006 (dual source DECT, Siemens AG, Forchheim, Germany),[10,11] the technology has significantly evolved and there are multiple scanning systems currently available for use in clinical practice.[7,8] Some DECT systems have been refined over time (and continue to be refined) to address important challenges including optimizing radiation dose, image quality, improving material decomposition and other postprocessing tasks, reducing postprocessing times, and addressing ease of use and a more workflow friendly implementation. The different DECT approaches and scanner types are reviewed next. A more detailed discussion of different DECT systems can also be found in other recently published reviews on this topic.[7–9]

Dual-Source Dual-Energy Computed Tomography

Dual-source DECT scanners consist of two source X-ray tubes combined with separate detector arrays (Siemens AG) (**Fig. 1**).[5,7,8,12] The tubes and detector layers are aligned at a perpendicular or near-perpendicular angle, so that the same volume is scanned with the high and low energy X-ray beams simultaneously. The main advantage of this system is the use of separate imaging chains for the acquisition of the low- and high-energy spectra, enabling independent adjustment of the tube voltage and current for each chain and facilitating balancing of the quanta emitted from the two tubes. This can help improve separation of the low- and high-energy spectra. Depending on the model, filters may also be applied at the source, further optimizing quality and decreasing

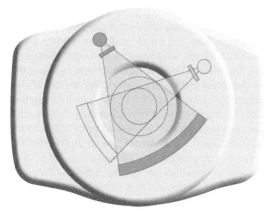

Fig. 1. Schematic diagram of a dual-source DECT, consisting of dual-source and detector combinations (Siemens AG, Forchheim, Germany). The two imaging chains are set in a nearly orthogonal plane, allowing for simultaneous scanning of the same area of the patient. Because there are two separate sources, filters can be placed at the source for additional beam optimization. Yellow is used to illustrate the low-energy spectrum and blue the high-energy spectrum. (*Courtesy of Reza Forghani, MD, PhD, Montreal, Quebec, Canada; and Bruno De Man, PhD, Niskayuna, NY.*)

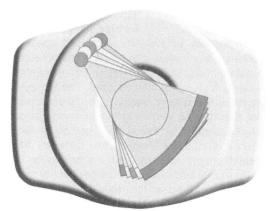

Fig. 2. Schematic diagram of a single-source DECT with rapid kilovolt peak switching (Gemstone spectral imaging; GE Healthcare, Waukesha, WI). These scanners consist of a single source–detector combination. The X-ray tube rapidly switches between low- and high-energy spectra that are recorded using the fast sampling capabilities of a garnet-based scintillator detector with low afterglow for spectral separation at each successive axial or spiral acquisition. Yellow is used to illustrate the low-energy spectrum and blue the high-energy spectrum. (*Courtesy of Reza Forghani, MD, PhD, Montreal, Quebec, Canada; and Bruno De Man, PhD, Niskayuna, NY.*)

image noise. Among the disadvantages, one is that a different part of the patient is scanned at any given time. Therefore, material decomposition can only be performed in the image domain, which is theoretically less robust. This also results in a small temporal skew or delay between the low- and high-energy acquisitions. There can also be cross-scatter between the two imaging chains resulting in data contamination, although different technical innovations are applied to at least partly reduce cross-scatter and make appropriate corrections during image reconstruction. Because of space limitations in the CT gantry, the second detector is smaller, resulting in a smaller field of view when used in DECT mode (eg, 27, 33, or 35 cm, depending on the model) versus full field of view of 50 cm in single-energy CT (SECT) mode.

Single-Source Dual-Energy Computed Tomography with Rapid Kilovolt Peak Switching (Gemstone Spectral Imaging)

Fast kilovolt peak switching scanners, also referred to as Gemstone spectral imaging, are based on a single X-ray source and detector combination (GE Healthcare, Waukesha, WI) (**Fig. 2**).[5,13,14] This is made possible by a highly specialized generator capable of rapid transitions between the 80 and 140 kVp voltages and the fast sampling capabilities of a proprietary garnet-based scintillator called Gemstone. The voltage

of the tube follows a nearly square waveform, alternating between low and high kilovolt peak on a view-by-view basis to obtain projection data. This results in a very short delay (or temporal skew) between the high- and low-energy acquisitions of 50 μs, with excellent spatiotemporal registration. Advantages of these systems are a cost-efficient design with excellent temporal and spatial registration that enables material decomposition to be performed directly in the projection domain. In addition, DECT scanning is at the full field of view of 50 cm. One of the disadvantages of this approach pertains to the adaptation of the current that can result in reduction of signal from the low-energy spectrum. However, this is at least in part mitigated by increasing the time allocated for the low-energy acquisition to help balance relative photon flux between the two energies. Another disadvantage is that the voltage does not have a purely rectangular shape, resulting in a spectral difference slightly lower than the nominal tube voltages. This is taken into account during image reconstruction.

Layered or "Sandwich" Detector Dual-Energy Computed Tomography

Layered detector DECT systems also consist of a single X-ray source and a single detector array but achieve spectral separation using highly specialized detectors (Philips Healthcare, Andover, MA) (**Fig. 3**).[5,7,15,16] A single CT scan is performed (usually at 120–140 kVp), and spectral separation is achieved at the level of the detector consisting of two scintillator layers with differential sensitivity for X-ray photon energies. The top layer absorbs lower energy photons, and the second layer absorbs the remaining higher energy photons. Advantages of this system include perfect temporal and spatial registration between the different energy spectra, and the capability to scan at the full field of view. Because spectral separation is achieved at the detector level, these scans are essentially always acquired in DECT mode. One of the disadvantages of this system is the lower energy separation between low- and high-energy spectrum, related to the absorption properties of the scintillator. Although these systems do not have the problems of cross-scatter discussed for dual-source scanners, they are susceptible to a different type of cross-scatter between the two detector layers.

Single-Source Dual-Energy Computed Tomography with Beam Filtration at the Source (TwinBeam Dual-Energy Computed Tomography)

This system is based on a single X-ray source and detector combination, with spectral separation at

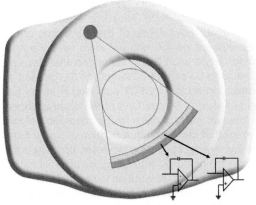

Fig. 3. Schematic diagram of a layered or "sandwich" detector DECT (Philips Healthcare, Andover, MA). In this single source–detector combination system, the polychromatic X-ray beam is generated at a single peak energy and spectral separation is achieved at the level of the detector arrays. Specialized detectors consisting of two layers with maximal sensitivity for low- and high-energy photons form the basis for spectral separation using these scanners. Yellow is used to illustrate the low-energy spectrum and blue the high-energy spectrum. (*Courtesy of* Reza Forghani, MD, PhD, Montreal, Quebec, Canada; and Bruno De Man, PhD, Niskayuna, NY.)

the level of the source achieved by prefiltering of the beam using two different materials, gold and tin. These two materials split the single X-ray beam into a high- and low-energy beam (Siemens AG) (**Fig. 4**).[17,18] The low- and high-energy spectra are detected by the corresponding halves of the detector. Advantages of this system include the ability to scan at the full field of view and less complex and less costly hardware design. The main disadvantage of this technique is that different parts of the patient are irradiated at low- and high-energy spectra per gantry rotation. This implies that helical acquisitions have to be performed to ensure scanning of the same area at low and high energies, resulting in decreased temporal resolution and registration between the low- and high-energy acquisitions. Because of the design, the central 2- to 3-mm portion of the beam has a mixed energy spectrum and there is also potential for cross-scatter between the two sides.

Dual-Energy Computed Tomography Scanning Using Sequential Acquisitions

The sequential acquisition approach is the least complex approach for DECT scanning from a hardware perspective (**Fig. 5**).[5,7,19,20] With these systems, the different energy data are obtained sequentially and combined to generate a DECT scan. The obvious major disadvantage of this approach is the significant potential for spatial misregistration caused by motion between the two different energy acquisitions and temporal delay between the two energy spectra. Some design innovations can reduce the time between the two acquisitions and partially mitigate these challenges, such as by alternating scanning at low and high peak kilovolt for each gantry rotation instead of the entire scan volume. Even then, these factors may limit successful application of this technology to certain niche areas, with less optimal results for processes requiring high temporal resolution, such as vascular or perfusion examinations.

FUNDAMENTALS OF DUAL-ENERGY COMPUTED TOMOGRAPHY TISSUE CHARACTERIZATION

CT attenuation depends on three different physical processes or interactions between X-rays and matter: (1) Compton scatter, (2) photoelectric effect, and (3) Rayleigh scatter (the latter typically considered negligible).[5,9] Compton scatter accounts for a large component of attenuation seen in CT scanning but shows little energy dependency. The photoelectric effect, which is highly dependent on an element's atomic number (Z), is

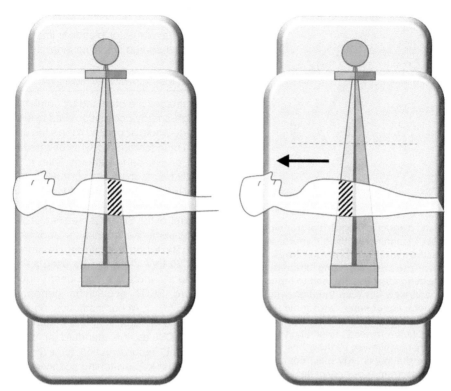

Fig. 4. Schematic diagram of single-source DECT with beam filtration at the source: TwinBeam DECT (Siemens AG). In this type of a single source–detector combination system, a split filter (containing gold and tin) is placed at the output of the tube to split the X-ray beam into low- and high-energy photons. The corresponding halves of the detector are then used for detection of the low- and high-energy spectra, respectively. (*Courtesy of* Reza Forghani, MD, PhD, Montreal, Quebec, Canada; and Bruno De Man, PhD, Niskayuna, NY.)

highly energy dependent and in general, the higher the atomic number of an element, the stronger the probability of photoelectric interactions. Therefore, although the Compton and photoelectric effect are both important for overall attenuation and material decomposition in DECT, the photoelectric effect is the main process underlying the energy dependent or "spectral" changes in attenuation seen with DECT. As a result, materials with higher atomic numbers are sometimes characterized as having strong "spectral" properties.

To understand the energy-dependent changes seen in DECT, one needs to be familiar with the concept of an element's K-edge. The probability of photoelectric interactions abruptly increases at the K-edge of an element and subsequently decreases with increasing photon energy. As a result, there is a rapid rise or spike in an element's attenuation at the K-edge, followed by a rapid drop in attenuation with further increase in energy above the K-edge. This explains the energy-dependent changes in the attenuation of elements with "strong" spectral properties, such as iodine (**Fig. 6**). Elements with a high atomic number, such as iodine (Z = 53), have strong energy

dependency of their attenuation. In addition to being present in the thyroid gland, iodine is the main constituent of most CT contrast agents, and the strong energy dependency of its attenuation can be exploited for tissue characterization and lesion visualization in the head and neck, as discussed later. Elements with low atomic number (eg, hydrogen [Z = 1], carbon [Z = 6], or oxygen [Z = 8]), common constituents of tissues in the human body, have weak photoelectric interactions, and may show little energy dependency of their attenuation (see **Fig. 6**). In general, if two elements or materials have significantly different atomic or effective atomic numbers, they may be distinguishable from one another based on their energy-dependent or spectral properties.

DUAL-ENERGY COMPUTED TOMOGRAPHY IMAGE RECONSTRUCTIONS AND MATERIAL DECOMPOSITION MAPS FOR THE EVALUATION OF THE NECK

There are various methods and algorithms for combining the data obtained from the low- and high-energy acquisitions from a DECT scan into

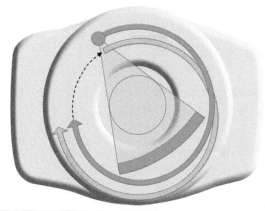

Fig. 5. Schematic diagram of sequential scanning approaches to DECT scanning. With this approach, the spectral data at the two different energies are acquired by scanning twice sequentially using different tube voltages. Some design features are used to reduce the delay or temporal skew between the high- and low-energy acquisitions. For example, with some systems, scanning at the two energies is performed sequentially for each gantry rotation, instead of scanning the entire volume at one energy followed by the other. Yellow is used to illustrate the low-energy spectrum and blue the high-energy spectrum. (*Courtesy of* Reza Forghani, MD, PhD, Montreal, Quebec, Canada; and Bruno De Man, PhD, Niskayuna, NY.)

an image set. Currently, the most commonly used reconstructions in head and neck radiology are virtual monochromatic images (VMIs) and material decomposition maps (**Fig. 7**).[2,3,9] The other

commonly obtained reconstruction is the weighted average (or blended) image (WA) if one has a dual-source DECT scanner.

Virtual Monochromatic Images

These images are obtained by combining the low- and high-energy acquisition data to simulate what an image would appear as if the scan was acquired using a monochromatic X-ray beam at a given predicted or prescribed energy level.[2,3,9] VMIs can typically be reconstructed from 40 to 140 keV but some DECT systems allow for reconstructions at even higher energy levels. The VMI is the "image correlate" of the SHUACs (see **Fig. 6**), which represent the numerical attenuation at different VMI energies. Based on the current literature, either the 65- or 70-keV VMIs can be used as a substitute for, and therefore are considered equivalent to a standard SECT acquisition performed at 120 kVp.[2,3,8,9,21–25] At our institution, 65-keV VMIs are sent to picture archiving and communication system (PACS) as the standard or default "SECT equivalent" reconstruction for every neck DECT using a fast kVp switching scanner, based on the studies showing the highest signal-to-noise ratio at this energy (slightly higher than 70 keV).[25,26]

In addition to the routine 65- or 70-keV VMIs, VMIs reconstructed at other energies have been demonstrated to be useful for specific applications in the neck. For example, low-energy VMIs, such as the 40-keV VMI, increase iodine attenuation

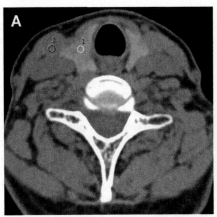
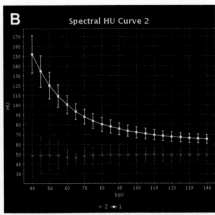

Fig. 6. Examples of weak and strong spectral or energy dependency of the attenuation of different tissues. (*A*) Axial noncontrast DECT image of the neck is shown, acquired using a fast kilovolt peak switching scanner. Region of interest analysis was performed comparing the SHUACs of muscle (*2, red*) and the thyroid gland (*1, yellow*). (*B*) The corresponding SHUACs of region of interest shown in A demonstrate differences in energy-dependent attenuation of muscle and thyroid gland. Most soft tissues, such as muscle, contain a large component of low Z elements, such as hydrogen, carbon, and oxygen. As a result, there is little change in the attenuation of muscle at different energies on a noncontrast CT. Tissues containing high atomic number elements, such as iodine (Z = 53) in the thyroid gland, however, have strong spectral properties. This is shown by the significant changes in the attenuation of the thyroid gland at different energies, with a marked increase in attenuation at lower energies approaching the K-edge of iodine (33.2 keV).

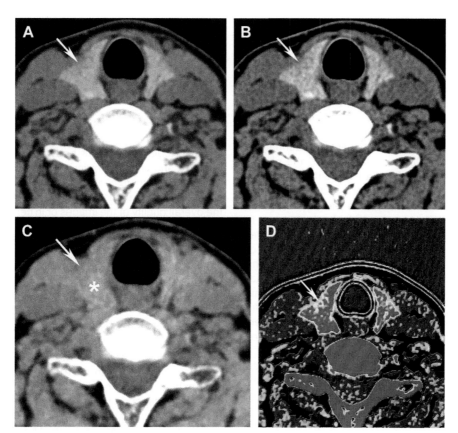

Fig. 7. Examples of DECT VMI and basis material decomposition maps using a noncontrast DECT of the neck acquired with a fast kilovolt peak switching scanner. (A) 65-keV VMI, (B) 40-keV VMI, (C) virtual noncontrast (water-iodine) material decomposition map, and (D) iodine map (iodine-water material decomposition map) are shown. Note the increase in the attenuation of the iodine containing thyroid gland (*arrow*) on the low-energy (40 keV; B) VMI compared with the 65-keV VMI (A), although this comes at the expense of increased image noise. For comparison purposes, the images are displayed using the same window-level settings. Material decomposition maps can be created to remove iodine from the images on virtual noncontrast images (C; eg, *asterisk* on the right thyroid lobe) or demonstrate iodine distribution and estimated concentration within tissues on iodine maps (D).

and therefore attenuation of enhancing lesions, such as tumor.[25–28] High-energy VMIs are used to reduce metallic or dental artifact and also can help distinguish nonossified thyroid cartilage (NOTC) from tumor.[24,29–34] These are discussed in detail in the upcoming section on DECT applications for the evaluation of head and neck cancer. However, some general principles should be kept in mind when using these reconstructions. For example, although iodine attenuation increases with decreasing VMI energy approaching 40-keV VMIs, this comes at the expense of image noise. VMIs reconstructed at energies much higher than the 65- or 70-keV VMIs can decrease artifact but also result in decreased iodine attenuation and soft tissue contrast. These are important trade-offs and partly the reason behind a recommended multiparametric scan interpretation approach in which different reconstructions complement one another for optimal diagnostic interpretation, akin to the use of different MR imaging sequences for interpretation.[3]

Weighted Average Images

This type of reconstruction is routinely generated with dual-source CT systems. WA images are created by blending of the data from the two energy acquisitions. Typically, images created using a combination 30% of the low and 70% of the high-energy data are considered equivalent to 120-kVp SECT images.[27,35–37] However, similar to VMIs, specific tissue characteristics and attenuation of materials of interest are accentuated by changing the proportion of the data blended or modifying the reconstruction algorithm, as discussed in the sections that follow.

Material Decomposition Maps

In addition to VMIs or WA images, another type of reconstruction possible with DECT that cannot be obtained with SECT is the basis material decomposition map.[7,9] In broad terms, basis material decomposition is based on the fact that the X-ray attenuation of any material can be represented as a linear combination of Compton scatter attenuation and photoelectric attenuation. Therefore, the Compton scatter and the photoelectric effect can form a material basis pair in which all materials are expressed, although for clinical DECT scanners, it is more common to express materials in a material basis pair that is more relatable to human tissues, such as water and iodine. Although a detailed discussion of how these maps are generated is beyond the scope of this article, it is important to be familiar with the strengths and weaknesses of this approach. Basis material decomposition is useful for characterization of a tissue or material of interest by cross-correlating its attenuation properties to known materials.

Through basis material decomposition, one can generate iodine overlay maps that provide an estimate of the tissue distribution and concentration of iodine (see **Fig. 7**D), or virtual noncontrast images (see **Fig. 7**C), among many other types of maps. These are powerful tools but one must be aware of their limitations for optimal application. Based on the description of how these are derived, one can deduce that these maps cannot be interpreted as the physical distribution of *pure* iodine or *pure* water. For example, bone or calcified tissue is bright on both the iodine and the water maps, which is the reason why osseous structures, such as vertebral bodies (or ossified part of the thyroid cartilage), have high "signal" on the iodine map (see **Fig. 7**D) that should not be confused with pure or high iodine content. Most of the time, this pitfall in interpretation is easily avoidable by comparing with standard images (eg, 65-keV VMIs). Less commonly, when the distinction is not clear and clinically important, other types of maps can be created to address a clinical question of interest, such as calcium maps or staining in brain imaging.[38] The presence of artifact, especially if severe, can also result in misclassification, again usually avoidable if the material decomposition maps are interpreted in conjunction with the standard images. This again highlights the importance of the previously suggested multiparametric approach of using different DECT images in combination for optimal diagnostic evaluation.[3] For interested readers, a more detailed discussion of basis material decomposition maps is found in a recent article by Forghani and colleagues[9] discussing different DECT reconstructions.

OVERVIEW OF RADIATION DOSE AND IMAGE QUALITY IN DUAL-ENERGY COMPUTED TOMOGRAPHY

Although increased patient radiation exposure was a concern with early applications of DECT, various studies in different body parts, including the head and neck, have demonstrated that modern DECT scanners enable scan acquisition at an acceptable, similar dose to SECT without reducing the overall quality of the images or in certain cases yielding an even better image quality.[21,25,35,39–41] As such, the additional reconstructions and advanced quantitative analytical capabilities of DECT represent an advantage compared with SECT. For those starting to implement DECT, it is nonetheless recommended that special attention be paid to the radiation dose using SECT scanners in their departments, and available society guidelines and recommendations where applicable, to ensure that the DECT protocols are optimized with radiation dose as low as reasonably achievable. Of course, the dose considerations also depend on the patient population and demographics. Minor dose adjustments in the head and neck cancer population, many of whom have radiation therapy as part of their therapeutic regimen, is unlikely to be of any significance and it is the author's philosophy that in such instances, the focus should be to obtain a high-quality diagnostic evaluation that enables confident diagnosis and staging, essential for appropriate patient management. The consideration is different in the pediatric population where much more aggressive dose reduction strategies may be required.

WORKFLOW IMPLICATIONS OF DUAL-ENERGY COMPUTED TOMOGRAPHY

DECT has specific workflow implications for the radiologist and the technologist that may affect patient scheduling and the productivity of the department.[42] For this reason, it is the author's suggestion that departments interested in routine clinical DECT scanning develop predetermined algorithms that dictate which scans should be acquired in DECT mode and what reconstructions should be automatically generated and sent to PACS so that they are readily available for use by the radiologist. Depending on the type of scanner and the reconstructions made at the CT workstation, DECT examinations may require additional time for image processing at the CT console compared with SECT acquisitions, and these factors need to be taken into account and planned for to minimize impact on CT department productivity, particularly in settings where the scanner is operating at full or near full capacity. On the radiologist side, automatically generating and sending specialized DECT reconstructions that have been shown to be useful for a given type of examination to PACS, such as low-energy VMIs for neck CTs (see later), increases their use.[42] In the long term, the ideal setting would be one where the most important reconstructions are ready for use in PACS and the radiologist also has direct access to advanced analytical DECT tools for complex cases requiring additional reconstructions or analysis through software integrated into PACS. For those interested in a more detailed discussion of workflow impact and potential solutions for workflow friendly implementation, the topic has been recently reviewed elsewhere in detail based on the experience of a site using a fast kilovolt peak switching scanner.[42]

DUAL-ENERGY COMPUTED TOMOGRAPHY APPLICATIONS FOR THE EVALUATION OF PATHOLOGY IN THE NECK

The final section of this article reviews different clinical applications of DECT in the neck, focusing on applications in head and neck oncology.

Evaluation of Head and Neck Squamous Cell Carcinoma and Its Boundaries

Imaging plays an essential role in the initial evaluation and staging of HNSCC and in surveillance for tumor recurrence.[43] At many institutions, CT is the first-line modality used for the work-up of most mucosal head and neck cancers, and it should be performed after administration of intravenous contrast unless contraindicated. The main advantages of CT accounting for its popularity are its widespread availability, its rapid acquisition time (within seconds), and its lower cost compared with MR imaging. In the head and neck cancer population in particular, and especially for cancers below the level of the hard palate, there is significant propensity for motion degradation. This is because many patients may have difficulty remaining supine for prolonged periods of time or clearing secretions. In this population, the advantages of the rapid acquisition time of CT for obtaining a high diagnostic quality examination compared with MR imaging may become even more apparent. At many institutions, MR imaging is typically used as a second-line examination for trouble shooting or specific applications, such as evaluation of perineural tumor spread, intracranial extension, evaluation of sinonasal tumors, or supplementary evaluation of nasopharyngeal carcinoma.[43]

During the initial tumor evaluation, one of the most important functions of imaging is to evaluate tumor extent, especially deep extent to areas that are not amenable to accurate characterization clinically, upstaging the initial clinical assessment. This in turn helps determine the tumor stage that forms the basis for optimal patient management. Using VMIs at energies lower than 65 keV increases iodine attenuation and the spectral properties of iodine within enhancing tissues, such as tumor, have been exploited for improving tumor visibility and contour delineation. On contrast-enhanced CT, the highest HNSCC attenuation is seen on 40-keV VMIs, although this comes at the expense of increased image noise (**Figs. 8** and **9**).[25–27] Even then, at least in some studies

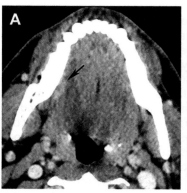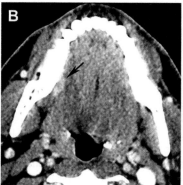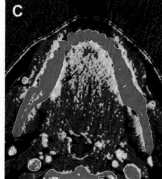

Fig. 8. Low-energy VMIs and iodine maps (iodine-water; IW maps) for the evaluation of oral tongue HNSCC. (*A*) 65-keV VMI (typically considered equivalent to a standard 120-kVp SECT acquisition), (*B*) 40-keV VMI, and (*C*) IW map demonstrate a subtle enhancing lesion along the right lateral margin of the oral tongue (*arrows*). Note improved visibility of the lesion on the 40-keV VMI. In this case, the lesion is also well seen on the IW map. The scan was acquired using a fast kilovolt peak switching scanner.

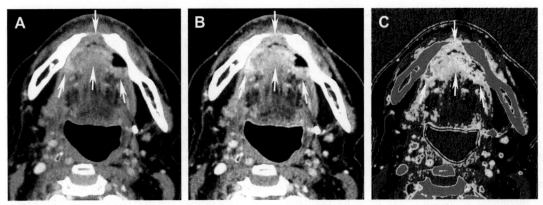

Fig. 9. Low-energy VMIs and iodine maps (iodine-water; IW maps) for the evaluation of HNSCC of the floor of the mouth. (*A*) 65-keV VMI, (*B*) 40-keV VMI, and (*C*) IW map demonstrate an ulcerated lesion centered in the anterior floor of mouth and extending to both sides of the midline with invasion of adjacent structures and spaces (*arrows*). Note improved tumor delineation and definition of the tumor margins on the 40-keV VMI compared with 65 keV. In this case, the tumor extent is also well delineated on the IW map.

using certain scanners or advanced forms of VMIs that reduce noise, the contrast-to-noise ratio is still highest with 40-keV VMIs.[3,28] At the author's institution where a fast kilovolt peak switching scanner is used, 40-keV VMIs are routinely reconstructed and sent to PACS for interpretation. These have been found to be a useful reconstruction for diagnostic evaluation based on a recent survey of head and neck radiologists interpreting these examinations (see **Figs. 8** and **9**).[42] For dual-source scanners, one report using an advanced type of monoenergetic reconstructions referred to as "Mono +" found that quantitatively, contrast-to-noise ratio of tumor was highest at 40 keV. Mono + VMIs were generated through algorithms that preferentially combine the high signal data at low energies with the superior noise properties at medium energies.[28]

Although most studies evaluating the utility of low-energy VMIs for HNSCC evaluation compared these VMIs with SECT equivalent VMIs or WA images generated from the DECT acquisition, at least one study directly compared these with SECT scans and found tumor attenuation and tumor-muscle attenuation difference on 40-keV VMIs to be superior to SECT.[25] It is also noteworthy that there is not consensus on the exact low-energy VMI that is optimal, especially based on subjective evaluation. In a study that included subjective evaluation using images from a fast kilovolt peak switching scanner, the raters consistently selected 40-keV VMIs as the best one for tumor evaluation, even though they did not find the images "as appealing" as the high signal-to-noise ratio, less noisy 65-keV VMIs.[25] However, two studies using dual-source scanners have reported that 55 or 60 VMIs were preferred

subjectively, even though one of the studies found that quantitatively, the contrast-to-noise ratio for tumor evaluation was highest at 40 keV.[27,28] The reason for the variation is not entirely clear. In our experience, it takes some time before the readers get comfortable in "reading through" the noisier 40-keV images and it is possible that this accounts for some of the discrepancy in the literature. Other factors potentially contributing to this could be technical differences between the scanners (the latter studies were performed using dual-source scanners) used or differences in scan radiation dose used, affecting overall image quality with the noise accentuated on the low-energy VMIs. It should also be noted that low-energy VMIs may not work as well in areas already prone to artifact, such as lower neck or thoracic inlet region (or in the presence of dental artifact). For the latter, one may rely on the 65-keV VMIs for evaluation or alternatively use a slightly higher VMI energy than 40 keV for the low-energy reconstructions. Like other things in medicine, there is likely some leeway in the exact energy used for the low-energy reconstructions for improving visibility of HNSCC.

Similar to the use of low-energy VMIs, alterations can be made in the WA images obtained using dual-source DECT scanners to improve visibility of HNSCC and its contours. For example, blending of 60% of the low-energy and 40% of the high-energy data has been shown to improve visibility and contour delineation of HNSCC compared with the default 30% to 70% reconstructions.[36] Another approach demonstrated to improve HNSCC visualization is through nonlinear blending of the different energy data (instead of linear blending).[28,44]

Dual-Energy Computed Tomography for the Evaluation of Head and Neck Squamous Cell Carcinoma Recurrence

Based on the few studies available, low-energy VMIs also seem to improve recurrent tumor visibility and therefore potentially improve detection and differentiation of recurrent tumor from benign posttreatment changes.[26,45] One study directly compared recurrent tumors with benign posttreatment changes and found statistically significant higher attenuation on 40-keV images and higher iodine content on iodine maps in tumor compared with posttreatment changes.[45] The latter suggests that iodine maps could also be useful for the evaluation of tumor or its extent in selected cases. Anecdotally, we have also observed that iodine maps sometimes better delineate the extent of HNSCC, including untreated tumors (see **Fig. 9**).

Determination of Thyroid Cartilage Invasion

One of the fundamental factors in laryngeal and hypopharyngeal HNSCC staging is the assessment of thyroid cartilage invasion, because it may influence the staging and therapeutic management of the patient.[2,3] CT and MR imaging are both useful for the evaluation of thyroid cartilage invasion, each with its own strengths and limitations. CT is generally good for evaluation of gross cartilage invasion but may become less reliable for the evaluation of partial or early cartilage invasion.[43,46,47] MR imaging may improve sensitivity for cartilage invasion but may result in overestimation or false-positive diagnosis of

thyroid cartilage invasion because of signal changes resulting from reactive changes and edema rather tumor invasion.[43,48–50] One of the challenges for the evaluation of thyroid cartilage on CT is the variable ossification of thyroid cartilage with unpredictable patterns, including islands of nonossification interspersed with ossified components.[43,50–53] On conventional SECT, NOTC can have attenuation similar to tumor.[24] This may make interpretation challenging when the tumor approaches or abuts a segment of cartilage that is partially ossified.

Although NOTC can have attenuation close to enhancing tumor on SECT or SECT equivalent DECT VMIs, NOTC has different energy-dependent attenuation characteristics compared with tumor (**Fig. 10**).[24] Specifically, at high energies, there is relative preservation of the intrinsically high attenuation of NOTC but relative suppression of iodine within enhancing tumor, resulting in increased density separation and improved distinction (see **Fig. 10; Fig. 11**).[24] Therefore, on these reconstructions, NOTC may be distinguishable from adjacent (or invading) tumor by its higher attenuation compared with the native tumor (see **Fig. 11**). Areas of thyroid cartilage invasion, however, would appear as a low-attenuation defect within the cartilage, with similar (low) attenuation as the tumor on the high-energy VMIs in areas with corresponding high attenuation on the standard 65-keV VMIs (**Fig. 12**). Based on one study, VMIs reconstructed at 95 keV or higher (140 keV) can achieve good separation between the attenuation of NOTC and

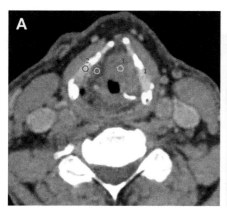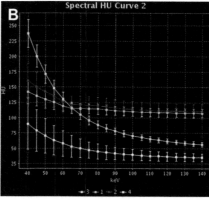

Fig. 10. Differences in energy-dependent attenuation characteristics of NOTC and enhancing tumor. (*A*) Region of interest analysis on a 140-keV DECT VMI with corresponding (*B*) SHAUCs is shown. Four regions of interest were placed on normal paraglottic tissue (*4, yellow*), contralateral normal NOTC (*2, red*), laryngeal tumor (*3, blue*), and ipsilateral NOTC (*1, pink*). Note the separation of SHUAC/energy-dependent attenuation of tumor (*blue*) compared with NOTC (*pink* and *red*) in the high-energy range. Note also the different SHUAC of tumor compared with normal paraglottic tissue. The quantitative differences in attenuation of NOTC compared with tumor on high-energy VMIs are appreciated qualitatively in A (140-keV VMI). The improved distinction on 140-keV compared with standard 65-keV VMIs is shown in **Fig. 11**.

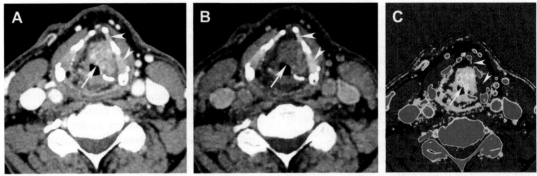

Fig. 11. High-energy VMIs and iodine maps for evaluation of thyroid cartilage. (*A*) 65-keV VMIs, (*B*) 140-keV VMIs, and (*C*) iodine (iodine-water) material decomposition map demonstrate a left laryngeal tumor (*arrow*; same case as in **Fig. 10**). There is partial ossification of the thyroid cartilage in this patient. On the left, the arrowheads point to the NOTC components. Note how on the SECT equivalent 65-keV VMI (*A*), the tumor has similar attenuation to NOTC. Anteriorly, the tumor abuts part of NOTC with loss of fat plane in between; it is not possible to differentiate the tumor-NOTC boundary or invasion on the 65-keV VMI in this location. However, on the high-energy 140-keV VMI, the attenuation of iodine within enhancing tumor is suppressed but there is relative preservation of the intrinsically high NOTC attenuation (*B*). Note how well the sharp interface and differences in attenuation between tumor and NOTC is appreciated on the 140-keV VMI, reflecting the differences seen on the spectral Hounsfield unit attenuation curves in **Fig. 10**. Iodine maps can also be used for characterization of NOTC, which should not have significant iodine signal on these maps, as shown in C, in contradistinction to iodine signal within tumor. Calcified/ossified tissue also has high signal on iodine maps and should not be mistaken with pure iodine signal. This pitfall is readily avoided by correlation with standard images, such as 65-keV VMIs.

tumor, with the separation being greatest at the highest (140 keV) VMIs.[24]

Iodine maps have also been shown to improve evaluation of thyroid cartilage invasion. In one study, it was shown that the addition of iodine maps to standard WA images obtained with a dual-source DECT scanner improved sensitivity and reduced interrater variability for detection of thyroid cartilage invasion.[54] Iodine maps help distinguish patches of NOTC from tumor because, unlike enhancing tumor, NOTC should not have significant iodine "signal" on these maps (see **Fig. 11**). It should be noted that calcified/ossified tissue has high signal on iodine maps that should not be misinterpreted as pure iodine signal on iodine maps (see **Fig. 11**). This pitfall is readily avoided by

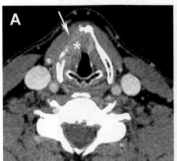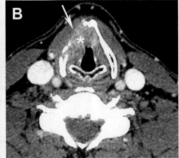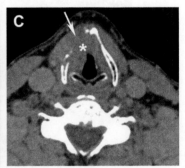

Fig. 12. Appearance of thyroid cartilage invaded by tumor on different energy VMIs. (*A*) 65-keV, (*B*) 40-keV, and (*C*) 140-keV VMIs demonstrate a large laryngeal tumor (*asterisk*) invading the right thyroid cartilage (*arrow*). Different energy VMIs (and iodine maps, not shown) are used in conjunction with one another for a full diagnostic evaluation. Note the improved tumor visibility on the 40-keV compared with 65-keV VMIs, with better visualization of the tumor invading the cartilage with extralaryngeal extension (*arrow*). On the high-energy 140-keV VMI, iodine attenuation is suppressed within enhancing tumor, with a low-attenuation defect that corresponds to high-attenuation areas on the 65- and 40-keV VMIs, consistent with cartilage invasion. If there was nonossified thyroid cartilage on the right instead of invasion, it would have higher attenuation than native tumor, as shown in **Fig. 11**.

correlation with standard images, such as the 65-keV VMIs. This again highlights the importance of interpreting different DECT reconstructions, whether different energy VMIs or material decomposition maps, in conjunction with one another for optimal diagnostic evaluation.[3] Based on current evidence, for purposes of thyroid cartilage evaluation to assess for tumor invasion, iodine maps are used to evaluate and distinguish the nonossified part of the thyroid cartilage from tumor.

Artifact Reduction

The presence of artifact from dental fillings or implants is a frequent problem on neck CT scans. When extensive, these can significantly limit assessment of the oral cavity or oropharyngeal tissues, potentially precluding accurate evaluation of tumor extent or even lesion visualization. Dental artifact is unpredictable and can vary based on the amount of material/size, shape, and its exact composition. High-energy DECT VMIs have been shown to variably reduce metallic and dental artifacts. There is no consensus on a specific energy that is optimal, and this is likely to vary between patients based on the extent of artifact and the specific application. However, VMIs reconstructed at 88 keV or higher (140 keV or beyond) have been shown achieve good artifact reduction in various studies (**Fig. 13**).[29–34] One of the pitfalls of high-energy VMIs is reduced iodine attenuation and soft tissue contrast. Therefore, if the objective is to evaluate an area or structure that has high intrinsic attenuation in the absence of contrast,

such as bone, then one may attempt VMIs in the extreme of the high-energy range, 130 to 140 keV or beyond for scanners allowing reconstruction of VMIs at energies higher than 140 keV. However, if the objective is to evaluate enhancing soft tissue, such as tumor in the oral cavity or oropharynx, more intermediate high-energy VMIs close to 95 keV may yield a better result.[31] It is noteworthy that high-energy VMIs can have a dual purpose for artifact reduction and thyroid cartilage assessment. Furthermore, the use of high-energy VMIs does not have to be limited to prosthetic artifact reduction. These could also be useful for reduction of artifact at the thoracic inlet secondary to bone or from dense venous contrast.[55]

Dual-Energy Computed Tomography Evaluation of Cervical Lymphadenopathy

Although there is currently limited evidence, DECT can potentially be useful for the evaluation of cervical lymphadenopathy. For instance, just like the primary tumor, low-energy VMIs can improve the visibility of nodal metastases and potentially nodal heterogeneity (**Fig. 14**).[2,26] In addition, recent studies performing quantitative analysis of nodal attenuation curves and iodine content suggest that DECT may help with the differentiation of various types of abnormal lymph nodes, including inflammatory lymphadenopathy, HNSCC nodal metastasis, papillary cancer metastasis, lymphoma, and salivary carcinoma.[56–58] Analysis of DECT SHUACs and iodine maps has also been

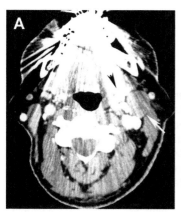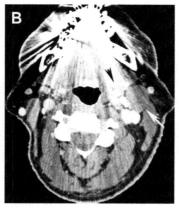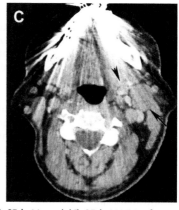

Fig. 13. Dental artifact reduction using high-energy VMIs. (*A*) 40-keV, (*B*) 65-keV, and (*C*) 95-keV VMIs from a contrast-enhanced neck CT with extensive dental artifact partially obscuring vessels (*short arrows*) and a pathologic lymph node (*long arrows*). 40-keV VMIs increase iodine attenuation and contrast but are particularly prone to degradation by these types of artifacts, as would be expected for the "low-energy" spectrum. Note artifact reduction on the 95-keV VMI compared with the SECT equivalent 65-keV VMI, enabling much better visualization of the vessels (*short arrow*) and reducing artifact in the area of the pathologic left level IIA lymph node. As observed here, artifact reduction on high-energy VMIs is achieved at the expense of decreased iodine attenuation and soft tissue contrast.

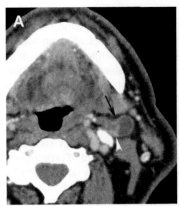
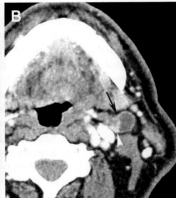
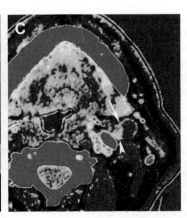

Fig. 14. Metastatic lymphadenopathy from HNSCC of the base of the tongue. Axial (*A*) 65-keV VMI, (*B*) 40-keV VMI, and (*C*) iodine (iodine-water) material decomposition map from a contrast-enhanced neck CT demonstrate a pathologic left level IIA lymph node with cystic internal change and necrosis (*black* and *white arrows*). Note the enhancing solid component (*arrowheads*) having a higher attenuation on the 40-keV VMI compared with the 65-keV VMIs. The iodine signal within the enhancing component and the internal heterogeneity is also well appreciated on the IW map.

used in a few studies to characterize and potentially differentiate between benign thyroid nodules and cancerous thyroid tissue.[59] These are interesting topics of future research and application.

Table 1 Summary of different reconstructions for multiparametric evaluation of the neck using DECT	
DECT Reconstruction	**Comments**
65- or 70-keV VMIs	Equivalent to SECT; use for routine evaluation and as reference standard
Low-energy VMIs: 40 keV (slightly higher energy VMIs than 40 keV may be acceptable alternatives)	Improve tumor visibility and soft tissue boundary delineation
High-energy VMIs (95/140 keV) Given the trade-offs in iodine attenuation and artifact reduction, it may be worthwhile to automatically reconstruct VMIs at both energies	Evaluation of thyroid cartilage invasion Dental and metallic artifact reduction
Iodine maps	Evaluation of thyroid cartilage invasion Possibly evaluation of tumor extent and boundary?

Multiparametric Approach for Head and Neck Squamous Cell Carcinoma Evaluation Using Dual-Energy Computed Tomography

As should be evident based on the discussion of underlying DECT principles and various applications, different DECT reconstructions have unique advantages and disadvantages. Therefore, it is likely that these are best used in conjunction with one another, in a multiparametric fashion, for optimal diagnostic evaluation.[3] This approach is similar to what radiologists routinely use for MR imaging, interpreting information from multiple MR imaging sequences for optimal diagnostic evaluation. **Table 1** provides a summary of current potentially useful reconstructions for the evaluation of neck using DECT.

SUMMARY

There is increasing availability and use of DECT, with multiple established or emerging applications in head and neck imaging. Increasing evidence supports advantages of DECT for tumor evaluation, and these are reviewed in detail in this article. It should be noted that currently, most if not all of the published literature on DECT applications for the evaluation of soft tissues of the neck is based on data acquired using fast kilovolt peak switching or dual-source DECT scanners. Given that the fundamental principles of DECT are the same, it is likely that these can be extrapolated to other scanner types. However, there are also significant differences in the acquisition and postprocessing techniques used with different DECT scanners. Therefore, for those using other scanner types, it is likely that some degree of optimization is required for optimal cross-platform application and results.

Spectral CT is an emerging and exciting technique that, if implemented appropriately, is likely to expand the already robust diagnostic capabilities of CT. Implementation of DECT into routine clinical practice can present some challenges but these can be overcome with appropriate planning, implementation, and future development of even more workflow-friendly systems in collaboration with different stakeholders in this technology. In addition, refinements in currently known clinical applications and development of new applications in the neck have the potential to increase diagnostic accuracy and potentially enable noninvasive tissue characterization in ways not previously possible. These include potential future use of experimental spectral CT systems, such as photon counting scanners or the use of texture or radiomic tools for an even more robust use of the rich quantitative DECT data, providing new horizons for research and advanced imaging in the future.

REFERENCES

1. Vogl TJ, Schulz B, Bauer RW, et al. Dual-energy CT applications in head and neck imaging. AJR Am J Roentgenol 2012;199(5 Suppl):S34–9.
2. Forghani R. Advanced dual-energy CT for head and neck cancer imaging. Expert Rev Anticancer Ther 2015;15(12):1489–501.
3. Lam S, Gupta R, Kelly H, et al. Multiparametric evaluation of head and neck squamous cell carcinoma using a single-source dual-energy CT with fast kVp switching: state of the art. Cancers (Basel) 2015; 7(4):2201–16.
4. Forghani R, Kelly H, Curtin HD. Applications of dual energy CT for the evaluation of head and neck squamous cell carcinoma. Neuroimaging Clin N Am 2017;27(3):445–59.
5. Johnson TRC, Kalender WA. Physical background. In: Johnson T, Fink C, Schönberg SO, et al, editors. Dual energy CT in clinical practice. Berlin: Springer-Verlag Berlin Heidelberg; 2011. p. 3–9.
6. Johnson TR. Dual-energy CT: general principles. AJR Am J Roentgenol 2012;199(5 Suppl):S3–8.
7. McCollough CH, Leng S, Yu L, et al. Dual- and multi-energy CT: principles, technical approaches, and clinical applications. Radiology 2015;276(3):637–53.
8. Forghani R, De Man B, Gupta R. Dual energy CT: physical principles, approaches to scanning, usage, and implementation - Part 1. Neuroimaging Clin N Am 2017;27(3):371–84.
9. Forghani R, De Man B, Gupta R. Dual energy CT: physical principles, approaches to scanning, usage, and implementation - Part 2. Neuroimaging Clin N Am 2017;27(3):385–400.
10. Flohr TG, McCollough CH, Bruder H, et al. First performance evaluation of a dual-source CT (DSCT) system. Eur Radiol 2006;16(2):256–68.
11. Johnson TR, Krauss B, Sedlmair M, et al. Material differentiation by dual energy CT: initial experience. Eur Radiol 2007;17(6):1510–7.
12. Krauss B, Schmidt B, Flohr TG. Dual source CT. In: Johnson T, Fink C, Schönberg SO, et al, editors. Dual energy CT in clinical practice. Berlin: Springer-Verlag Berlin Heidelberg; 2011. p. 10–20.
13. Chandra N, Langan DA. Gemstone detector: dual energy imaging via fast kVp switching. In: Johnson T, Fink C, Schönberg SO, et al, editors. Dual energy CT in clinical practice. Berlin: Springer-Verlag Berlin Heidelberg; 2011. p. 35–41.
14. Xu D, Langan DA, Wu X, et al. Dual energy CT via fast kVp switching spectrum estimation. Paper presented at: Medical Imaging 2009: Physics of Medical Imaging. Lake Buena Vista (FL), March 14, 2009.
15. Alvarez RE, Seibert JA, Thompson SK. Comparison of dual energy detector system performance. Med Phys 2004;31(3):556–65.
16. Vlassenbroek A. Dual layer CT. In: Johnson T, Fink C, Schönberg SO, et al, editors. Dual energy CT in clinical practice. Berlin: Springer-Verlag Berlin Heidelberg; 2011. p. 21–34.
17. Euler A, Parakh A, Falkowski AL, et al. Initial results of a single-source dual-energy computed tomography technique using a split-filter: assessment of image quality, radiation dose, and accuracy of dual-energy applications in an in vitro and in vivo study. Invest Radiol 2016;51(8):491–8.
18. Kaemmerer N, Brand M, Hammon M, et al. Dual-energy computed tomography angiography of the head and neck with single-source computed tomography: a new technical (split filter) approach for bone removal. Invest Radiol 2016;51(10):618–23.
19. Alvarez RE, Macovski A. Energy-selective reconstructions in X-ray computerized tomography. Phys Med Biol 1976;21(5):733–44.
20. Millner MR, McDavid WD, Waggener RG, et al. Extraction of information from CT scans at different energies. Med Phys 1979;6(1):70–1.
21. Matsumoto K, Jinzaki M, Tanami Y, et al. Virtual monochromatic spectral imaging with fast kilovoltage switching: improved image quality as compared with that obtained with conventional 120-kVp CT. Radiology 2011;259(1):257–62.
22. Patel BN, Thomas JV, Lockhart ME, et al. Single-source dual-energy spectral multidetector CT of pancreatic adenocarcinoma: optimization of energy level viewing significantly increases lesion contrast. Clin Radiol 2013;68(2):148–54.
23. Pinho DF, Kulkarni NM, Krishnaraj A, et al. Initial experience with single-source dual-energy CT

abdominal angiography and comparison with single-energy CT angiography: image quality, enhancement, diagnosis and radiation dose. Eur Radiol 2013;23(2):351–9.

24. Forghani R, Levental M, Gupta R, et al. Different spectral Hounsfield unit curve and high-energy virtual monochromatic image characteristics of squamous cell carcinoma compared with nonossified thyroid cartilage. AJNR Am J Neuroradiol 2015; 36(6):1194–200.

25. Forghani R, Kelly H, Yu E, et al. Low-energy virtual monochromatic dual-energy computed tomography images for the evaluation of head and neck squamous cell carcinoma: a study of tumor visibility compared with single-energy computed tomography and user acceptance. J Comput Assist Tomogr 2017;41(4):565–71.

26. Lam S, Gupta R, Levental M, et al. Optimal virtual monochromatic images for evaluation of normal tissues and head and neck cancer using dual-energy CT. AJNR Am J Neuroradiol 2015;36(8): 1518–24.

27. Wichmann JL, Noske EM, Kraft J, et al. Virtual monoenergetic dual-energy computed tomography: optimization of kiloelectron volt settings in head and neck cancer. Invest Radiol 2014;49(11):735–41.

28. Albrecht MH, Scholtz JE, Kraft J, et al. Assessment of an advanced monoenergetic reconstruction technique in dual-energy computed tomography of head and neck cancer. Eur Radiol 2015;25(8):2493–501.

29. Bamberg F, Dierks A, Nikolaou K, et al. Metal artifact reduction by dual energy computed tomography using monoenergetic extrapolation. Eur Radiol 2011; 21(7):1424–9.

30. Komlosi P, Grady D, Smith JS, et al. Evaluation of monoenergetic imaging to reduce metallic instrumentation artifacts in computed tomography of the cervical spine. J Neurosurg Spine 2015;22(1):34–8.

31. Nair JR, DeBlois F, Ong T, et al. Dual energy CT: balance between iodine attenuation and artifact reduction for the evaluation of head and neck cancer. J Comput Assist Tomogr 2017. [Epub ahead of print].

32. Srinivasan A, Hoeffner E, Ibrahim M, et al. Utility of dual-energy CT virtual keV monochromatic series for the assessment of spinal transpedicular hardware-bone interface. AJR Am J Roentgenol 2013;201(4):878–83.

33. Stolzmann P, Winklhofer S, Schwendener N, et al. Monoenergetic computed tomography reconstructions reduce beam hardening artifacts from dental restorations. Forensic Sci Med Pathol 2013;9(3): 327–32.

34. Tanaka R, Hayashi T, Ike M, et al. Reduction of dark-band-like metal artifacts caused by dental implant bodies using hypothetical monoenergetic imaging after dual-energy computed tomography.

Oral Surg Oral Med Oral Pathol Oral Radiol 2013; 115(6):833–8.

35. Tawfik AM, Kerl JM, Razek AA, et al. Image quality and radiation dose of dual-energy CT of the head and neck compared with a standard 120-kVp acquisition. AJNR Am J Neuroradiol 2011;32(11):1994–9.

36. Tawfik AM, Kerl JM, Bauer RW, et al. Dual-energy CT of head and neck cancer: average weighting of low- and high-voltage acquisitions to improve lesion delineation and image quality-initial clinical experience. Invest Radiol 2012;47(5):306–11.

37. Graser A, Johnson TR, Hecht EM, et al. Dual-energy CT in patients suspected of having renal masses: can virtual nonenhanced images replace true nonenhanced images? Radiology 2009;252(2):433–40.

38. Hu R, Daftari Besheli L, Young J, et al. Dual-energy head CT enables accurate distinction of intraparenchymal hemorrhage from calcification in emergency department patients. Radiology 2016; 280(1):177–83.

39. Schenzle JC, Sommer WH, Neumaier K, et al. Dual energy CT of the chest: how about the dose? Invest Radiol 2010;45(6):347–53.

40. Kamiya K, Kunimatsu A, Mori H, et al. Preliminary report on virtual monochromatic spectral imaging with fast kVp switching dual energy head CT: comparable image quality to that of 120-kVp CT without increasing the radiation dose. Jpn J Radiol 2013; 31(4):293–8.

41. Hwang WD, Mossa-Basha M, Andre JB, et al. Qualitative comparison of noncontrast head dual-energy computed tomography using rapid voltage switching technique and conventional computed tomography. J Comput Assist Tomogr 2016;40(2):320–5.

42. Perez-Lara A, Levental M, Rosenbloom L, et al. Routine dual energy CT scanning of the neck in clinical practice: a single institution experience. Neuroimaging Clin N Am 2017;27(3):523–31.

43. Forghani R, Johnson JM, Ginsberg LE. Imaging of head and neck cancer. In: Myers J, Hanna E, Myers EN, editors. Cancer of the head and neck. 5th edition. Philadelphia: Wolters Kluwer; 2017. p. 92–148.

44. Scholtz JE, Husers K, Kaup M, et al. Non-linear image blending improves visualization of head and neck primary squamous cell carcinoma compared to linear blending in dual-energy CT. Clin Radiol 2015;70(2):168–75.

45. Yamauchi H, Buehler M, Goodsitt MM, et al. Dual-energy CT-based differentiation of benign posttreatment changes from primary or recurrent malignancy of the head and neck: comparison of spectral Hounsfield units at 40 and 70 keV and iodine concentration. AJR Am J Roentgenol 2016; 206(3):580–7.

46. Mafee MF, Schild JA, Michael AS, et al. Cartilage involvement in laryngeal carcinoma: correlation of

CT and pathologic macrosection studies. J Comput Assist Tomogr 1984;8(5):969–73.

47. Becker M, Burkhardt K, Dulguerov P, et al. Imaging of the larynx and hypopharynx. Eur J Radiol 2008; 66(3):460–79.

48. Becker M. Neoplastic invasion of laryngeal cartilage: radiologic diagnosis and therapeutic implications. Eur J Radiol 2000;33(3):216–29.

49. Becker M, Zbaren P, Casselman JW, et al. Neoplastic invasion of laryngeal cartilage: reassessment of criteria for diagnosis at MR imaging. Radiology 2008;249(2):551–9.

50. Kuno H, Onaya H, Fujii S, et al. Primary staging of laryngeal and hypopharyngeal cancer: CT, MR imaging and dual-energy CT. Eur J Radiol 2014; 83(1):e23–35.

51. Archer CR, Yeager VL. Evaluation of laryngeal cartilages by computed tomography. J Comput Assist Tomogr 1979;3(5):604–11.

52. Hermans R. Staging of laryngeal and hypopharyngeal cancer: value of imaging studies. Eur Radiol 2006;16(11):2386–400.

53. Dadfar N, Seyyedi M, Forghani R, et al. Computed tomography appearance of normal nonossified thyroid cartilage: implication for tumor invasion diagnosis. J Comput Assist Tomogr 2015;39(2):240–3.

54. Kuno H, Onaya H, Iwata R, et al. Evaluation of cartilage invasion by laryngeal and hypopharyngeal squamous cell carcinoma with dual-energy CT. Radiology 2012;265(2):488–96.

55. Perez-Lara A, Forghani R. Dual energy CT of the neck: a pictorial review of normal anatomy and pathology using different energy reconstructions and material decomposition maps. Neuroimaging Clin N Am 2017;27(3):499–522.

56. Tawfik AM, Razek AA, Kerl JM, et al. Comparison of dual-energy CT-derived iodine content and iodine overlay of normal, inflammatory and metastatic squamous cell carcinoma cervical lymph nodes. Eur Radiol 2014;24(3):574–80.

57. Liang H, Li A, Li Y, et al. A retrospective study of dual-energy CT for clinical detecting of metastatic cervical lymph nodes in laryngeal and hypopharyngeal squamous cell carcinoma. Acta Otolaryngol 2015;135(7):722–8.

58. Yang L, Luo D, Li L, et al. Differentiation of malignant cervical lymphadenopathy by dual-energy CT: a preliminary analysis. Sci Rep 2016;6:31020.

59. Li M, Zheng X, Li J, et al. Dual-energy computed tomography imaging of thyroid nodule specimens: comparison with pathologic findings. Invest Radiol 2012;47(1):58–64.

Perfusion and Permeability Imaging for Head and Neck Cancer
Theory, Acquisition, Postprocessing, and Relevance to Clinical Imaging

Adam J. Davis, MD[a],*, Razia Rehmani, MD[b],
Ashok Srinivasan, MD[c],
Girish M. Fatterpekar, MBBS, DNB, MD[d]

KEYWORDS

- Head and neck cancer • Perfusion • Permeability • MR imaging • CT

KEY POINTS

- Perfusion imaging is the study of tissue circulation at the capillary level.
- Perfusion and permeability imaging are closely related but assess different characteristics of the movement of contrast tracers from the intravascular plasma to the tissue interstitial space and back again.
- The analysis of perfusion and permeability clinical imaging data relies on algorithms designed to model the underlying physiologic processes. The analysis of the acquired imaging data depends greatly on the assumptions of the model chosen.
- The acquisition protocols should be carefully designed and matched to the type of perfusion and/or permeability imaging performed and must obtain the data necessary to satisfy the requirements of the model chosen.
- Perfusion and permeability imaging provide powerful clinical information affecting the diagnosis, prognosis, and treatment of head and neck cancer.

INTRODUCTION

Radiologists are exposed to 2 different paradigms within the practice of perfusion imaging. First, they are occupied with perfusion imaging for central nervous system (CNS) pathologic conditions, most commonly ischemic stroke and tumors. These pathologic conditions occur within a system protected by a blood-brain barrier (BBB) that dictates the type of perfusion models that can be applied. The BBB represents the impermeability of the vessel wall to large molecules, including contrast agents. These pathologic conditions disrupt the normal physiologic mechanisms and structural barriers that create the BBB and result in both a characteristic radiographic appearance and a perfusion dynamic that generates diagnostic information. Conversely, the head and neck soft tissue structures, like the rest of the body, are governed by a different set of physiologic mechanisms and, consequently, a different perfusion model, typically referred to as permeability, which is

[a] Image Processing Lab, Department of Radiology, New York University School of Medicine, New York University Langone Medical Center, 660 First Avenue, New York, NY 10016, USA; [b] St Barnabas Healthcare System, Albert Einstein College of Medicine, 4422 Third Avenue, Bronx, NY 10457, USA; [c] Division of Neuroradiology, Department of Radiology, University of Michigan, 1500 East Medical Center Drive, Ann Arbor, MI 48109, USA; [d] Division of Neuroradiology, NYU Langone Medical Center, 660 First Avenue, New York, NY 10016, USA
* Corresponding author.
E-mail address: Adam.Davis@nyumc.org

Magn Reson Imaging Clin N Am 26 (2018) 19–35
http://dx.doi.org/10.1016/j.mric.2017.08.002

defined by the passage of these same large molecules across the capillary wall and into the interstitial space (IS). It has been demonstrated that studying the perfusion characteristics of head and neck tumors improves historadiologic diagnosis, correlates with response to treatment, and predicts the potential for recurrence. How clinicians acquire radiographic images and model these physiologic processes, and how data are analyzed, profoundly alters the resultant data and the interpretation of the study. Consequently, diagnostic and prognostic opinion depends on the initial acquisition and postprocessing choices. This article focuses on the theoretic and technical processes that are fundamental to perfusion, and particularly on permeability imaging, using an explanatory method without the use of complicated mathematics.

PERFUSION FUNDAMENTALS
Perfusion Imaging Basics

In essence, perfusion imaging is the study of the microcirculation at the capillary level. There is, unfortunately, confusion created by the nomenclature. Perfusion is often used as a unifying term to describe the entire medical discipline of the study of dynamic contrast-enhanced (DCE) imaging. When it is applied to simple systems in which only the vasculature can be measured (eg, the brain), it is termed perfusion. When applied to the remainder of the body, where there is passage of contrast into the extracellular extravascular space (EES) also known as the Interstitial Space (IS), it is termed permeability. Care must be taken not to confuse the general term perfusion with the more specific term perfusion or its counterpart permeability.

In medicine, a tracer (or indicator) is defined as a detectable substance introduced into a dynamic biological system that acts in a physiologic manner to provide information about the function of the system. Within clinical imaging there is a myriad selection of tracers, including iodinated contrast agents, gadolinium-based contrast agents, nuclear isotope tagged molecules, and the like. The total amount of the indicator within a given volume of tissue is termed the concentration of the indicator. For imaging purposes, it is typically normalized to a given volume of tissue in milliliters, using the nomenclature concentration of tissue (Ct). This should not be confused with the concentration of an indicator at a given amount of time (C[t]).

Within the brain parenchyma, the impermeable BBB creates a simplified system because contrast material remains within the vascular network and does not pass into the EES. The vascular space may be divided into the cellular component, which is most pragmatically represented by hematocrit (Hct) and the plasma, in which the contrast material is contained. The extravascular space may be considered the IS and the intracellular space. Brain models of perfusion are typically perfusion only; there is no passage of contrast to the IS to complicate the analysis.

For the measurement of contrast within the vascular space, or if the BBB is disrupted, the EES is represented either by signal intensity change (for MR imaging) or Hounsfield unit (HU) attenuation change (for computed tomography [CT]). The measurement produces a time concentration curve that represents the tissue blood flow (BFt), tissue blood volume (BVt), and mean transit time (MTT). BFt is the total amount of blood delivered to a given amount of tissue and is expressed in milliliters of blood per minute per 100 mL of tissue. In some models it is simply expressed as flow (F) of blood to the tissue or blood flow (BF). BVt is the total intravascular volume of blood within a given amount of tissue and is expressed in mL/100 mL of tissue. BVt is sometimes abbreviated BV.

Depending on the mode of acquisition and the model being used, the necessary data to quantify perfusion require the contrast concentration of the arterial input to the tissues (arterial input function [AIF]), the concentration of the contrast in the tissues themselves (Ct) and the venous outflow concentration (venous outflow function [VOF]). This last measurement is typically used not for BF purposes but to provide a standard of voxel contrast concentration for normalization of the AIF, which reduces artifact from volume averaging if a small artery is chosen for the AIF that fails to fill the entire voxel adequately.

The concentration curve of contrast in the arteries has a characteristic morphology (Fig. 1). It consists of the baseline before vessel opacification, a rapid increase in concentration terminating in a peak, and an initially rapid and then more gradual decline in the magnetic resonance (MR) signal intensity or CT HU attenuation as the contrast leaves the voxel and is cleared systemically by the body. A second small peak in the arterial concentration curve (the AIF) is caused by blood that has passed through the circulatory system and is now reentering the arterial inflow, although it is markedly diluted by the rest of the body BV (recirculation).

The measurement of the Ct of contrast produces a different appearance than the AIF due to dispersion of contrast through the much larger BV of the capillary network, as well as the decreased perfusion pressure with slower velocity. This physiologic phenomenon is critical because it allows for micromolecular passage

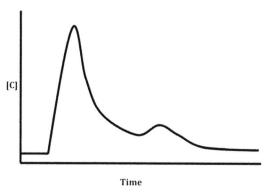

Fig. 1. Contrast concentration curve of the AIF.

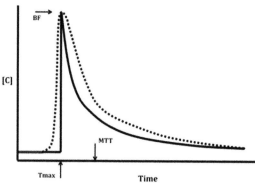

Fig. 2. Theoretic and actual residue function of AIF and Ct deconvolution. The deconvolution of the AIF and the Ct results in a residue function. The theoretic result (*solid line*) is a perfect vertical slope followed by a gradual decline. The time delay between the AIF and the Ct is the Tmax, represented by the vertical line. Longer Tmax has been used as a marker of decreased tissue perfusion. The height of the vertical line represents the BF. The greater the BF, the larger the delivery of contrast and the greater the measured MR imaging signal intensity or CT HU attenuation. Theoretically, the height of the line in the residue function can be thought of as the instantaneous delivery of contrast into the voxel. It is followed by the gradual downward slope representing the efflux of contrast from the voxel. The weighted mean time under this curve is the MTT. Solving mean MTT for BF results in the BV or, alternatively, the AUC. In real practice, the residue function is more gradual (*dotted line*) and has small fluctuations around each point in the curve due to noise and other measurement error (not shown). This introduces error into the results.

across the capillary wall to ensure that oxygen and nutrients pass to the cells for respiration and waste products are removed.

The simplest quantitative models assume the AIF defines the tissue perfusion. The slope of the initial AIF curve represents the cerebral BF and the area under the curve (AUC) represents the BV. Solving one variable for the other provides MTT (cerebral blood flow [CBF] = cerebral blood volume [CBV] × mean transit time [MTT]). Unfortunately, this leads to erroneous results. The upslope of the curve depends on injection parameters, including the speed of injection, the viscosity of the contrast, and the use of a saline chaser.[1] Physiologic factors, such as cardiac output, further influences the upslope. The AUC is imprecise because most concentration curves are truncated before reaching their final baseline and are contaminated by recirculation. Furthermore, the contrast curves within the tissue are physiologically different than within the arteries, usually more delayed in initiation and more gradual in rise and downslope. The delay between the AIF and the Ct causes significant problems with the usefulness of the initial slope and AUC method. Some models interpret a delay in perfusion as indicating diminished perfusion. However, a delay in contrast arrival does not necessarily indicate poor tissue perfusion but simply a consequence of time needed for BF to reach the tissues due to a collateral circulation pattern. The more gradual and lower intensity (Ct) is a normal physiologic process, which produces a different AUC than the AIF AUC, but this is not necessarily pathologic.

To diminish these challenges, more advanced mathematical algorithms are used. Deconvolution methods are mathematical equations used to solve 2 functions simultaneously over time to produce a novel third equation. In the case of perfusion, deconvolution is used to simultaneously solve the AIF and the Ct curves to produce a new function, termed the residue function (**Fig. 2**).

The residue function is a mathematical construct and has no real physiologic correlate, although the values of the residue function curve help to more precisely reflect the true BF, BV, and MTT. In a perfect scenario without noise or other distortion, the time between initiation of contrast injection and the rapid vertical increase of MR signal intensity or CT HU attenuation is termed the time to maximum (Tmax) residue function. Tmax has no true physiologic correlate but roughly corresponds to the time it takes to deliver the contrast from the artery to the tissues. The height of the peak is the BF because greater BF delivery results in a greater signal intensity or HU. The mean (weighted average) of the downslope of the residue function curve indicates the MTT and reflects the microcirculation or capillary flow. Solving BF and MTT results in the BV (CBF/CBV=MTT).

The residue function results in more accurate values but is also degraded during the actual radiographic measurement of true physiologic values. The sharp vertical peak is in practice more rounded (see **Fig. 2**) and the depiction of the smooth curve is in reality more irregular because the measurement of the MR signal intensity or CT HU attenuation curve of the AIF or Ct is degraded by noise during acquisition, within the imaging chain or from external artifact.

The problem of the delay between the AIF and the Ct still persists because, ideally, clinicians want to measure the AIF in the smallest arteriole just before the tissue capillaries. However, practically, only the larger arteries at the surface of the organ or tissue of interest can be measured (eg, brain, lymph nodes, tumor). Nonoscillating (or circulant) decomposition methods try to correct for this. Other mathematical applications, including Bayesian techniques, impose a truer physiologic model to the data measurements and correct for some of the uncertainty due to noise. Furthermore, it diminishes the inherent problem of measurement at the extremes of very low or very high BF, for which accuracy tends to deteriorate.

Permeability Imaging Basics

The fundamental difference between perfusion and permeability models is that permeability models account for the passage of macromolecules from the intravascular space (VS) to the IS. Excellent reviews are available.[2–5] The IS is synonymous with the EES. The total volume of the IS (Ve) is typically represented by the notation Ve. Contrast agents pass freely from the plasma to the IS at a rate that depends on the type of contrast (size and charge of the molecule) and the difference in concentration between the plasma and the IS. The state of the vascular wall endothelium contributes to the rate of passage.

The permeability of the vascular wall to contrast is also termed leakage. The total passage of contrast from the plasma to the IS is determined by the product of the permeability of the vascular wall to the contrast agent and the surface area of the endothelium within the capillaries. The product is referred to as the permeability surface (PS) factor. It is the outflux of the tracer from the plasma to the IS. PS is often erroneously referred to as Ktrans (see below Models and Interpretation of Data), but it is not truly representative of this physiologic modeling constant, which also depends on the tissue perfusion rate, the actual physiologic conditions of the endothelium, and the concentration and type of indicator used. The value of the measured Ktrans constant is influenced by the acquisition. When the delivery of the tracer, typically contrast, is limited by F, then Ktrans equals the BF rate. When the permeability of the endothelial transport is the limiting factor, then Ktrans equals permeability. Usually, the true value lies somewhere in between.

From a clinical perspective, the amount of contrast within a given volume of IS measured radiographically is referred to as the degree of enhancement. The rate and duration of this enhancement depends on the physiologic conditions of the tissue. A swollen IS with high hydrostatic pressure will demonstrate less enhancement than a normal tissue IS.

The contrast within the capillary vascular space (indicating the plasma component because the Hct component carries no tracer) will increase and peak during the initial bolus and rapidly diminish as the first bolus passes. This is similar to the typical AIF that occurs during perfusion imaging but, as previously discussed, occurs more slowly and appears more muted. The contrast concentration within the vascular space simultaneously replenishes itself due to recirculation, which gradually decreases due to systemic renal clearance. The contrast within the IS, however, continues to slowly accumulate. When the plasma concentration of contrast diminishes to less than that of the IS, the contrast agent slowly diffuses back again into the vascular space. The rate at which contrast diffuses back to the vascular space is referred to as the Kep (Fig. 3). It is a constant much like Ktrans but defines the reverse phenomenon. This dynamic is central to the information provided by permeability imaging.

The total tissue enhancement is a combination of the contrast within the vascular space (plasma) of the capillaries and the more slowly accumulating contrast within the IS of the tissues. To differentiate these 2 processes, the permeability models use algorithms to represent the physiologic processes that are occurring. Commonly used values include F; the fraction of the tissue occupied by the VS reflected by either the plasma fraction (vp) or the volume of the plasma space (Vp); the fraction of the tissue occupied by the EES reflected by the fraction of the interstitial space (ve); and the rate of passage of contrast molecules between them (Ktrans from the plasma to the EES and Kep from the EES to the plasma). It should be remembered that the EES and IS are used interchangeably.

Typically used clinical contrast agents (gadolinium or iodine-based) pass quickly from the VS to the EES and are quickly cleared systemically by the kidneys. These contrast agents provide the best estimate of permeability. Conversely, blood pool contrast agents are either large molecular size or bind to blood proteins to create a macromolecule and, consequently, do not readily diffuse through the endothelium. Iron oxide microparticles perform similarly. They are used for determining the Vp. It is important to remember that these definitions apply to normal physiologic conditions. Leaky vasculature or tumor neovascularity may allow large molecules to pass from the VS to the IS.

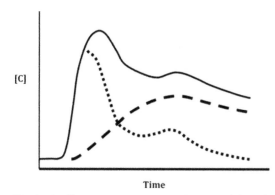

Fig. 3. Capillary contrast concentration curve (*dotted*), IS contrast concentration curve (*dashed*), and resulting measured composite voxel contrast concentration curve (*solid*): the 2-compartment model. The dotted line represents the concentration of contrast in the vascular space (capillary plasma), which has a configuration similar to the AIF. The dashed line is the concentration of contrast in the IS of the tissues. The IS concentration curve is more gradual and delayed due to the need for movement across the endothelium. The sum of these 2 curves is the composite curve within the tissue voxel and is the actual result obtained. The 2 contributing capillary and interstitial curves are theoretic and can only be modeled, not directly measured. However, the AIF may be used to represent the capillary space. The shape and slope of the composite curve gives information regarding the passage of tracer (contrast) between the capillary and IS: Ktrans and Kep.

Models and Interpretation of Data

The conversion of the C(t) into a quantifiable amount is fundamental to perfusion imaging. Clinicians' data are the MR imaging signal intensity or CT HU attenuation as a function of time, typically notated as signal per time (S[t]). The relationship between iodinated contrast concentration and the CT HU attenuation is precisely linear. The measurement is simplified and robust. Similarly, the conversion of gadolinium concentration to signal intensity is linear or nearly so for MR imaging DCE sequences based on T1-weighted relaxation. Degradation of the accuracy of MR imaging DCE sequences may be due to several factors, including coherent fluid (blood) inflow signal intensity changes and the geometry of the slice profile, which creates variability of the flip angle within the acquisition. Precontrast T1-weighted mapping may be necessary to normalize the results of the gadolinium-enhanced dynamic images. T1-weighted DCE sequences include dynamic acquisition sequences, such as volumetric interpolated breath hold examination (VIBE) or golden angle radial sparse parallel (GRASP) technique. (Siemens Healthineers, Forcheim, Germany). By extension, these same principles may be applied

to other modalities that have a linear conversion of indicator agent to signal intensity, including PET, single photon emission computerized tomography (SPECT), and MR imaging arterial spin labeling. MR imaging dynamic susceptibility contrast techniques are T2-weighted gradient echo-based sequences and the interpretation of the acquired data is complicated by the logarithmic relationship between the measured signal intensity and the degree of gadolinium enhancement.

Unfortunately, even for CT or MR imaging DCE, the conversion of the signal into CT HU attenuation or MR signal intensity representing C(t) requires mathematical assumptions. The mathematical equation is

$$C(t) = S(t) / S \text{ (baseline)} \times \ln K$$

This simply means that the contrast concentration the imaging modality produces equals the signal detected at any given time divided by the baseline signal (for equilibration purposes) times the natural log of a constant, termed K.

The value of K for any particular imaging study is difficult to determine because it depends on the contrast delivery, the vascular architecture, the acquisition parameters, and the equipment itself. Consequently, K is unknown and only estimated for any given patient. As a result, true quantitative values are rarely possible in routine clinical imaging unless special measurements are made, including blood analysis to determine the actual concentration of contrast. It is for this reason that practical clinical imaging tends to use relative values of enhancement, comparing the signal detected within a region of interest with the detected signal within a reference tissue. The actual measured contrast enhancement value within a region of interest is typically not used.

The interpretation of permeability imaging data may be simple or complex, depending on the requirements of the study, the sophistication of the imager, the available postprocessing resources, and/or the time constraints placed on the reader. Simple qualitative analysis relies on the reader's visual interpretation of the curve. Typically, 3 phases are recognized similar to those defined within the AIF: the slope of the initial contrast accumulation (washin), the height of the maximum accumulation (peak), and the slope and shape of the diminishing or accumulating contrast concentration (washout, plateau, and/or slow enhancement). It is important to remember that there are 2 simultaneous processes occurring in the tissue: the intravascular (plasma) capillary enhancement and the EES or IS enhancement. It is the sum of these 2 curves that provides the entire tissue enhancement pattern (see **Fig. 3**).

Radiologists may recognize a typical contrast curve pattern and, in combination with the morphologic characteristics of the tissue, render a diagnosis. A typical pattern of malignancy is rapid intense contrast enhancement followed by a rapid washout (ie, in the case of arteriovenous shunting) or a more rapid diminution of contrast enhancement than in neighboring normal tissue. This is thought to be due to tumor angiogenesis. At the senior author's institution, simple curve recognition is used successfully for the diagnosis of breast and prostate cancer diagnosis. However, this practice is limited by the lack of reproducibility of the results due to the differences in personal interpretation and precludes comparison between different studies, different patients, and different equipment.

Sometimes these basic parameters are further quantified to add greater specificity; the most commonly used parameters are the slope of the washin curve or of the washout phase. The AUC may be determined within a certain time limit, such as 60 seconds (AUC_{60}) or 90 seconds (AUC_{90}) to allow a more reproducible comparison with other studies.

More complicated permeability models are available to provide greater detail about the underlying physiologic processes and anatomic compartments, as well as a more robust and reproducible analysis. Many of the details of these multicompartmental models are beyond the scope of this article, as well as beyond the mathematical abilities of the corresponding author. Regardless, clinicians can generally understand the physiologic parameters these are based on and choose models that best fit the clinical imaging needs.

The earliest models of permeability, including those created by Tofts and Kermode,[6,7] Kety,[8] Patlak and colleagues,[9] and Larsson and colleagues[4] were 1-compartment and did not distinguish between the intravascular capillary space and the IS. Some were developed specifically for the study of BBB disruption in patients with multiple sclerosis.[4,6,10] These are based on only 2 parameters, the Ktrans and the Ve, and model the passage of tracers into the IS. By ignoring many of the known physiologic processes, these models were robust and reproducible and became widely disseminated. These first models assumed a negligible and insignificant size of the intravascular space. Although appropriate for brain tissue, it is less appropriate for non-CNS tissue permeability studies in which the percentage of vascular volume (VS),

including both the Hct and plasma (Vp) is much larger, exceeding 13% in lymph nodes[11] and even greater within many tumors. The Tofts-Kety model improved on this, accounting for the VS, and remains among the most widely used permeability models today.

Later modifications, including the work of St Lawrence and Lee,[12] Brix and colleagues,[13] and Balvay and colleagues,[14] assumed a more complex construct in which the AIF and the Ct are considered separately as 2 compartments (**Fig. 4**). Depending on the particular model, the following physiologic processes and anatomic components may be included:

- Quantity or concentration of contrast within the entire voxel = Ct
- Quantity or concentration of contrast within the plasma space = Cp
- Volume of the plasma space = Vp or its fraction vp
- Hematocrit (contrast concentration = 0) = Hct
- Quantity or concentration of contrast in the IS = C_{EES}, Ce
- Volume of the interstitial space = EES, Ve; the fraction = ve
- Intracellular space (contrast concentration = 0)
- Blood flow (or more accurately plasma) in and out of the voxel = F
- Permeability surface product = PS
- Transfer constant from the plasma (Vp) to the extravascular extracellular space (EES), also known as the interstitium (Ve), = Ktrans
- Transfer constant from the EES or Ve to the Vp = Kep
- Extraction constant, the fraction of the indicator (contrast) that passes from the plasma to the EES in the first bolus pass = E
- Tc, the time until the contrast leaves the capillary and only contrast in the EES persists.

There are multiple mathematical constructs that can be used to solve these complex equations on a per voxel basis to arrive at the most accurate result. Computer analysis may be performed to continuously test the modeled curve with the actual measured signal. The parameters of the model are continuously altered so that it eventually arrives at a best fit with the measured values using a least square regression analysis. Alternatively deconvolution methods may be used. Both techniques may be used for more complicated models that measure both perfusion and permeability, including adiabatic models (St Lawrence and Lee[12]) and quality of fit models (Balvay and colleagues[14]). The St Lawrence and Lee[12] model is widely used and considers 5 primary parameters;

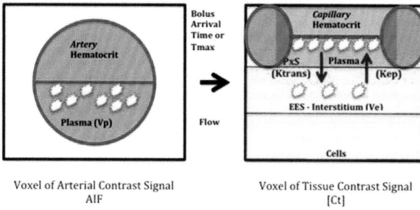

Voxel of Arterial Contrast Signal
AIF

Voxel of Tissue Contrast Signal
[Ct]

Fig. 4. The 2-compartment permeability model. The 2 boxes represent voxels corresponding to the artery AIF and the Ct. The artery may or may not fill the entire voxel (as shown here) and normalization with a VOF (described in the article) would be needed. The contrast is separate from the cellular component (Hct) and resides within the plasma component (Vp) even though in reality these 2 compartments are heterogeneously mixed. The delay between arrival of the contrast even within the artery and the tissue is the bolus arrival time or when deconvolution mathematical algorithms are used it is termed the Tmax (time to maximum residue function). The tissue voxel is separated into the vascular space (the capillary) comprised of the Hct component and the plasma component similar to the larger arteries. Again, the contrast resides within the plasma component, the volume of which is Vp. The extravascular tissue may be divided into the cellular component and the EES, also known as the IS. The volume of the EES is the Ve. Solving the AIF and the (Ct) through various mathematical methods allows the determination of the rate of transfer of contrast from the plasma to the EES, and the slower return from the EES to the plasma. The rate of the first is determined by the permeability of the endothelium and its surface area PS. The rate constant is termed Ktrans. Conversely the rate constant for the return of contrast from the EES to the plasma is termed Kep.

F, E, Ve, PS, and Tc. It makes reasonable physiologic assumptions to simplify the mathematics, including slower equilibrium of contrast from the EES back to the plasma. The 2-compartment model is shown to work well for brain permeability using MR imaging T1-weighted DCE techniques.[15] Adiabatic models have been shown to have the best fit with actual data for laryngeal tumors.[16] Bayesian models may further improve the accuracy of the results.[17]

The strength of these models lie in their ability to produce results that more closely mimic the true physiologic processes, and are quantified and more reproducible than the subjective evaluation of contrast concentration curves. The use of models allows for different studies from the same patient to be compared over time and allows for the collection of data with large numbers of patients.

It should be apparent that inherent problems exist. These models make assumptions that may not be appropriate for a given clinical situation, the tissue of interest, or the imaging acquisition used. Physiologic parameters may be assumed by the model that are not available within the dataset or, conversely, measurements may be available that are not accounted for by using a simplified model. Algorithmic accuracy does not necessarily equate with clinical accuracy and

attention should be paid to the model selected and the imaging acquisition applied. Care should be taken not to compare information obtained with different models, different modalities, or acquired with different protocols. Furthermore, poor signal-to-noise ratio, inappropriate selection of the AIF or tissue of interest, or imaging related artifact may corrupt the analysis.

ACQUISITION PROTOCOLS AND OPTIMIZATION
Contrast Concentration to Data

Although CT and MR imaging are wholly different in the foundation of their imaging signal, both CT electron attenuation and MR imaging T1-weighted signal intensity share a (nearly) linear relationship between the concentration of contrast in a voxel and the detected attenuation or signal. Consequently, the same perfusion and permeability algorithms may be applied to both modalities.

Protocols

The injection parameters and acquisition protocols for CT and MR imaging T1 DCE share similar characteristics and are extremely important for good quality studies. Many excellent theoretic and practical reviews are available.[18–21] Contrast administration needs to assume a bolus configuration using a power injector with a rapid rate of BF to ensure a single, discrete, high-concentration column of contrast within the vasculature. This provides the best representation of the true BF. For CT perfusion (CTp) studies, a rate of 4, 5, or 6 cc per second is recommended, as permitted by the intravenous access and the cardiac output. A normal saline chaser of 40 mL at the same rate should be used to move the contrast from the peripheral to the central venous vasculature and keep the configuration of the contrast bolus tight. For MR imaging studies, a power injector is also necessary, with similar bolus considerations, although the amount of contrast is considerably less. An inadequate long, slow bolus tends to be diluted and will widen and flatten the arterial contrast concentration curve and distort the AIF determination.

The acquisition requirements for each modality share similarities in their temporal characteristics. Perfusion imaging and, particularly, the measurement of the AIF require a short-interval acquisition so that the contrast bolus concentration curve can be adequately sampled. Ischemic stroke imaging literature demonstrates a need for acquisition intervals of approximately 3 to 4 seconds to insure accurate results.[22] Other investigators support a slightly faster interval for DCE tissue perfusion,[23] whereas an even faster time interval is required for myocardial MR perfusion.[24] Similar but not greater sampling intervals may be considered for head and neck soft tissue perfusion.

The arrival, duration, and intensity of the arterial first pass bolus are variable, depending on the individual physiology, particularly the cardiac output and the organ system studied. The capillary phase begins rapidly after the arterial opacification and is of only slightly longer duration. Generally, rapid sampling over the first 30 to 60 seconds will provide an adequate time frame to capture this arterial, capillary bolus perfusion phase. A delay of acquisition after injection is typically used in CT so that little radiation exposure is accrued before the contrast reaching its target. However, the acquisition must start early enough so that a non-contrast baseline is established, which is mandatory for the postprocessing.

The duration of the acquisition is equally important so that enough data are available to define the more gradual transport of contrast from the plasma into the IS and the even longer transfer back to the plasma. These contrast curves provide the data for the permeability coefficients of the models and are of utmost importance. Truncating the acquisition risks biasing the permeability results by relying on the early washout phase before equilibrium is established. At least 1 minute and, depending on the tissues studied, upwards of 3.5 minutes may be required for a robust determination. Brain perfusion studies demonstrate that the Patlak model, a simplified 2-compartment construct, requires 210 seconds for accurate BBB permeability determination.[25]

The complete protocol information for both CT and MR perfusion and permeability imaging for head and neck tumors at the senior author's institution are contained within **Table 1**. At this institution, variable interval CT acquisition for neck perfusion is performed. A time interval of 1.5 seconds is used for the first 20 acquisitions, followed by an interval of 3.0 seconds for the remaining 10 acquisitions, not including baseline measurements. This ensures capture of the arterial bolus and the early washout phase, which is of particular importance in tumors with a rapid transit time compared with normal soft tissue.

Acquisition interval for MR imaging is more complex. T1-weighted radial acquisition GRASP is used in a single 4-minute acquisition and then divided into discrete intervals with off-line postprocessing. Acquisition intervals as short as 2.4 seconds are possible, though typically longer intervals of 8 seconds are used. The long duration allowed by MR imaging is excellent for permeability studies, although the considerable postprocessing and bulky datasets produced with short-interval reconstruction make it less desirable for studying the AIF perfusion characteristics.

Radiation dose, particularly to radiosensitive organs such as the thyroid and the lens, is a constant concern and has been responsible for much of the hesitation to use CTp in head and neck imaging. Newer generation scanners, however, provide considerable dose reduction due to increased detector efficiency and dose modulation. At this institution, acquisition of CT soft tissue neck perfusion is customized in an effort to reduce dose but retain high temporal information. Using a 70 kilovolt (peak) (kV[p]) tube voltage instead of the more typical 100 or 140 kV(p), to more closely approximate the K-edge of iodine provides greater attenuation and higher contrast conspicuity with considerable dose reduction. The authors' current perfusion study covers 22 cm of anatomy, and delivers an approximate dose length product of 706 mGy-cm. In comparison, the traditional multiphase contrast-enhanced CT, which has subsequently been abandoned, delivered a radiation dose of 579 mGy-cm. This modest increase in dose provides perfusion and permeability information that was previously unavailable. This improves diagnosis, prediction of therapeutic efficacy, and estimation of prognosis.

Table 1
Protocols for computed tomography and magnetic resonance perfusion of the soft tissue neck

Perfusion CT of the Soft Tissue Neck with Contrast: New York University Langone Medical Center

Dynamic Multi 4D Single tube acquisition on 3rd-generation dual source scanner	
Voltage Tube A	70 kV
mAs Tube A	100
Gantry Rotation time	0.25 s
Detector Acquisition	48 detector × 1.2 mm
Care Dose kV	Off
Pitch	1
CTDIvol (32 cm)	∼34.46 mGy
DLP	705.1 mGy cm
FoV	380 mm
Range	∼224 mm
Time	∼43.9 s
Slice Thickness	5mm
Increment	5mm
Scan Intervals	1.5 s × 20, 3.0 s × 5
Delay	5 s
Contrast Dose	50 cc
Injection Rate	5 cc/s
Normal Saline Chaser	40 cc at 5 cc/s

MR imaging Neck Perfusion Protocol: New York University Langone Medical Center

1.5-T Multichannel GRASP Sequence: Radial Acquisition	
FoV	256 mm
FoV Phase	100.0%
Slice Thickness	2.0 mm
Base Resolution	256
Radial Views	600
Slice Resolution	72% (2.78 mm)
TR	4.62 ms
TE	2.06 ms
FA	12 deg
Averages	1
Fat Suppression	Q-fat sat
Lines/Shot	83
Slabs	1
Slices/Slab	144

(continued on next page)

Table 1
(continued)

MR imaging Neck Perfusion Protocol: New York University Langone Medical Center

Gap	None
Phase-Encoding Direction	Anterior posterior

Abbreviations: CTDI, CT dose index volume; DLP, dose length product; FA, flip angle degree; FoV, field of view; Q-fat sat, fat saturation; TE, echo time; TR, repetition time.

Selection of Modality

CTp has inherent advantages compared with MR imaging, including higher resolution, faster perfusion acquisition intervals eliminating swallowing and phonation artifacts, faster overall acquisition time, diminished artifact from blood products, and lack of MR-related safety issues (eg, implants, electronic medical devices). Additionally, CT scanners may allow for dual-energy technique, which provides diagnostic information not attainable with MR imaging. This includes virtual noncontrast, iodine quantification, monoenergetic spectral analysis, calcium identification and quantification, bone subtraction, and tissue atomic density, which are all potentially important characteristics for tumor evaluation, which may be obtained at the same time as perfusion imaging.

The complete absence of ionizing radiation remains a considerable advantage of MR imaging perfusion. Consequently, the decision to use CT or MR imaging perfusion is often based on the clinical situation, the pretest suspicion for tumor, and the modality preference of the requesting referrer. CTp tends to be used for the characterization of a known soft tissue neck mass when radiation exposure is less of a consideration.

PREPROCESSING AND POSTPROCESSING
Preprocessing, Preconditioning, or the Cleaning of Data

The acquired images are typically preprocessed to provide a better image quality before applying the mathematical models that allow for analysis of perfusion and permeability characteristics. Deconvolution methods are particularly sensitive to noise and multiple techniques are used to improve the ratio of signal intensity or attenuation change compared with baseline noise. Compression or truncation of the signal is performed first to define the signal intensity range, whether the modality is MR imaging or CT. Noise filters are applied to improve the signal to noise ratio. Motion correction, typically using rigid coregistration, removes artifacts. For cerebral imaging, the entire image is generally well-corrected; however, for imaging of the neck, complex multidirectional movements of the soft tissue, vasculature, and spine make this more difficult. Segmentation followed by motion correction of only the region of interest may be required.

Determination of the Arterial Input Function

The AIF is a fundamental component of the algorithms used to determine perfusion and permeability characteristics of the tissue. Consequently, accurate data are needed to avoid producing erroneous results. There is considerable variability in technique, depending on the anatomic region of interest, particularly the organ system being studied, the modality used, the postprocessing software available, or the preferences of the practitioner. Using population-based AIF is a well-established technique but does not account for the hemodynamics of the individual patient, which may be quite variable, not only across different patients but even the same patient at different times. Consequently, it may contribute to erroneous results although the bias is consistent.

Direct measurement of the arterial BF within each study is preferred. It is most desirable to measure the AIF as close to the tissue of interest as possible to diminish the delay between AIF and Ct. Theoretically, measuring the precapillary arteriole itself would be best but is not possible due to its small size and the limited resolution of CT and MR imaging. Generally, a single large artery within the region of interest is selected when performed manually. Typically, for head and neck imaging, the common, internal, or external carotid arteries are selected.

Some postprocessing software automatically assesses all of the voxels within the study and identifies those that have characteristics of the arterial bolus concentration curve (Olea Sphere, La Ciotat, France). This subset is averaged together to create a single composite curve that is termed a local AIF as opposed to a single global AIF. The advantage is that this averaged value tends to bring the AIF measurement closer to that of the true AIF of the tissue within the region of interest and diminishes delay. Brain perfusion studies show that this improves the accuracy of the results.[26] The exact impact on soft tissue imaging of the neck is not precisely known. It has been demonstrated that perfusion and permeability results are not affected by the artery selected for the AIF, regardless whether it is ipsilateral or contralateral to the lesion or whether it is internal versus external carotid artery.[27]

For head and neck perfusion imaging, utilization of the carotid vasculature is usually adequate to provide a robust measurement of the AIF. There are added difficulties if a small artery close to or within the tissue of interest is selected in an effort to diminish delay or bolus arrival time. Volume averaging may be a problem when determining the AIF of a small vessel. If the artery does not fill the voxel completely and nonarterial tissue is included, then the signal intensity or attenuation value may be diminished, affecting the determination of permeability. Consequently, a large vessel VOF is used to standardize the measured AIF. The logic is that the entire BF in and out of the organ is equal so that the AUC of the AIF and VOF should be equal.

Analysis

Most readily available commercial software intended for clinical use provides color-coded multiparametric maps to display the results of the perfusion or permeability analysis. Typically, each map is dedicated to 1 parameter and is displayed in a voxel by voxel format. This allows for a visual assessment of the entire study by scrolling through the different sections obtained and allows for ease of comparison between different permeability parameters. This technique allows for easy visual identification of the lesion of interest and its boundaries, and allows for the easy detection of clusters of voxels that may be abnormal or in some way different from the surrounding tissue.

The voxel-by-voxel technique is susceptible to poor signal-to-noise ratio and, consequently, may produce erroneous results if the size of the voxel is too small. Increasing MR imaging field strength, time of acquisition, or CT radiation dose may overcome this limitation but is often neither feasible nor desirable. Consequently, most perfusion imaging studies are limited in their inherent resolution because they must be balanced with the need for adequate slice thickness to average the signal.

Further quantification of the results may be obtained by using a region of interest. Averaging the values of the individual voxels provides a more robust measurement and may be used to compare the characteristics of each parameter between regions of interest. Additionally, it allows for quantitative ratios between tumor and surrounding normal tissue. Results may be displayed numerically or as a histogram of the voxels, depending on preference. Histograms allow for a visual analysis of the change in maximum or minimum values, as well as easy identification of a shift of the number of voxels to a lower or higher value.

CLINICAL APPLICATIONS OF PERFUSION PERMEABILITY IMAGING TO HEAD AND NECK CANCER

The advantage of perfusion permeability imaging compared with conventional MR and CT imaging is the ability to provide information regarding vascular physiology. Tumor angiogenesis is considered to be an essential requirement for the growth and metastatic potential of head and neck tumors.[28,29] This results in abnormal perfusion and permeability characteristics of head and neck tumors compared with normal surrounding tissue.

CTp was long recognized as an adjunctive component of head and neck tumor imaging to provide physiologic information.[18,30,31] Excellent clinical reviews are available.[21,32] Clinically, both CT and MR imaging provide similar results with statistically significant correlations and may be used interchangeably.[33] Results are robust and reproducible.[34]

Since there are other articles in this issue which have focused on MR permeability and perfusion of head and neck tumors, we will limit the subsequent discussion to CT perfusion in such malignancies. Specific applications follow.

Distinction of Head and Neck Cancer from Benign Tissue

Head and neck cancers demonstrate significantly lower MTT and elevated BV, BF, and PS (PS area product) levels when compared with adjacent normal tissue.[27,28,35]

Determine Local Extension of Head and Neck Cancer

It is crucial to detect the exact extent of the tumor for staging purposes. CTp parameters can complement conventional cross-sectional imaging and suggest possible tumor infiltration into adjacent soft tissues allowing for better demarcation of tumor extent (Fig. 5).[36]

Distinction of Benign Versus Malignant Tumor

It is possible to differentiate between benign and malignant lesions based on MTT values during CTp. According to several studies, malignant tumors demonstrate significantly lower MTT compared with benign tumors. Lesions with MTT less than 3.5 are almost always malignant, whereas lesions with MTT greater than 5.5 are never malignant.[31] There is also overall increased BV and BF with malignant tumors. This may be secondary to higher cellularity stromal grade in benign rather than malignant tumors, as well as areas of necrosis in malignant tumors.[37]

Metastatic Cervical Lymph Nodes

Accurate tumor staging depends on identifying presence or absence of metastatic lymph nodes. This remains challenging on routine cross-sectional anatomic and functional imaging. One study showed that metastatic lymph nodes have higher perfusion than benign nodes, although the difference was not significant.[38] Another study demonstrated significantly higher BF, BV, and PS values for metastatic lymph nodes in hypopharyngeal and laryngeal carcinoma compared with benign cervical lymph nodes.[39]

Guidance for Biopsy

CTp can serve as a tool to decrease sampling errors by avoiding the necrotic or nonviable portion of the tumor from viable portion. High BV and BF are seen in viable regions of malignancy, whereas low BV and BF are seen in nonviable regions (Fig. 6).[40]

Biomarker of Angiogenesis

CTp may be used for monitoring molecular biomarkers because a significant correlation exists between CTp parameters and epidermal growth factor (EGFR) overexpression in head and neck squamous cell carcinoma (HNSCC). EGFR is a marker for disease-specific death and recurrence in HNSCC. Another study showed a significant correlation between interleukin-8 and relative BF measured by CTp. Interleukin-8 is a biomarker of increased angiogenesis. CTp can be used to predict tumor angiogenesis and, hence, its aggressiveness, which in turn can influence better patient management.[41–43]

Recurrent Tumor Versus Posttherapeutic Changes

Differentiating between residual or recurrent tumor from posttherapeutic change is challenging on routine CT due to similar degree of enhancement. Recurrent tumor has been shown to demonstrate increased BV, BF, and PS as compared with post therapeutic changes (Fig. 7).[44]

Prediction of Response to Radiotherapy and Chemotherapy

CTp can be used to predict response to induction chemotherapy and radiotherapy based on the principle of detection of tissue perfusion and local oxygen delivery. Higher pretreatment tumor BF and capillary permeability correlate with better oxygen or drug delivery, and have been observed more often in patients with superior locoregional control than in those with treatment failure. On the other hand, low perfusion of HNSCC is associated with higher rates of failure of radiation therapy.[45–48]

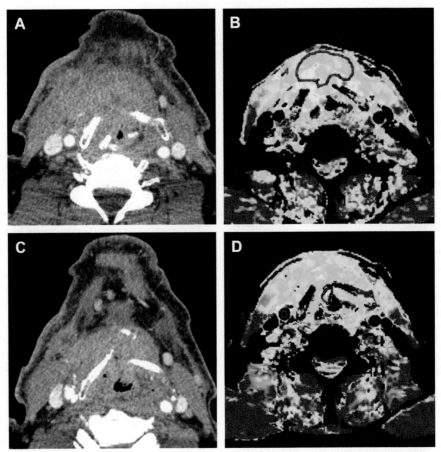

Fig. 5. A 63-year-old man with laryngeal carcinoma. (*A*) Contrast-enhanced CT scan demonstrates laryngeal carcinoma with extralaryngeal spread. (*B*) CTp study demonstrates an elevated BV measuring up to 11.8 mL/100 g of tissue. (*C*) Posttreatment (following 2 cycles of chemotherapy) contrast-enhanced CT scan demonstrates interval decrease in the size of the previously noted mass. (*D*) Corresponding CTp study demonstrates interval decrease in the BV (measuring up to 9.6 mL/100g), suggesting interval response to treatment.

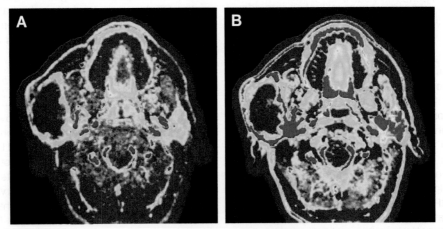

Fig. 6. (*A*) BF and (*B*) BV maps of a right parotid lesion. The sites of increased BV should be targeted for biopsy for maximal yield. Biopsy-proven case of carcinoma ex pleomorphic adenoma.

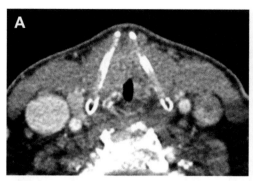
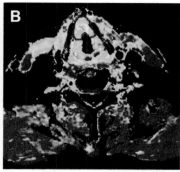

Fig. 7. A 54-year-old man with a treated case of laryngeal carcinoma with new hoarseness of voice. (*A*) Contrast-enhanced CT scan through the neck demonstrates soft tissue in the region of the anterior commissure. Based strictly on conventional images it is difficult to suggest whether this soft tissue represents a posttreatment change or recurrence. (*B*) Corresponding CTp study demonstrates increased BV measuring 10.1 to 11.5 mL/100g, suggestive of tumor recurrence (proven on pathologic testing).

Hence, CTp parameters are independent predictors of local failure in irradiated patients in HNSCC. The response to radiation therapy or chemotherapy would allow clinicians to identify patients with poorly perfused tumors, who in turn are likely to demonstrate poor response to chemotherapy-radiotherapy, which would allow them to be directed to alternative treatments.[49] In a study of 17 subjects, Zima and colleagues[50] demonstrated that elevated pretreatment values of BF (*P*<.03) and BV (*P*<.004) showed a significant correlation with response to induction chemotherapy evaluated endoscopically. In a series of 4 to 5 subjects with HNSCC treated with definitive radiotherapy, some associated with adjacent chemotherapy, Hermans and colleagues[46] concluded that CTp parameters are independent predictors of local control together with the tumor stage. In particular, patients with a low perfusion pretreatment value, which is presumed to be due to a higher degree of hypoxia, showed significantly higher local failure than those with a high perfusion value (*P*<.05), resulting in low radiosensitivity. Bisdas and colleagues,[44] showed that pretreatment CTp has been shown to predict response to induction chemotherapy. It also provides prognostic value in predicting postchemotherapy and postsurgical outcomes for squamous cell carcinoma of the oral cavity, hypopharynx, and oropharynx. Also, tumor volume and BF can predict progression-free survival in advanced squamous cell cancer of the oropharynx.[44]

Treatment Response Monitoring During and After Treatment

The gold standard for therapy monitoring for HNSCC after therapy includes endoscopic examination integrated by biopsy and cross-sectional imaging. Changes produced by radiochemotherapy

agents and tumor vascularity can be identified by changes in CTp parameters (**Fig. 8**). Treatment response manifested by reduction of microvessels inside the tumor could be reflected as a decrease in BV values. A decrease in BF could indicate reduction of low-resistance BF arteriovenous shunts in the microvasculature. The reduction of hyperpermeable capillary bed could be expressed with a decrease of PS values.[51] Variable degree of decrease in BF, BV, and PS values, and increase in MTT values, are seen in responders after induction chemotherapy. Gandhi and colleagues[52] showed correlation between pretherapy increased BV to endoscopic tumor response. They also found that reduction in BV greater than or equal to 20% after 3 weeks of therapy is able to predict more than 50% reduction of cancer volume. Petralia and colleagues[53] supported CTp in monitoring response to the therapy. They found positive correlation between the percentage change in BV and BF values, and the percentage reduction of tumor volume, after 3 cycles of induction chemotherapy. CTp results are more reliable because the use of tumor volume alone assessed by CT and standard endoscopy are operator-dependent techniques for response quantification. CTp has been used to provide information about the periodic changes in tumor oxygenation during the course of radiotherapy, according to a study by Truong and colleagues.[49] Higher pretreatment tumor BF was demonstrated in subjects who achieved locoregional control compared with those with locoregional failure (*P* = .004), consistent with the findings of Hermans and colleagues.[46] The investigators established that higher BF in tumor tissue at the baseline and during the early course of chemotherapy predicts a better tumor control. Surlan-Popovic and colleagues,[54] in a series 24 subjects with locally advanced HNSCC demonstrated that variations in CTp parameters during the course

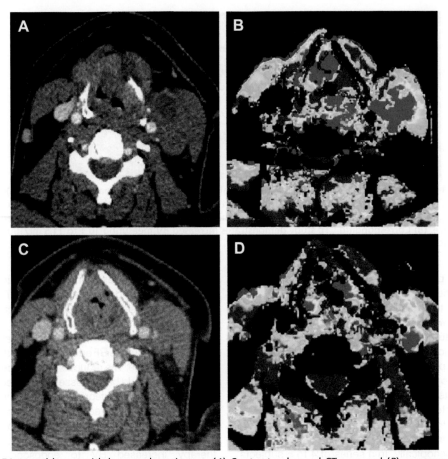

Fig. 8. A 54-year-old man with laryngeal carcinoma. (*A*) Contrast-enhanced CT scan and (*B*) corresponding CTp study demonstrate laryngeal carcinoma with left level III metastatic lymphadenopathy with increased BV at the primary tumor site, as well as in the region of metastatic lymphadenopathy. A PS of 26 mL/100 g/min was obtained from the lymph nodes. (*C*) Post-treatment contrast-enhanced CT scan and (*D*) corresponding CTp study demonstrate interval decrease in the size of the lesion, lymphadenopathy with interval decrease in PS (measuring up to 6.1 mL/100 g/min), suggesting interval response to treatment (1 cycle of chemoradiation).

of treatment may predict tumor response to cisplatin-based chemoradiotherapy. This study demonstrated that responders demonstrated significant reduction of BF values after 40 Gy (*P* = .04), which were further pronounced after 70 Gy (*P* = .01), along with a significant reduction in BV values after 40 Gy, with a plateau after 70 Gy (*P* = .04). MTT and PS values showed nonsignificant modifications. On the contrary, nonresponders showed a nonsignificant increase in BF, BV, and PS values after 40 Gy. This is explained by the cytotoxic effects of the radiotherapy to the vascular endothelium, which is more effective than the antivascular action of cisplatin-based chemotherapy. As far as increased perfusion parameters in nonresponders, it is hypothesized that ionizing radiation therapy may produce upregulation of vascular endothelial growth factor, which promotes survival of endothelial cells within the residual tumor tissue and, consequently, leads to radiation resistance.[55]

Lymphoma

CTp parameters have a unique role in both Hodgkin and non-Hodgkin lymphoma, which are often seen in the head and neck. Low MTT and elevated BF, BV, and PS have been observed in primary sphenoid sinus lymphoma.[56] Similar parameters have been used to distinguish untreated (low MTT, high BV, BF, PS) versus treated lymphoma. Higher perfusion was shown in active lymphoma compared with inactive lymphoma, as well as with transformation of inactive to active lymphoma on serial examinations.[57]

SUMMARY

Perfusion and permeability imaging applied to head and neck cancer provides a powerful diagnostic and prognostic tool for clinicians. Understanding the basics of these techniques allows the radiologist to make informed decisions regarding the use of modeling algorithms, acquisition parameters, and postprocessing techniques. This helps to ensure that studies are acquired, analyzed, and reported appropriately, and erroneous results are avoided. These techniques are highly automated, widely available, and can be easily and safely incorporated into daily imaging workflow.

REFERENCES

1. Schindera ST, Nelson RC, Howle L, et al. Contrast media dynamics without and with a saline chaser. Eur Radiol 2008;18(8):1683–9.
2. Cuenoda CA, Balvay D. Perfusion and vascular permeability: basic concepts and measurement in DCE-CT and DCE-MRI. Diagn Interv Imaging 2013; 94:1187–204.
3. Chen H, Liu N, Li Y, et al. Permeability imaging in cerebrovascular diseases: applications and progress in research. Neurovascular Imaging 2016;2:1.
4. Larsson HB, Stubgaard M, Frederiksen JL, et al. Quantitation of blood-brain barrier defect by magnetic resonance imaging and gadolinium-DTPA in patients with multiple sclerosis and brain tumors. Magn Reson Med 1990;16:117–31.
5. Sourbron SP, Buckley DL. Tracer kinetic modelling in MRI: estimating perfusion and capillary permeability. Phys Med Biol 2012;57:R1–33.
6. Tofts PS, Kermode AG. Blood-brain barrier permeability in multiple sclerosis using labelled DTPA with PET, CT and MRI. J Neurol Neurosurg Psychiatry 1989;52:1019–20.
7. Tofts PS, Kermode AG. Measurement of the blood-brain barrier permeability and leakage space using dynamic MR imaging. 1. Fundamental concepts. Magn Reson Med 1991;17:357–67.
8. Kety SS. Regional cerebral blood flow: estimation by means of nonmetabolized diffusible tracers — an overview. Semin Nucl Med 1985;15(4):324–8.
9. Patlak CS, Blasberg RG, Fenstermacher JD. Graphical evaluation of blood-to-brain transfer constants from multiple-time uptake data. J Cereb Blood Flow Metab 1983;3(1):1–7.
10. Pozzilli C, Bernardi S, Mansi L, et al. Quantitative assessment of blood-brain barrier permeability in multiple sclerosis using 68-Ga-EDTA and positron emission tomography. J Neurol Neurosurg Psychiatry 1988;51:1058–62.
11. Kanick SC, van der Leest C, Djamin RS, et al. Characterization of mediastinal lymph node physiology in vivo by optical spectroscopy during endoscopic ultrasound-guided fine needle aspiration. J Thorac Oncol 2010;5(7):981–7.
12. St Lawrence KS, Lee TY. An adiabatic approximation to the tissue homogeneity model. J Cereb Blood Flow Metab 1998;18(12):1365–77.
13. Brix G, Bahner ML, Hoffmann U, et al. Regional blood flow, capillary permeability, and compartmental volumes: measurement with dynamic CT - initial experience. Radiology 1999;210(1):269–76.
14. Balvay D, Frouin F, Calmon G, et al. New criteria for assessing fit quality in dynamic contrast-enhanced T1-weighted MRI for perfusion and permeability imaging. Magn Reson Med 2005;54: 868–77.
15. Larsson HBW, Courivaud F, Rostrup E, et al. Measurement of brain perfusion, blood volume, and blood-brain barrier permeability, using dynamic contrast-enhanced T1-weighted MRI at 3 Tesla. Magn Reson Med 2009;62:1270–81.
16. Oosterbroek J, Bennink E, Philippens MEP, et al. Comparison of DCE-CT models for quantitative evaluation of Ktrans in larynx tumors. Phys Med Biol 2015;60:3759–73.
17. Brochot C, Bessoud B, Balvay D, et al. Evaluation of antiangiogenic treatment effects on tumors' microcirculation by Bayesian physiological pharmacokinetic modeling and magnetic resonance imaging. Magn Reson Imaging 2006;24: 1059–67.
18. Faggioni L, Neri E, Bartolozzi C. CT perfusion of head and neck tumors: how we do it. AJR Am J Roentgenol 2010;194:62–9.
19. Kassner A, Thornhill R. Measuring the integrity of the human blood–brain barrier using magnetic resonance imaging. In: Nag S, editor. The blood-brain and other neural barriers: reviews and protocols. Methods in molecular biology, vol. 686. New York: Humana Press; 2011. p. 229–45.
20. Chassidim Y, Veksler R, Lublinsky S. Quantitative imaging assessment of blood brain barrier permeability in humans. Fluids Barriers CNS 2013;10(9): 1–8.
21. Razek AA, Tawfik AM, Elsorogy LG, et al. Perfusion CT of head and neck cancer [review]. Eur J Radiol 2014;83:537–44.
22. Wintermark M, Smith WS, Ko NU, et al. Dynamic perfusion CT: optimizing the temporal resolution and contrast volume for calculation of perfusion CT parameters in stroke patients. AJNR Am J Neuroradiol 2004;25(5):720–9.
23. Brix G, Zwick S, Kiessling F, et al. Pharmacokinetic analysis of tissue microcirculation using nested models: multimodel inference and parameter identifiability. Med Phys 2009;36(7):2923–33.
24. Jerosch-Herold M. Quantification of myocardial perfusion by cardiovascular magnetic resonance. J Cardiovasc Magn Reson 2010;12(57):1–16.
25. Hom J, Dankbaar JW, Schneider T, et al. Optimal duration of acquisition for dynamic perfusion CT assessment of blood-brain barrier permeability using the Patlak model. AJNR Am J Neuroradiol 2009;30:1366–70.

26. Willats L, Christensen S, Ma HK, et al. Validating a local arterial input function method for improved perfusion quantification in stroke. J Cereb Blood Flow Metab 2011;31:2189–98.

27. Tawfik A, Razek AAKA, Elsorogy LG, et al. Perfusion CT of head and neck cancer: effect of arterial input selection. AJR Am J Roentgenol 2011;196:1374–80.

28. Srinivasan A, Mohan S, Mukherji SK. Biologic imaging of head and neck cancer: the present and the future. AJNR Am J Neuroradiol 2012;33:586–94.

29. Jansen J, Koutcher J, Dave A. Non-invasive imaging of angiogenesis in head and neck squamous cell carcinoma. Angiogenesis 2010;13:149–60.

30. Mukherji SK, Castelijns JA. CT perfusion of head and neck cancer: why we should care versus why should we care! AJNR Am J Neuroradiol 2010;31:391–3.

31. Rumboldt Z, Al-Okaili R, Deveikis JP. Perfusion CT for head and neck tumors: pilot study. AJNR Am J Neuroradiol 2005;26:1178–85.

32. Preda L, Calloni SF, Moscatelli MEM, et al. Role of CT perfusion in monitoring and prediction of response to therapy of head and neck squamous cell carcinoma. Biomed Res Int 2014;2014:917150.

33. Bisdas S, Medov L, Baghi M, et al. A comparison of tumor perfusion assessed by deconvolution-based analysis of dynamic contrast-enhanced CT and MR imaging in patients with squamous cell carcinoma of the upper aerodigestive tract. Eur Radiol 2008; 18:843–50.

34. Bisdas S, Surlan-Popovic K, Didanovic V, et al. Functional CT of squamous cell carcinoma in the head and neck: repeatability of tumor and muscle quantitative measurements, inter- and intra-observer agreement. Eur Radiol 2008;18:2241–50.

35. Hermans R, Op de Beeck K, van den Bogaert W, et al. The relation of CT-determined tumor parameters and local and regional outcome of tonsillar cancer after definitive radiation treatment. Int J Radiat Oncol Biol Phys 2001;50:37–45.

36. Petralia G, Preda L, D'Andrea G, et al. CT perfusion in solid body tumours. Part I: technical issues. Radiol Med 2010;83:537–44.

37. Bisdas S, Baghi M, Wagenblast J, et al. Differentiation of benign and malignant parotid tumors using deconvolution-based perfusion CT imaging: feasibility of the method and initial results. Eur J Radiol 2007;64:258–65.

38. Bisdas S, Baghi M, Smolarz A, et al. Quantitative measurements of perfusion and permeability of oropharyngeal and oral cavity cancer, recurrent disease, and associated lymph nodes using first-pass contrast-enhanced computed tomography studies. Invest Radiol 2007;42:172–9.

39. Trojanowska A, Trojanowski P, Bisdas S, et al. Squamous cell cancer of hypopharynx and larynx – evaluation of metastatic nodal disease based on computed tomography perfusion studies. Eur J Radiol 2012;81:1034–9.

40. Miles KA, Griffiths MR. Perfusion CT: a worthwhile enhancement? Br J Radiol 2003;251:422–8.

41. Ash L, Tekons TN, Gandhi D, et al. Head and neck squamous cell carcinoma: CT perfusion can help noninvasively predict intratumoral microvessel density. Radiology 2009;251:422–8.

42. Hoefling N, McHugh J, Light E, et al. Human papillomavirus, p16, and epidermal growth factor receptor biomarkers and CT perfusion values in head and neck squamous cell carcinoma. AJNR Am J Neuroradiol 2013;34:1062–6.

43. Jo SY, Wang PI, Nör JE, et al. CT perfusion can predict overexpression of CXCL8 (interleukin-8) in head and neck squamous cell carcinoma. AJNR Am J Neuroradiol 2013;34:2338–42.

44. Jin G, Su D, Liu L, et al. The accuracy of computed tomographic perfusion in detecting recurrent nasopharyngeal carcinoma after radiation therapy. J Comput Assist Tomogr 2011;35:26–30.

45. Bisdas B, Rumboldt Z, Wagenblast J, et al. Response and progression-free survival in oropharynx squamous cell carcinoma assessed by pretreatment perfusion CT: comparison with tumor volume measurements. AJNR Am J Neuroradiol 2009;30:793–9.

46. Hermans R, Meijerink M, Van den Bogaert W, et al. Tumor perfusion rate determined noninvasively by dynamic computed tomography predicts outcome in head-and-neck cancer after radiotherapy. Int J Radiat Oncol Biol Phys 2003;57:1351–6.

47. Bisdas S, Nguyen SA, Anand SK, et al. Outcome prediction after surgery and chemoradiation of squamous cell carcinoma in the oral cavity, oropharynx, and hypopharynx: use of baseline perfusion CT microcirculatory parameters versus tumor volume. Int J Radiat Oncol Biol Phys 2009;73:1313–8.

48. Cao Y, Popovtzer A, Li D, et al. Early prediction of outcome in advanced head and-neck cancer based on tumor blood volume alterations during therapy: a prospective study. Int J Radiat Oncol Biol Phys 2008;72:1287–90.

49. Truong M, Saito N, Ozonoff A, et al. Prediction of locoregional control in head and neck squamous cell carcinoma with serial CT perfusion during radiotherapy. AJNR Am J Neuroradiol 2011;32:1195–201.

50. Zima A, Carlos R, Gandhi D, et al. Can pretreatment CT perfusion predict response of advanced squamous cell carcinoma of the upper digestive tract treated with induction chemotherapy? AJNR Am J Neuroradiol 2007;28:328–34.

51. Bellomi M, Viotti S, Preda L, et al. Perfusion CT in solid body-tumours. Part II: clinical applications and future development. Radiol Med 2010;115:858–74.

52. Gandhi D, Chepeha B, Miller T, et al. Correlation between initial and early follow-up CT perfusion parameters with endoscopic tumor response in patients with advanced squamous cell carcinomas of the oropharynx treated with organ-preservation therapy. AJNR Am J Neuroradiol 2006;27:101–6.

53. Petralia G, Preda L, Giugliano G, et al. Perfusion computed tomography for monitoring induction chemotherapy in patients with squamous cell carcinoma of the upper digestive tract: correlation between changes in tumor perfusion and tumor volume. J Comput Assist Tomogr 2009;33:552–9.

54. Surlan-Popovic K, Bisdas S, Rumboldt Z, et al. Changes in perfusion CT of advanced squamous cell carcinoma of the head and neck treated during the course of concomitant chemoradiotherapy. AJNR Am J Neuroradiol 2010;31:570–5.

55. Gupta VK, Jaskowiak NT, Beckett MA, et al. Vascular endothelial growth factor enhances endothelial cell survival and tumor radioresistance. Cancer J 2002; 8:47–54.

56. Bisdas S, Fetscher S, Feller A, et al. Primary B cell lymphoma of the sphenoid sinus: CT and MRI characteristics with correlation to perfusion and spectroscopic imaging features. Eur Arch Otorhinolaryngol 2007;264:1207–13.

57. Dugdale PE, Miles KA, Bunce I, et al. CT measurement of perfusion and permeability within lymphoma masses and its ability to assess grade, activity, and chemotherapeutic response. J Comput Assist Tomogr 1999;23:540–7.

PET–Computed Tomography in Head and Neck Cancer
Current Evidence and Future Directions

Yin Jie Chen, MD[a], Tanya Rath, MD[b], Suyash Mohan, MD, PDCC[c],*

KEYWORDS

- Head and neck • Squamous cell carcinoma • HNSCC • FDG • PET • PET-CT

KEY POINTS

- ^{18}F-fluorodeoxyglucose (FDG) PET–computed tomography (CT) provides more accurate staging in head and neck cancers (HNCs) and is critical for treatment planning.
- FDG PET-CT is more useful than conventional imaging in detection of unknown primary HNC and secondary primary malignancies, which affects therapy.
- FDG PET-CT has tremendous value for staging in advanced HNC, prognostication, assessing treatment response, as well as for long-term surveillance.
- Novel non-FDG PET tracers are under investigation and have great potential in improving personalized care for HNC in the future.

INTRODUCTION

According to the American Cancer Society, almost 50,000 new cases of head and neck cancer (HNC) occur each year in the United States, with approximately 10,000 attributable deaths.[1] HNC most commonly arises in the oral cavity, oropharynx, and larynx; followed by nasopharynx and nasal cavity, and other less common sites. From a histopathologic perspective, squamous cell carcinoma (SCC) accounts for more than 90% to 95% of HNC; therefore, head and neck SCC (HNSCC) is the focus of this article.[2] Over recent years, although there has been decreasing incidence of HNC associated with the carcinogens tobacco and alcohol, there has been increasing incidence of HNC related to human papillomavirus (HPV).[3]

The tumor-node-metastasis (TNM) staging system of the American Joint Committee on Cancer is most commonly used to predict prognosis and guide therapy for HNSCC.[4] Early-stage HNSCC may be managed by radiation or surgery alone, whereas locally advanced HNSCC may require a combination of surgery, radiation, and chemotherapy or targeted-therapy. Accurate staging at initial diagnosis, as well as posttherapy assessment, is of vital importance in optimizing outcomes. Although contrast-enhanced computed

Disclosure Statement: The authors have nothing to disclose.

[a] Department of Radiology, Perelman School of Medicine, University of Pennsylvania, Hospital of the University of Pennsylvania, 1 Silverstein, 3400 Spruce Street, Philadelphia, PA 19104, USA; [b] Departments of Radiology and Otolaryngology, University of Pittsburgh School of Medicine, Radiology Administration, PUH Suite E204, 200 Lothrop Street, Pittsburgh, PA 15213, USA; [c] Department of Radiology, Perelman School of Medicine, University of Pennsylvania, Hospital of the University of Pennsylvania, 219 Dulles Building, 3400 Spruce Street, Philadelphia, PA 19104, USA
* Corresponding author.
E-mail address: Suyash.Mohan@uphs.upenn.edu

tomography (CT) and MR imaging remain critical in the management of HNSCC, recently, PET with ^{18}F-fluorodeoxyglucose (FDG) has become increasingly important in the care of patients with HNSCC.[5] This article focuses on the utility of FDG PET–CT in HNSCC at initial diagnosis and treatment, assessing therapeutic response, and long-term surveillance. This is followed by an overview of novel non-FDG PET tracers for HNSCC as the future direction of molecular imaging and personalized medicine.

BASICS OF 18F-FLUORODEOXYGLUCOSE PET–COMPUTED TOMOGRAPHY

PET can provide quantitative evaluation of physiologic processes by combining positron-emitting radioisotopes with ligands that target the biochemical processes of interest. PET radioisotopes emit a positron that travels a short distance of a few millimeters in tissue before colliding with an electron, leading to an annihilation event and emission of 2 511 keV photons, 180° apart, detectable by the PET scanner. FDG is the most commonly used PET tracer clinically and is vital to the management of many solid malignancies.[6] FDG is an analogue of glucose that becomes irreversibly trapped in a cell after phosphorylation and is, therefore, a measure of glycolysis, which tends to be higher in tumors. Increased FDG uptake is not specific for malignancy. Benign processes, including inflammation, can also be FDG-avid. In clinical practice, FDG PET is generally combined with CT. The CT can be low-dose used for attenuation correction and anatomic localization. Alternatively, if the appropriate workflow is in place, the CT portion can be done similar to diagnostic CTs with inclusion of intravenous contrast, which can be especially useful in necrotic tumors.[7] For HNSCC, FDG PET-CT is commonly acquired from skull base or vertex of the skull to the proximal thighs. Some institutions also acquire separate dedicated head and neck images with longer bed time and smaller field of view, which may offer better assessment of locoregional disease, although the incremental utility of these dedicated head and neck images has been questioned. For example, Yamamoto and colleagues[8] showed that, although the dedicated head and neck PET-CT was more sensitive than whole body imaging, the findings did not reach statistical significance. Recent advancements in PET-CT scanners, including time of flight, has led to improved lesion detection and further research may be warranted to assess the added utility of dedicated head and neck PET-CT in current clinical practice.

Tumor metabolism can be measured semiquantitatively on FDG PET-CT using standard uptake value (SUV), which normalizes the photon counts in a region of interest to the administered radiotracer dose and patient's weight (or, alternatively, lean body mass or body surface area). Clinically, the most commonly used SUV measure is the maximal SUV value (SUVmax) value, which can be sensitive to noise, reconstruction algorithms, and other acquisition parameters. Therefore, changes in SUVmax should be interpreted with caution when 2 PET-CT studies are acquired from different scanners without cross-calibration, and strict cutoffs in SUVmax should not be used given the variability in tumor FDG uptake and technical parameters. Another measure is the metabolic tumor volume (MTV) more commonly seen in the radiation oncology literature, which measures tumor volume using a percentage of SUVmax to define boundaries. Total lesion glycolysis (TLG) is also commonly encountered and defined as mean SUV multiplied by MTV. Despite its shortcomings, SUVmax remains the predominantly used measure of FDG uptake by tumors clinically due to its ease of use.

UTILITY OF 18F-FLUORODEOXYGLUCOSE PET–COMPUTED TOMOGRAPHY IN INITIAL DIAGNOSIS AND TREATMENT
Initial Staging

Accurate staging of HNSCC has significant impact on prognosis and treatment planning.[4] The T component in the TNM staging system is based on primary tumor size and extent of local disease involvement, which differs for various regions in head and neck, and is beyond the scope of this article. Although PET has inferior resolution and anatomic details compared with CT and MR imaging, studies have shown that FDG PET-CT has higher sensitivity in depicting primary HNSCC.[9,10] One example in which FDG PET-CT is more useful in demonstrating the primary tumor is in the oral cavity adjacent to dental hardware, an area that remains obscured from streak artifacts on CT and susceptibility artifacts on MR imaging (**Fig. 1**). Combining FDG PET with contrast-enhanced CT, Krabbe and colleagues[9] reported sensitivity and specificity of FDG PET-CT for detecting primary tumor of greater than 90%. Due to the spatial resolution of PET, small lesions of a few millimeters may not be detected, especially along superficial mucosal surfaces.[11] This limitation in spatial resolution is compounded by physiologic FDG uptake in the head and neck, such as lymphoid tissues in Waldeyer ring, vocal cords, and muscles. In addition, necrotic primary tumors may not exhibit

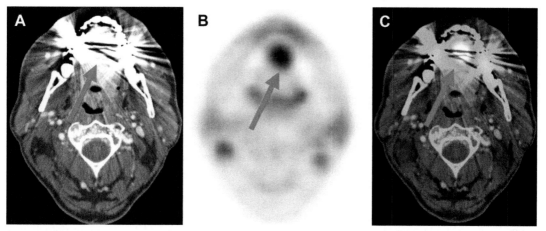

Fig. 1. Oral cavity SCC. A 50-year-old man with oral tongue and floor-of-mouth SCC that was obscured by dental amalgam streak artifacts (*arrow* in *A*) but easily identified on PET due to intense FDG avidity (*arrows* in *B* and *C*). Physiologic brown fat FDG avidity is seen in the posterior triangles bilaterally and should not be mistaken for nodal uptake. (*A*) Contrast-enhanced CT. (*B*) FDG PET. (*C*) Fused PET-CT.

FDG uptake above background (**Fig. 2**). In these situations, contrast-enhanced PET-CT can be especially useful for improving diagnostic accuracy by distinguishing normal muscles and other anatomic structures from pathologic cystic and necrotic tumors.

The N component in the TNM staging system refers to the metastatic regional lymph nodes, among the most important prognostic factors in HNSCC.[12] On CT and MR imaging, size and morphology are used to assess for metastatic involvement, such as maximum cross-sectional dimension greater than 10 to 15 mm or central necrosis.[13] In contrast, FDG PET-CT can be useful in detecting pathologic lymphadenopathy in smaller morphologically normal lymph nodes. However, given the shortcomings of SUVmax, numeric thresholds in SUVmax for determining metastatic involvement should be viewed with caution, especially because reactive lymph nodes can have variable FDG avidity. Studies have demonstrated high sensitivity and specificity of FDG PET-CT in detection of cervical lymph nodes involved by metastatic HNSCC. For example, Su and colleagues[14] reported a meta-analysis showing pooled sensitivity of 84% and pooled

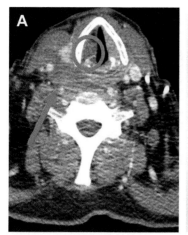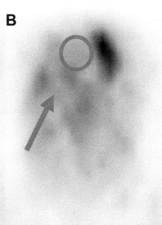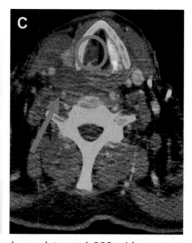

Fig. 2. Non-FDG–avid primary tumor. A 63-year-old man with locally advanced treated SCC with recurrent necrotic non-FDG–avid tumor involving the right tracheoesophageal groove and invading the right thyroid lobe, which is well-delineated on contrast-enhanced CT (*arrow* in *A*) but PET occult (*arrow* in *B*). There is absent physiologic FDG avidity in the associated paralyzed right true vocal cord (all *circles*) and normal physiologic FDG avidity in the contralateral left true vocal cord, which should not be mistaken for tumor. (*A*) Contrast-enhanced CT. (*B*) FDG PET. (*C*) Fused PET-CT.

specificity of 93% of FDG PET-CT for detecting cervical lymph node metastases. In a prospective study of 473 subjects with oral cavity SCC, Liao and colleagues[15] reported sensitivity of 78% and specificity of 58% of FDG PET-CT in demonstrating cervical lymph node metastases compared with histopathologic confirmation. The investigators concluded that the lower observed sensitivity and specificity of FDG PET could be related to microscopic disease in lymph nodes or poor uptake in metastatic nodes from low-grade primary tumors. Studies have also shown superior sensitivity and specificity of PET-CT in detecting cervical lymph node involvement compared with CT and MR imaging. For example, Kyzas and colleagues,[16] in a meta-analysis of 32 studies including 1236 subjects showed pooled sensitivity of 79% and specificity of 86% of FDG PET. The investigators also reported that sensitivity and specificity of FDG PET were 80% and 86% compared with 75% and 79% for CT or MR imaging, respectively. Due to its low sensitivity for micrometastasis related to resolution limitations, FDG PET-CT is usually not useful in the workup of clinically N0 neck, with studies reporting sensitivity 50% to 60% and specificity of 80% to 90%.[17,18] In addition, FDG PET-CT may fail to detect cystic necrotic lymph nodes that are more easily seen on contrast-enhanced CT or MR imaging (**Figs. 3** and **4**).[19,20] In these situations, combining diagnostic quality contrast-enhanced CT with PET can be particularly useful in identifying necrotic pathologic lymph nodes.

The M component in the TNM staging system refers to distant metastasis (**Fig. 5**). Studies have shown incidence of distant metastasis of 9% to 10% in HNSCC within a few years of initial diagnosis, with lung, bone, and liver being the most common sites.[21,22] FDG PET-CT plays an important role in determining the M stage in HNSCC. In a study of 299 subjects with HNSCC, Haerle and colleagues[23] reported sensitivity of 98% and specificity of 95% of FDG PET-CT for detecting distant metastatic disease, with a low false-negative rate of 3%. In a study of 103 subjects with oropharyngeal and hypopharyngeal SCC, Chan and colleagues[24] showed a consistent trend in the higher sensitivity of FDG PET-CT compared with whole body 3 T MR imaging for detection of distant metastasis.

Given the superior performance of FDG PET-CT, studies have shown that the incorporation of FDG PET-CT in initial workup led to changes in disease staging and therapy plans.[25–27] For example, in a multicenter prospective study with 233 HNSCC subjects, Lonneux and colleagues[27] showed the FDG PET-CT led to upstaging in 30% and downstaging in 13% of subjects, with alteration in treatment plan in 13.7% of subjects.

Most studies in the literature on FDG PET in HNSCC included either an unenhanced CT or PET only. As emphasized previously, the use of contrast-enhanced PET-CT as combined diagnostic quality CT and diagnostic quality PET can reduce radiation dose and improve diagnostic accuracy, especially for identifying cystic

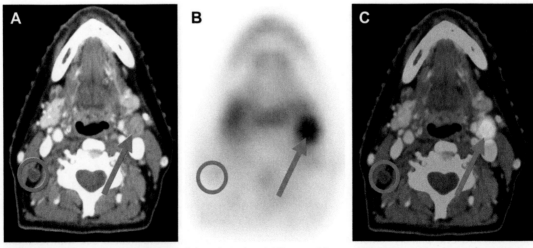

Fig. 3. FDG-avid and non-FDG–avid neck lymph nodes. A 54-year-old man with HPV-positive base of tongue cancer and bilateral metastatic neck lymph nodes. The solid FDG-avid left level II lymph node is well-delineated on contrast-enhanced CT and PET (all *arrows*). The metastatic non-FDG–avid cystic right level II B lymph node (*circle*) is PET occult but well delineated on contrast-enhanced CT portion of this radiation treatment planning scan. (*A*) Contrast-enhanced CT. (*B*) FDG PET, (*C*) Fused PET-CT.

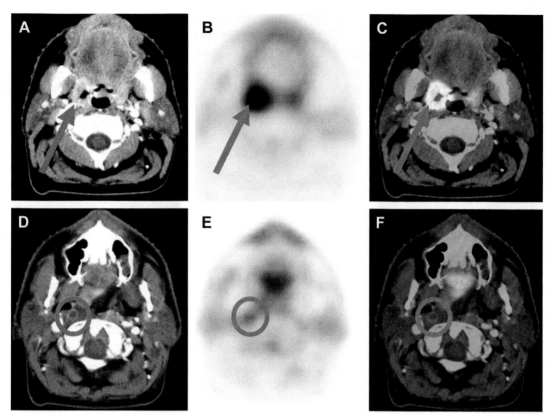

Fig. 4. FDG-avid primary and non-FDG–avid lymph node. A 60-year-old man with FDG-avid right tonsillar cancer (all *arrows*). The cystic metastatic right retropharyngeal lymph node is only faintly FDG avid (all *circles*) but is clearly seen on contrast-enhanced CT. The PET and CT are complementary in characterizing the full extent of disease. (*A, D*) Contrast-enhanced CT. (*B, E*) FDG PET. (*C, F*) Fused PET-CT.

and necrotic tumors and lymph nodes, and avoiding pitfalls arising from normal physiologic findings.[9,28]

Unknown Primary

Around 5% of HNC present with lymph node metastasis with an unknown primary.[29] FDG PET-CT is useful in revealing the site of primary malignancy.[30–32] For example, Rusthoven and colleagues[31] reported in a meta-analysis that FDG PET-CT revealed the site of primary HNSCC in 24.5% of cases of unknown primary after standard work-up, which could include panendoscopy with mucosal biopsies. When performed before panendoscopy, FDG PET-CT has been shown to detect site of primary HNC in 44.2% of subjects in a retrospective series (**Fig. 6**).[32] Therefore, FDG PET-CT can be used to guide endoscopic biopsy and increase diagnostic yield.

Secondary Primary

Patients with HNSCC are also at increased risk for secondary primary cancers, such as lung,

esophageal, or second HNC (**Fig. 7**). Douglas and colleagues[33] showed that 14% of subjects with HNC developed lung cancer, 31% of which were synchronous. FDG PET-CT can play an important role in the detection of secondary primaries.[34,35] For example, Strobel and colleagues[34] reported that in HNSCC subjects, synchronous second primary occurred in 9.5%, of which 84% were detected by FDG PET-CT, resulting in alteration of therapy in 80% of those subjects.

Impact on Radiation Plan

FDG PET-CT has a critical role in planning radiation therapy.[36] Accurate identification of primary tumor and involved lymph nodes is of vital importance in delineating the radiation therapy portal, particularly for intensity-modulated radiotherapy (IMRT), so that normal tissue can be spared while malignant sites are not missed or undertreated.[37] For IMRT, the gross tumor volume (GTV) is an important factor in determining the contour of the radiation field, and FDG PET-CT has been shown

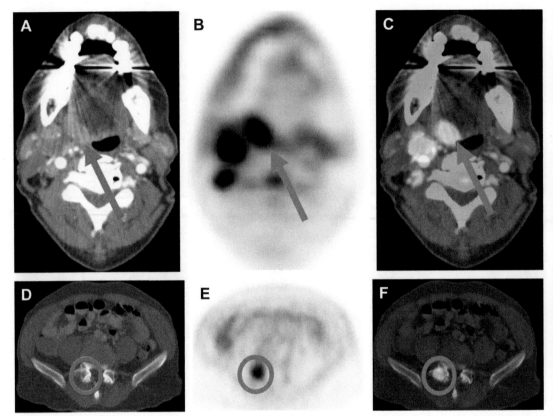

Fig. 5. HNSCC metastatic on staging PET-CT. A 68-year-old man with HPV-negative base-of-tongue SCC (all *arrows*) and FDG-avid right level II cervical metastatic lymph nodes. On staging PET-CT, the patient was also found to have abnormal FDG avidity in the right posterior elements of L5 that was occult on CT, which on biopsy showed metastatic SCC (all *circles*). (*A, D*) Contrast-enhanced CT. (*B, E*) FDG PET. (*C, F*) Fused PET-CT.

to be superior to CT in measuring GTV. For example, Paulino and colleagues[38] showed when using GTV based on CT, 25% of subjects did not receive an optimal radiation dose compared with FDG PET-CT. However, FDG PET-CT can be falsely negative in areas of necrotic tumor, which highlights the importance of using contrast-enhanced PET-CT in radiation planning.[39]

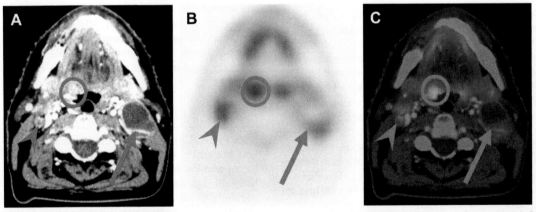

Fig. 6. Unknown primary detected on PET-CT. A 60-year-old man with palpable biopsy proven HPV-positive left level II lymphadenopathy (all *arrows*) and a clinically occult primary. A right level II FDG-avid metastatic lymph node with early necrosis is also present (all *arrowheads*). The unknown primary site was correctly localized on PET-CT with asymmetric FDG uptake at the right glossotonsillar sulcus with minor asymmetry abnormality on CT (all *circles*). (*A*) Contrast-enhanced CT. (*B*) FDG PET. (*C*) Fused PET-CT.

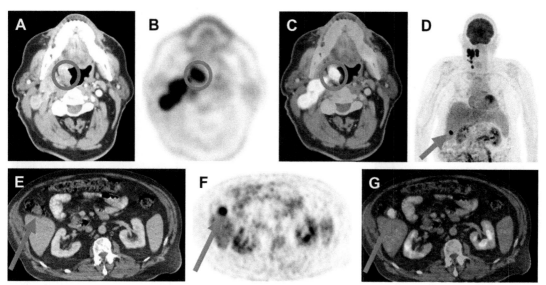

Fig. 7. Secondary primary malignancy on staging PET-CT for HNSCC. A 73-year-old man with right tonsillar SCC (all *circles*) with FDG-avid right level II metastatic lymph nodes. An FDG-avid soft tissue mass at the hepatic flexure was biopsy-confirmed colon cancer (all *arrows*). (*A, E*) Contrast-enhanced CT. (*B, F*) FDG PET. (*C, G*) Fused PET-CT. (*D*) MIP.

Prediction of Prognosis

Many studies have examined the relationship between survival and measures of FDG uptake (eg, SUVmax, MTV, and TLG). A recent systematic review by Castelli and colleagues[40] provides a good summary of the evidence on the prognostic utility of FDG PET-CT. In general, although studies have reported a correlation of SUVmax with outcome measures, there is wide range in reported cutoff value for SUVmax, likely attributable to the sensitivity of SUVmax to technical parameters and variable tumor FDG avidity. In addition, although MTV and TLG have been shown to have higher predictive value in prognostication than SUVmax, the reproducibility of MTV and TLG is limited by their intrinsic reliance on a SUV threshold for contour definition.[40,41]

UTILITY OF 18F-FLUORODEOXYGLUCOSE PET–COMPUTED TOMOGRAPHY AFTER INITIAL TREATMENT
Treatment Response and Early Follow-up

Optimal assessment of treatment response in HNSCC can guide patients toward additional therapies when warranted and avoid unnecessary interventions. FDG PET-CT is thought to be superior to CT and MR imaging for response assessment because FDG PET-CT does not rely solely on size or morphology, and because changes in tumor metabolism typically occur earlier than anatomic changes.[6,42] The presence

of inflammation and fibrosis in the posttreatment head and neck complicates the determination of metabolically active residual tumor on FDG PET-CT.[43] Moreover, compensatory and reactive physiologic changes related to treatment can lead to pitfalls in interpretation (**Figs. 8** and **9**). In a meta-analysis, Gupta and colleagues[44] reported that FDG PET-CT performed at least 12 weeks after definitive therapy had higher diagnostic accuracy than those done earlier than 12 weeks. To further clarify the optimal time frame, Leung and colleagues[45] found that there was no difference in diagnostic accuracy for response assessment when FDG PET-CT was performed at 8 weeks or 12 weeks.

In recent years, various criteria for qualitative treatment response assessment in HNSCC on FDG PET-CT have been proposed, such as the Hopkins criteria[46] and the Deauville criteria.[47] Both the Hopkins criteria and the Deauville criteria are 5-point visual scales comparing FDG uptake in tumor to blood pool and liver background. Both scales were found to correlate with outcome measures, and the Hopkins criteria showed a positive predictive value (PPV) of 71.1% and a negative predictive value (NPV) of 91.1%, versus Deauville criteria with PPV of 68.7% and NPV of 86.4%.

Multiple studies have reported high diagnostic performance of FDG PET-CT in response assessment for HNSCC. In a meta-analysis of 51 studies encompassing 2335 subjects, Gupta and colleagues[44] reported sensitivity of 79.9%, specificity of 87.5%, PPV of 58.6%, and NPV of 95.1% for the

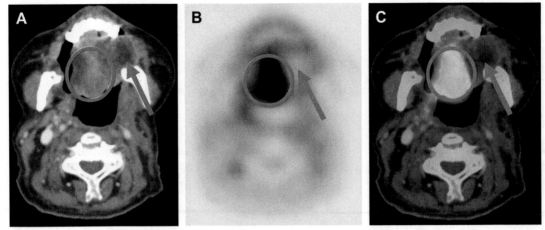

Fig. 8. Physiologic tongue FDG uptake posttherapy. A 55-year-old woman status after chemoradiation and surgery for left tongue carcinoma. Posttherapy PET-CT shows left hemitongue fatty atrophy (all *arrows*) and intense physiologic FDG avidity in the right hemitongue (all *circles*), which should not be mistaken for tumor. The contrast-enhanced CT delineates the normal muscle morphology of the right hemitongue in this posttreatment neck. (*A*) Contrast-enhanced CT. (*B*) FDG PET. (*C*) Fused PET-CT.

primary site, and sensitivity of 72.7%, specificity of 87.6%, PPV of 52.1%, and NPV of 94.5% for the neck. Similar findings were reported by Isles and colleagues[48] in a meta-analysis of 27 studies with sensitivity of 94%, specificity of 82%, PPV of 75%, and NPV of 95% for detection of recurrent or residual HNSCC after definitive therapy. The consistently high NPV of FDG PET-CT in treatment response assessment may allow the safe

avoidance of neck dissections following chemoradiation.[49,50] A recent prospective, randomized study by Mehanna and colleagues[51] showed that survival following chemoradiation was similar among patients in the FDG PET-CT surveillance group and those in the neck dissection group, with fewer operations and lower cost in the FDG PET-CT surveillance group. The comparatively lower PPV of FDG PET-CT in this setting is

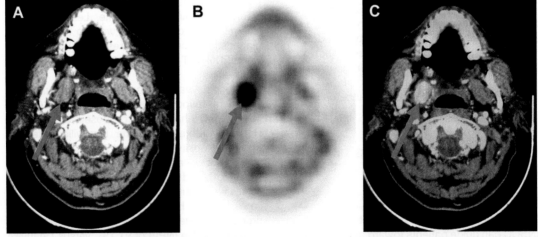

Fig. 9. Physiologic muscle FDG uptake posttherapy. A 66-year-old man with tumor involving the right neck treated with chemoradiation. Posttherapy PET-CT shows intense asymmetric physiologic FDG activity within the right pterygoid muscle (all *arrows*), which maintains a normal morphologic appearance on contrast-enhanced CT and should not be misinterpreted as tumor. Variable patterns of physiologic FDG avidity in the neck can be seen in muscles that are contracting or tensed during the uptake phase and can be asymmetric, particularly following treatment when normal mechanics in the neck have been altered. The contrast-enhanced CT is critical to characterizing a normal appearance of the musculature and avoiding a false-positive interpretation. (*A*) Contrast-enhanced CT. (*B*) FDG PET. (*C*) Fused PET-CT.

attributable to posttherapy inflammatory changes; therefore, tissue confirmation should be pursued to clarify suspicious findings before modifying the treatment plan.

Studies have also examined the role of FDG PET-CT obtained during chemoradiation therapy in guiding early treatment adjustment. A recent study by Wong and colleagues[52] examined the predictive value of FDG PET-CT and diffusion-weighted MR imaging after 1 cycle of induction chemotherapy in 23 subjects with stage III to IVa HNSCC. The investigators found significantly more reduction in MTV and TLG after 1 cycle of induction chemotherapy in responders than in nonresponders. The optimal timing of FDG PET-CT during therapy to guide treatment modification is unclear and remains an active area of research.

Long-Term Prognosis and Surveillance

FDG PET-CT has been shown to have long-term prognostic implications when performed for therapy assessment. For example, Sheikhbahaei and colleagues,[53] in a meta-analysis of 26 studies, reported that intratherapy or posttherapy FDG PET-CT significantly predicted the 2-year and the 3-year to 5-year risk of death or disease progression, with a positive PET result associated with greater than 6-fold increase in the risk of death within 2 years, which was attenuated but remained significant with longer follow-up.

In long-term surveillance, early detection of recurrence is critical for timely institution of additional therapy and optimizing clinical outcome. FDG PET-CT plays a vital role in surveillance of recurrent HNSCC because many recurrences are asymptomatic (**Fig. 10**). Beswick and colleagues[54] examined patterns of HNSCC recurrences after definitive chemoradiation in 388 subjects. Recurrences occurred in 110 of the 388 subjects, of which 66% were asymptomatic. Among the 73 asymptomatic subjects, 45% of the recurrences occurred within 6 months, 79% within 12 months, 92% within 18 months, and 95% within 24 months after chemoradiation. Based on these findings, the investigators concluded that routine FDG PET-CT surveillance after the first 24 months may have limited value in subjects without clinical suspicion for recurrence. In another study, Paidpally and colleagues[55] evaluated the added value of FDG PET-CT in follow-up of 134 HNSCC subjects with 227 FDG PET-CT examinations with a median follow-up period of 40 months. The investigators found that 18% of the follow-up FDG PET-CT examinations were positive for tumor. Overall, recurrence was identified in 5% of examinations performed

without clinical suspicion, and recurrence was excluded in 51.5% of examinations performed for evaluation of clinical suspicion or uncertainty of recurrence.

The value of FDG PET-CT in posttherapy surveillance in HNSCC arises from its high sensitivity and NPV, allowing detection of recurrences missed on physical examination and endoscopy. For example, Kim and colleagues[56] prospectively evaluated 143 subjects with HNSCC who underwent definitive therapy with regular clinical follow-up (using physical examination and endoscopy) and FDG PET-CT at 3 to 6 months and 12 months. The investigators found higher sensitivity and NPV of FDG PET-CT compared with regular clinical follow-up at both 3 to 6 months (sensitivity of 96% and NPV of 99% for FDG PET-CT compared with 11% and 80% for clinical follow-up, respectively) and at 12 months (sensitivity of 93% and NPV of 98% for FDG PET-CT compared with 19% and 80% for clinical follow-up, respectively). The high accuracy of FDG PET-CT in detecting recurrent HNSCC is confirmed in meta-analyses. For example, Sheikhbahaei and colleagues,[57] in a meta-analysis of 23 studies encompassing 2247 FDG PET-CT examinations reported pooled sensitivity of 92% and specificity of 87% in detecting recurrences.

The high sensitivity and NPV of FDG PET-CT in HNSCC recurrence surveillance suggests that relatively longer imaging intervals may be appropriate for certain patients. McDermott and colleagues[58] sought to clarify the utility of NPV of FDG PET-CT in this setting by adopting a surveillance protocol in which FDG PET-CT was performed at 2, 5, 8, and 14 months after therapy. Among 214 subjects with at least 1 negative examination, 19 subjects had recurrences leading to NPV of 91%. In contrast, among 114 subjects with 2 consecutive negative examinations, only 2 had recurrences resulting in NPV of 98%. The investigators concluded that recurrence surveillance in HNSCC with FDG PET-CT may be terminated in patients with 2 negative examinations within 6 months. In a retrospective study with long-term follow-up, Ho and colleagues[59] examined the value of subsequent surveillance in subjects with negative FDG PET-CT at 3-month posttherapy. The investigators found that, in clinically negative subjects, FDG PET-CT detected recurrence in 4% at 3 months, 9% at 12 months, and 4% at 24 months. Therefore, the investigators suggested that subjects with negative FDG PET-CT at 3 months may gain limited benefit from surveillance by FDG PET-CT in the absence of clinical suspicion for recurrence. These studies highlight

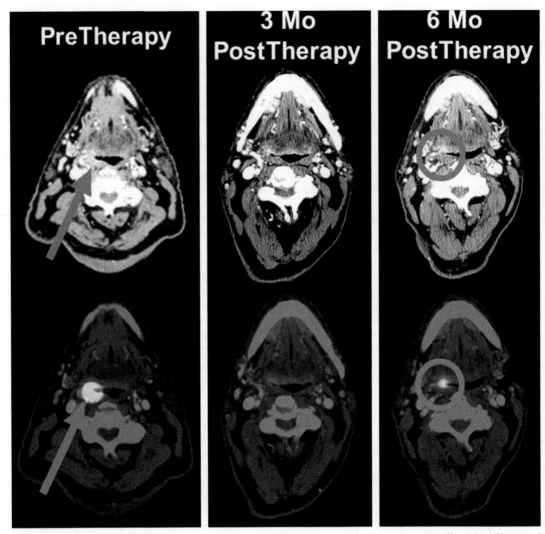

Fig. 10. Clinically occult locally recurrent HNSCC. A 79-year-old man with right glossotonsillar SCC (all *arrows*), treated with definitive radiotherapy. On the 3-month posttherapy PET-CT, there was low-level FDG avidity in the right glossotonsillar sulcus with no discrete mass on examination, so follow-up PET-CT in 3 months was recommended. On the 6-month posttherapy PET-CT, the interval increased FDG avidity in the right glossotonsillar sulcus with subtle enhancement (all *circles*) raised concern for recurrent tumor, which was clinically occult. Directed biopsy in the right glossotonsillar sulcus confirmed recurrent SCC. Top row, contrast-enhanced CT; bottom row, fused PET-CT.

the need for prospective trials to further clarify the value of FDG PET-CT in long-term surveillance for HNSCC patients.

Non–18F-FLUORODEOXYGLUCOSE PET: THE FUTURE OF MOLECULAR IMAGING AND PERSONALIZED MEDICINE

Most research efforts for novel PET tracers in HNSCC have been in hypoxia imaging because hypoxia in tumors is known to be associated with disease progression and resistance to radiation.[60] Among the hypoxia PET tracers under

development, ^{18}F-misonidazole (FMISO) was among the first to be developed.[61,62] The mechanism of action of FMISO involves passive diffusion into cells due to its lipophilicity, followed by reduction into radicals by nitroreductase. In the presence of oxygen, this is reversible and allows FMISO to diffuse back into the extracellular environment. In contrast, under hypoxic conditions, FMISO becomes progressively trapped in cells. FMISO does have slow kinetics of tracer accumulation in hypoxic cells, which causes low tumor to background ratios and complicates interpretation. Studies have shown the utility of hypoxia imaging for prognosis and therapy planning in HNSCC. For example, Rajendran and colleagues[63] demonstrated prognostic utility of pretherapy FMISO PET by showing correlation with overall survival. For chemotherapy guidance, Rischin and colleagues[64] showed that, in subjects with stage III to IV HNSCC, tumor hypoxia as indicated by FMISO PET was associated with higher risk of locoregional failure when subjects were treated with a chemoradiation regimen not containing tirapazamine compared with subjects treated a tirapazamine-containing chemoradiation regimen. This is likely because tirapazamine is only activated to a radical form in hypoxic conditions. This study highlighted the importance of determining hypoxia status in treatment regimen planning for HNSCC. The use of FMISO PET to identify hypoxic areas in tumors also allows dose escalation in IMRT specifically targeting those hypoxic areas with the goal of overcoming resistance to radiation.[65] Other novel hypoxia PET tracers are under investigation for HNSCC and other cancers, for which interested readers are referred to a recent review by Lopci and colleagues.[62]

SUMMARY

HNC is among the most common malignancies in the world with significant associated morbidity and mortality. More than 90% to 95% of HNC are SCC, which are treated with a combination of radiation, surgery, and chemotherapy, depending on the disease stage. Accurate staging at time of diagnosis allows optimal treatment plan and improves outcomes. Over the last decade, FDG PET-CT has become increasingly important in the care of HNSCC patients for diagnosis, staging, treatment planning, prognostication, and response assessment, as well as long-term surveillance. Novel non-FDG PET tracers are also under active investigation with great potential for improving patient care in this era of personalized medicine.

REFERENCES

1. Siegel RL, Miller KD, Jemal A. Cancer statistics, 2017. CA Cancer J Clin 2017;67(1):7–30.
2. Daley T, Darling M. Nonsquamous cell malignant tumours of the oral cavity: an overview. J Can Dent Assoc 2003;69(9):577–82.
3. Pezzuto F, Buonaguro L, Caponigro F, et al. Update on head and neck cancer: current knowledge on epidemiology, risk factors, molecular features and novel therapies. Oncology 2015;89(3):125–36.
4. Lydiatt WM, Patel SG, O'Sullivan B, et al. Head and Neck cancers-major changes in the American Joint Committee on cancer eighth edition cancer staging manual. CA Cancer J Clin 2017;67(2):122–37.
5. VanderWalde NA, Salloum RG, Liu TL, et al. Positron emission tomography and stage migration in head and neck cancer. JAMA Otolaryngol Head Neck Surg 2014;140(7):654–61.
6. Wahl RL, Jacene H, Kasamon Y, et al. From RECIST to PERCIST: Evolving Considerations for PET response criteria in solid tumors. J Nucl Med 2009; 50(Suppl 1):122s–50s.
7. Escott EJ. Positron emission tomography-computed tomography protocol considerations for head and neck cancer imaging. Semin Ultrasound CT MR 2008;29(4):263–70.
8. Yamamoto Y, Wong TZ, Turkington TG, et al. Head and neck cancer: dedicated FDG PET/CT protocol for detection–phantom and initial clinical studies. Radiology 2007;244(1):263–72.
9. Krabbe CA, Balink H, Roodenburg JL, et al. Performance of 18F-FDG PET/contrast-enhanced CT in the staging of squamous cell carcinoma of the oral cavity and oropharynx. Int J Oral Maxillofac Surg 2011;40(11):1263–70.
10. Hannah A, Scott AM, Tochon-Danguy H, et al. Evaluation of 18 F-fluorodeoxyglucose positron emission tomography and computed tomography with histopathologic correlation in the initial staging of head and neck cancer. Ann Surg 2002;236(2):208–17.
11. Zafereo ME. Evaluation and staging of squamous cell carcinoma of the oral cavity and oropharynx: limitations despite technological breakthroughs. Otolaryngol Clin North Am 2013;46(4):599–613.
12. Joo YH, Yoo Ie R, Cho KJ, et al. Relationship between extracapsular spread and FDG PET/CT in oropharyngeal squamous cell carcinoma. Acta Otolaryngol 2013;133(10):1073–9.
13. Curtin HD, Ishwaran H, Mancuso AA, et al. Comparison of CT and MR imaging in staging of neck metastases. Radiology 1998;207(1):123–30.
14. Su N, Li C, Shi Z, et al. Positron emission tomography/computed tomography for detecting cervical nodule metastases of oral and maxillofacial cancer. Hua Xi Kou Qiang Yi Xue Za Zhi 2012;30(1):36–9, 44, [in Chinese].
15. Liao CT, Wang HM, Huang SF, et al. PET and PET/CT of the neck lymph nodes improves risk prediction in patients with squamous cell carcinoma of the oral cavity. J Nucl Med 2011;52(2):180–7.
16. Kyzas PA, Evangelou E, Denaxa-Kyza D, et al. 18F-fluorodeoxyglucose positron emission tomography to evaluate cervical node metastases in patients with head and neck squamous cell carcinoma: a meta-analysis. J Natl Cancer Inst 2008;100(10):712–20.
17. Krabbe CA, Dijkstra PU, Pruim J, et al. FDG PET in oral and oropharyngeal cancer. Value for confirmation of N0 neck and detection of occult metastases. Oral Oncol 2008;44(1):31–6.

18. Murakami R, Uozumi H, Hirai T, et al. Impact of FDG-PET/CT imaging on nodal staging for head-and-neck squamous cell carcinoma. Int J Radiat Oncol Biol Phys 2007;68(2):377–82.

19. Haerle SK, Strobel K, Ahmad N, et al. Contrast-enhanced (1)(8)F-FDG-PET/CT for the assessment of necrotic lymph node metastases. Head Neck 2011;33(3):324–9.

20. Saindane AM. Pitfalls in the staging of cervical lymph node metastasis. Neuroimaging Clin N Am 2013;23(1):147–66.

21. Garavello W, Ciardo A, Spreafico R, et al. Risk factors for distant metastases in head and neck squamous cell carcinoma. Arch Otolaryngol Head Neck Surg 2006;132(7):762–6.

22. Xu GZ, Guan DJ, He ZY. (18)FDG-PET/CT for detecting distant metastases and second primary cancers in patients with head and neck cancer. A meta-analysis. Oral Oncol 2011;47(7):560–5.

23. Haerle SK, Schmid DT, Ahmad N, et al. The value of (18)F-FDG PET/CT for the detection of distant metastases in high-risk patients with head and neck squamous cell carcinoma. Oral Oncol 2011;47(7):653–9.

24. Chan SC, Wang HM, Yen TC, et al. (1)(8)F-FDG PET/CT and 3.0-T whole-body MRI for the detection of distant metastases and second primary tumours in patients with untreated oropharyngeal/hypopharyngeal carcinoma: a comparative study. Eur J Nucl Med Mol Imaging 2011;38(9):1607–19.

25. Dietl B, Marienhagen J, Kuhnel T, et al. The impact of FDG-PET/CT on the management of head and neck tumours: the radiotherapist's perspective. Oral Oncol 2008;44(5):504–8.

26. Deantonio L, Beldi D, Gambaro G, et al. FDG-PET/CT imaging for staging and radiotherapy treatment planning of head and neck carcinoma. Radiat Oncol 2008;3:29.

27. Lonneux M, Hamoir M, Reychler H, et al. Positron emission tomography with [18F]fluorodeoxyglucose improves staging and patient management in patients with head and neck squamous cell carcinoma: a multicenter prospective study. J Clin Oncol 2010; 28(7):1190–5.

28. Subramaniam RM, Agarwal A, Colucci A, et al. Impact of concurrent diagnostic level CT with PET/CT on the utilization of stand-alone CT and MRI in the management of head and neck cancer patients. Clin Nucl Med 2013;38(10):790–4.

29. Jereczek-Fossa BA, Jassem J, Orecchia R. Cervical lymph node metastases of squamous cell carcinoma from an unknown primary. Cancer Treat Rev 2004;30(2):153–64.

30. Dong MJ, Zhao K, Lin XT, et al. Role of fluorodeoxyglucose-PET versus fluorodeoxyglucose-PET/computed tomography in detection of unknown primary tumor: a meta-analysis of the literature. Nucl Med Commun 2008;29(9):791–802.

31. Rusthoven KE, Koshy M, Paulino AC. The role of fluorodeoxyglucose positron emission tomography in cervical lymph node metastases from an unknown primary tumor. Cancer 2004;101(11):2641–9.

32. Waltonen JD, Ozer E, Hall NC, et al. Metastatic carcinoma of the neck of unknown primary origin: evolution and efficacy of the modern workup. Arch Otolaryngol Head Neck Surg 2009;135(10):1024–9.

33. Douglas WG, Rigual NR, Loree TR, et al. Current concepts in the management of a second malignancy of the lung in patients with head and neck cancer. Curr Opin Otolaryngol Head Neck Surg 2003;11(2):85–8.

34. Strobel K, Haerle SK, Stoeckli SJ, et al. Head and neck squamous cell carcinoma (HNSCC)–detection of synchronous primaries with (18)F-FDG-PET/CT. Eur J Nucl Med Mol Imaging 2009;36(6):919–27.

35. Hujala K, Sipila J, Grenman R. Panendoscopy and synchronous second primary tumors in head and neck cancer patients. Eur Arch Otorhinolaryngol 2005;262(1):17–20.

36. Garg MK, Glanzman J, Kalnicki S. The evolving role of positron emission tomography-computed tomography in organ-preserving treatment of head and neck cancer. Semin Nucl Med 2012;42(5):320–7.

37. Dornfeld K, Simmons JR, Karnell L, et al. Radiation doses to structures within and adjacent to the larynx are correlated with long-term diet- and speech-related quality of life. Int J Radiat Oncol Biol Phys 2007;68(3):750–7.

38. Paulino AC, Koshy M, Howell R, et al. Comparison of CT- and FDG-PET-defined gross tumor volume in intensity-modulated radiotherapy for head-and-neck cancer. Int J Radiat Oncol Biol Phys 2005; 61(5):1385–92.

39. Subramaniam RM, Truong M, Peller P, et al. Fluorodeoxyglucose-positron-emission tomography imaging of head and neck squamous cell cancer. AJNR Am J Neuroradiol 2010;31(4):598–604.

40. Castelli J, De Bari B, Depeursinge A, et al. Overview of the predictive value of quantitative 18 FDG PET in head and neck cancer treated with chemoradiotherapy. Crit Rev Oncol Hematol 2016;108:40–51.

41. Pak K, Cheon GJ, Nam HY, et al. Prognostic value of metabolic tumor volume and total lesion glycolysis in head and neck cancer: a systematic review and meta-analysis. J Nucl Med 2014;55(6):884–90.

42. Suenaga Y, Kitajima K, Ishihara T, et al. FDG-PET/contrast-enhanced CT as a post-treatment tool in head and neck squamous cell carcinoma: comparison with FDG-PET/non-contrast-enhanced CT and contrast-enhanced CT. Eur Radiol 2016;26(4):1018–30.

43. King KG, Kositwattanarerk A, Genden E, et al. Cancers of the oral cavity and oropharynx: FDG PET with contrast-enhanced CT in the posttreatment setting. Radiographics 2011;31(2):355–73.

44. Gupta T, Master Z, Kannan S, et al. Diagnostic performance of post-treatment FDG PET or FDG PET/CT imaging in head and neck cancer: a systematic review and meta-analysis. Eur J Nucl Med Mol Imaging 2011;38(11):2083–95.

45. Leung AS, Rath TJ, Hughes MA, et al. Branstetter BFt. Optimal timing of first posttreatment FDG PET/CT in head and neck squamous cell carcinoma. Head Neck 2016;38(Suppl 1):E853–8.

46. Marcus C, Ciarallo A, Tahari AK, et al. Head and neck PET/CT: therapy response interpretation criteria (Hopkins Criteria)-interreader reliability, accuracy, and survival outcomes. J Nucl Med 2014; 55(9):1411–6.

47. Sjovall J, Bitzen U, Kjellen E, et al. Qualitative interpretation of PET scans using a Likert scale to assess neck node response to radiotherapy in head and neck cancer. Eur J Nucl Med Mol Imaging 2016; 43(4):609–16.

48. Isles MG, McConkey C, Mehanna HM. A systematic review and meta-analysis of the role of positron emission tomography in the follow up of head and neck squamous cell carcinoma following radiotherapy or chemoradiotherapy. Clin Otolaryngol 2008;33(3):210–22.

49. Porceddu SV, Pryor DI, Burmeister E, et al. Results of a prospective study of positron emission tomography-directed management of residual nodal abnormalities in node-positive head and neck cancer after definitive radiotherapy with or without systemic therapy. Head Neck 2011;33(12):1675–82.

50. Prestwich RJ, Subesinghe M, Gilbert A, et al. Delayed response assessment with FDG-PET-CT following (chemo) radiotherapy for locally advanced head and neck squamous cell carcinoma. Clin Radiol 2012;67(10):966–75.

51. Mehanna H, Wong WL, McConkey CC, et al. PET-CT surveillance versus neck dissection in advanced head and neck cancer. N Engl J Med 2016; 374(15):1444–54.

52. Wong KH, Panek R, Welsh L, et al. The predictive value of early assessment after 1 cycle of induction chemotherapy with 18F-FDG PET/CT and diffusion-weighted MRI for response to radical chemoradiotherapy in head and neck squamous cell carcinoma. J Nucl Med 2016;57(12):1843–50.

53. Sheikhbahaei S, Ahn SJ, Moriarty E, et al. Intratherapy or posttherapy FDG PET or FDG PET/CT for patients with head and neck cancer: a systematic review and meta-analysis of prognostic studies. AJR Am J Roentgenol 2015;205(5):1102–13.

54. Beswick DM, Gooding WE, Johnson JT. Branstetter BFt. Temporal patterns of head and neck squamous cell carcinoma recurrence with positron-emission tomography/computed tomography monitoring. Laryngoscope 2012;122(7):1512–7.

55. Paidpally V, Tahari AK, Lam S, et al. Addition of 18F-FDG PET/CT to clinical assessment predicts overall survival in HNSCC: a retrospective analysis with follow-up for 12 years. J Nucl Med 2013;54(12): 2039–45.

56. Kim JW, Roh JL, Kim JS, et al. (18)F-FDG PET/CT surveillance at 3-6 and 12 months for detection of recurrence and second primary cancer in patients with head and neck squamous cell carcinoma. Br J Cancer 2013;109(12):2973–9.

57. Sheikhbahaei S, Taghipour M, Ahmad R, et al. Diagnostic accuracy of follow-up FDG PET or PET/CT in patients with head and neck cancer after definitive treatment: a systematic review and meta-analysis. AJR Am J Roentgenol 2015;205(3):629–39.

58. McDermott M, Hughes M, Rath T, et al. Negative predictive value of surveillance PET/CT in head and neck squamous cell cancer. AJNR Am J Neuroradiol 2013;34(8):1632–6.

59. Ho AS, Tsao GJ, Chen FW, et al. Impact of positron emission tomography/computed tomography surveillance at 12 and 24 months for detecting head and neck cancer recurrence. Cancer 2013;119(7): 1349–56.

60. Brizel DM, Sibley GS, Prosnitz LR, et al. Tumor hypoxia adversely affects the prognosis of carcinoma of the head and neck. Int J Radiat Oncol Biol Phys 1997;38(2):285–9.

61. Grierson JR, Link JM, Mathis CA, et al. A radiosynthesis of fluorine-18 fluoromisonidazole. J Nucl Med 1989;30(3):343–50.

62. Lopci E, Grassi I, Chiti A, et al. PET radiopharmaceuticals for imaging of tumor hypoxia: a review of the evidence. Am J Nucl Med Mol Imaging 2014;4(4): 365–84.

63. Rajendran JG, Schwartz DL, O'Sullivan J, et al. Tumor hypoxia imaging with [F-18] fluoromisonidazole positron emission tomography in head and neck cancer. Clin Cancer Res 2006;12(18): 5435–41.

64. Rischin D, Hicks RJ, Fisher R, et al. Prognostic significance of [18F]-misonidazole positron emission tomography-detected tumor hypoxia in patients with advanced head and neck cancer randomly assigned to chemoradiation with or without tirapazamine: a substudy of Trans-Tasman Radiation Oncology Group Study 98.02. J Clin Oncol 2006; 24(13):2098–104.

65. Lee NY, Mechalakos JG, Nehmeh S, et al. Fluorine-18-labeled fluoromisonidazole positron emission and computed tomography-guided intensity-modulated radiotherapy for head and neck cancer: a feasibility study. Int J Radiat Oncol Biol Phys 2008; 70(1):2–13.

Neck Imaging Reporting and Data System

Ashley H. Aiken, MD*, Patricia A. Hudgins, MD

KEYWORDS

- NI-RADS • Contrast-enhanced computed tomography • Radiology • Head and neck cancer • CT
- PET/CT • Cancer surveillance • Imaging • Squamous cell carcinoma

KEY POINTS

- NI-RADS is a practical and clinically useful imaging surveillance template.
- It is designed to guide appropriate imaging follow up and next management steps.
- The standardization of linked management recommendations and correlation with patient outcomes has the potential to validate performance of the template and highlight the radiologists' significant value in patient care.

INTRODUCTION

The Neck Imaging Reporting and Data System (NI-RADS) was originally developed for surveillance contrast-enhanced computed tomography (CECT) imaging with or without PET in patients with treated head and neck (H&N) cancer.[1] The template is easily adaptable to other modalities such as MR imaging. The standard nomenclature promotes shared databases across institutions and is critical to the American College of Radiology (ACR) charge to reengineer the radiology enterprise to be patient-centered, data- driven, and outcomes-based.[2] The Breast Imaging Reporting and Data System demonstrated the success of a standardized mammography report because it simplifies communication, clearly directs management, and facilitates radiologic-pathologic correlation to continually refine and improve cutpoints for desired sensitivity, specificity, and accuracy. Similarly, a standardized reporting template in H&N cancer surveillance serves several important purposes:

- Easily understandable with numerical scores for levels of suspicion to guide patient care

- Linked management recommendations, which reflect a multidisciplinary consensus to standardize approach
- Data-minable reports will pave the way to address optimal surveillance imaging algorithms and timing, imaging accuracy, reader performance, interobserver variability, and so forth
- Opens avenues for direct patient reporting and highlights the radiologist's added value in patient care.

This article is a practical guide for using NI-RADS to reduce report-generation time for radiologists and create useful reports for referring clinicians and patients. After a review of the report template and legend, a case-based and pictorial review instructs readers on the proper assignment of NI-RADS categories.

Neck Imaging Reporting and Data System Template and Legend

The body of the report template is brief and focuses on the primary site and cervical metastatic adenopathy, with a brief description of

Disclosure: Drs A.H. Aiken and P.A. Hudgins serve as co-chairs of ACR NI-RADS committee.
Department of Radiology and Imaging Sciences, Emory University School of Medicine, Emory University Hospital, 1364 Clifton Road NE, Atlanta, GA 30322, USA
* Corresponding author.
E-mail address: ashley.aiken@emoryhealthcare.org

Magn Reson Imaging Clin N Am 26 (2018) 51–62
https://doi.org/10.1016/j.mric.2017.08.004

posttreatment change (**Box 1**). In a patient without suspicious findings, the radiologist can tab through these fields with little to no extra dictation to finalize a report. Changes related to chemotherapy or radiation therapy often include laryngeal mucosal edema, subcutaneous stranding, or intensely enhancing submandibular glands; and can generally be summed up in one sentence, which is built into the template. Radiologists can add a sentence to state the expected postsurgical changes from resection with or without a flap reconstruction. If there are suspicious findings, the templates are easily modifiable to add the specific finding both in the findings and impression sections.

Both the primary tumor site and neck are assessed for recurrence and assigned a category from 1 to 4 based on imaging suspicion. The categories of suspicion and management recommendations are based on current best practices, multidisciplinary consensus, and the ultrasound and computed tomography (CT)-guided biopsy experience of the NI-RADS originators,[1] and revised by the ACR NI-RADS committee:

- Category 1: no evidence of recurrence
- Category 2: low suspicion, defined as ill-defined areas of abnormality with only mild differential enhancement and/or mild fluoro-deoxyglucose (FDG) uptake. The linked management recommendation is direct inspection for mucosal abnormalities or short-interval follow-up with CECT or an additional PET.
- Category 3: high suspicion, defined as a discrete, new or enlarging lesion with marked enhancement and/or intense focal FDG uptake. The linked recommendation is biopsy.
- Category 4: Definitive recurrence, defined as pathologically proven or definite radiologic or clinical progression.

A reporting template must offer more than just efficiency. Early experience showed the NI-RADS reporting performance in a mixed cohort of both PET and PET-CECT surveillance for H&N squamous cell carcinoma (SCC) at different time points.[3] This study was performed to determine the accuracy of the NI-RADS system for predicting recurrent tumor. The initial performance was good with discrimination between the groups, with a NI-RADS 1 positive disease rate of 3.5%, a NI-RADS 2 positive disease rate of 17%, and a NI-RADS 3 positive disease rate of 59.4%.[3] As future studies look at the predictive value of these NI-RADS categories at specific time points, the positive predictive value will vary at different time points and each NI-RADS category will likely have a larger range of positive rate disease.

Notably, although the body of the template is the same for CECT alone and a CECT as part of a PET-CECT, the legend and specific management recommendations vary slightly (**Boxes 2** and **3**). The legends are included at the bottom of each report, although, after several months of use, referring clinicians become very comfortable and familiar with the 4 levels of suspicion and the linked management recommendations (**Table 1**). In fact, referring clinicians often ask for a NI-RADS level of suspicion for MR imaging surveillance (even though it was originally developed for CECT with or without PET). The authors have found anecdotally that NI-RADS can also be applied to MR imaging with the same 4 categories of suspicion but slightly different linked management recommendations (**Box 4**).

Box 1
Report template for posttreatment neck

Indication: [ ]

  Subsite and human papillomavirus status: [ ]

  Surgery and chemoradiation: [ ]

Technique:

Comparison: [<None.>]

Findings:

  [<No evidence of recurrent disease is demonstrated at the primary site.>]

  [<No pathologically enlarged, necrotic, or otherwise abnormal lymph nodes.>]

  Expected posttreatment changes are noted including [<supraglottic mucosal edema and thickening of the skin and subcutaneous soft tissues.>]

  There are no findings to suggest a second primary in the imaged aerodigestive tract.

  Evaluation of the visualized portions of brain, orbits, spine, and lungs show no aggressive lesions suspicious for metastatic involvement.

Impression:

  Primary: [1]. [<Expected posttreatment changes in the neck without evidence of recurrent disease in the primary site.>]

  Neck: [1]. [<No evidence of abnormal lymph nodes.>]

From ACR NI-RADS. Available at: https://www.acr.org/Quality-Safety/Resources/NIRADS. Accessed June 2017; with permission.

Box 2	Box 3
Contrast-enhanced computed tomography surveillance legend	**PET with contrast-enhanced computed tomography surveillance legend**

Box 2

Contrast-enhanced computed tomography surveillance legend

Primary

1. No evidence of recurrence: routine surveillance

2. Low suspicion

   a. Superficial abnormality (skin, mucosal surface): direct visual inspection

   b. Ill-defined deep abnormality: short-interval follow-up[a] or PET

3. High suspicion (new or enlarging discrete nodule or mass): biopsy

4. Definitive recurrence (path-proven or clinical progression): no biopsy needed

Nodes

1. No evidence of recurrence: routine surveillance

2. Low suspicion (ill-defined): short-interval follow-up or PET

3. High suspicion (new or enlarging lymph node): biopsy if clinically needed

4. Definitive recurrence (path-proven or clinical progression): no biopsy needed

[a]Short-interval follow-up: 3 months at the authors' institution.

From ACR NI-RADS. Available at: https://www.acr.org/Quality-Safety/Resources/NIRADS. Accessed June 2017; with permission.

Box 3

PET with contrast-enhanced computed tomography surveillance legend

Primary

1. No evidence of recurrence: routine surveillance, CECT

2. Low suspicion

   a. Superficial abnormality (eg, skin, mucosal surface): direct visual inspection

   b. Ill-defined deep abnormality with only mild FDG uptake-short-interval follow-up[a] or repeat PET-CECT at routine follow-up

3. High suspicion (new or enlarging discrete nodule or mass with intense FDG uptake): biopsy

4. Definitive recurrence (path-proven or clinical progression): no biopsy needed

Nodes

1. No evidence of recurrence: routine surveillance

2. Low suspicion (residual nodal soft tissue with only mild or intermediate FDG): short-interval follow-up or repeat PET-CECT at routine follow-up

3. High suspicion (new, enlarging with intense FDG uptake): biopsy

4. Definitive recurrence (biopsy proven or clinical progression): no biopsy needed

[a]Short-interval follow-up: 3 months at the authors' institution.

From ACR NI-RADS. Available at: https://www.acr.org/Quality-Safety/Resources/NIRADS. Accessed June 2017; with permission.

SURVEILLANCE IMAGING ALGORITHM

Even after standardized and appropriate treatment, 30% to 50% of patients with H&N cancer experience locoregional recurrence, typically during the first 2 years after treatment.[4,5] Therefore, patients undergo posttreatment clinical and radiologic surveillance but, unfortunately, there are no standard surveillance imaging algorithms for H&N cancer. PET combined with CECT has been shown to overcome inherent obstacles in posttreatment surveillance imaging; however, the optimal timing and frequency has not been standardized.[6–9] Furthermore, the 2015 National Comprehensive Cancer Network (NCCN) guidelines suggest imaging within 6 months of treatment of tumor stage (T)-3 and T4 and/or node stage (N)-2 or N3 disease but only advocate additional imaging follow-up for new signs or symptoms and areas inaccessible to clinical inspection.[10] Although the NCCN recommendations are vague regarding additional surveillance,

79% of referring clinicians do report using PET-CT for asymptomatic patients.[11] Currently, the benefit of surveillance imaging is not clearly defined, despite studies showing good sensitivity and moderate specificity with PET-CT. No studies demonstrate a survival advantage.[12] Given this universal lack of knowledge regarding treatment follow-up, it is reasonable to develop an institutional multidisciplinary consensus based on best available data, local patient population, and clinician preference. At the authors' institution, the routine surveillance protocol for advanced H&N SCC is

1. Posttreatment baseline PET-CECT at 10 to 12 weeks after surgery and/or the completion of chemoradiation therapy (CRT)

2. If negative, then CECT of the neck and chest 6 months later

Table 1
Neck Imaging Reporting and Data System category descriptors, imaging features and management

	Category	Imaging Findings	Management
No evidence of recurrence	1	• Expected posttreatment changes • Non-mass-like distortion of soft tissues • Low-density mucoid mucosal edema • No abnormal FDG uptake • Diffuse linear mucosal enhancement after radiation	Routine surveillance
Low suspicion	2a	• Focal mucosal enhancement but non-mass-like • Focal mucosal FDG uptake	Direct visual inspection
	2b	• Deep, ill-defined soft tissue mass • Borderline FDG uptake	Short-interval follow-up (3 mo), repeat PET
High suspicion	3	• New or definite enlarging primary mass or lymph node • Discrete nodule or mass with differential enhancement • Intense focal FDG uptake	Image guided or clinical biopsy
Definitive recurrence	4	• Pathologically proven or definite radiologic and clinical progression	Clinical management

From ACR NI-RADS. Available at: www.acr.org/Quality-Safety/Resources/NIRADS. Accessed June 2017; with permission.

Box 4
Neck Imaging Reporting and Data System lexicon

Non-mass-like soft tissue

• Nonenhancing or minimally enhancing distortion of soft tissue and fat planes (1)

Masses

• Morphology: ill-defined (2) versus discrete (3)

• Enhancement: mild (2) versus intense (3)

• FDG avidity: mild (2) versus intense (3)

Mucosal abnormality

• Low density submucosal edema (1)

• Diffuse linear enhancement: benign radiation mucositis (1)

• Focal or mass-like mucosal enhancement or FDG uptake (2a)

Lymph nodes:

• Residual nodal tissue plus no FDG (1)

• Residual nodal tissue plus mild FDG (2)

• Residual nodal tissue plus intense FDG (3)

• Lymph node, increasing size, without definite morphologically abnormal features, along with expected nodal drainage (2)

• Lymph node, increasing size, with morphologically abnormal features (3)

• Lymph node of increasing size plus intense FDG (3)

3. If that study is negative, then CECT of the neck only 6 months later
4. If negative, then CECT of the neck and chest 12 months later.

Patients with sinonasal tumors, nasopharyngeal carcinoma, parotid masses, or other skull base tumors with a propensity for perineural spread will often be followed with MR imaging to assess intracranial, perineural, and/or orbital disease. It is very important to establish a consensus surveillance imaging algorithm before a surveillance template so that recommendations can be optimized in context. For example, the suggested management options for NI-RADS 2 lesions are most often shorter imaging follow-up (3 months) or additional PET-CECT at follow-up rather than CECT only.

NECK IMAGING REPORTING AND DATA SYSTEM 1: NO EVIDENCE OF RECURRENCE → ROUTINE SURVEILLANCE
Diagnostic Criteria Box

• Expected posttreatment changes with non-mass-like soft tissue distortion.
• No abnormal FDG uptake.

Neck Imaging Reporting and Data System 1 descriptors: low density submucosal edema, low-density effacement of fat planes, distortion, hypoenhancing
Neck Imaging Reporting and Data System category 1 has a 3% rate of positive disease

Primary NI-RADS primary category 1 should have no residual FDG uptake or hyperenhancing soft tissue at the primary site (**Figs. 1** and **2**). After complicated surgical resection and flap reconstruction, especially for oral cavity SCC, PET false-positives are more likely. Readers should be familiar with common PET pitfalls (see later discussion) and rely on the diagnostic CECT and knowledge of the expected appearance of the flap reconstruction to avoid this pitfall (**Fig. 3**).[13]

Neck NI-RADS nodal category 1 should have no residual FDG uptake on the posttreatment 12-week baseline study. In this setting after CRT, the decision to perform a salvage neck dissection is needed, so it is critical for radiologists to be as definitive as possible. If there is no FDG uptake, a NI-RADS 1 category can be assigned even if residual nodal tissue is present (see **Fig. 1**).[14] In the authors' experience, if the initial node was large, matted, or there was extracapsular extension of tumor, the adequately treated node will be smaller, but there is almost always nonenhancing soft tissue at the site. Previous prospective studies have shown that H&N SCC patients with residual CECT nodal abnormalities after definitive CRT could be spared a salvage neck dissection if PET was negative.[15–17] For subsequent surveillance studies, stable nodal soft tissue can also be categorized as a NI-RADS 1.

Pearls and pitfalls
Recognition of posttreatment CECT and PET pitfalls is important. Areas of enhancement or FDG uptake may represent nonneoplastic posttreatment change and not tumor persistence or recurrence. If faced with a complicated postsurgical bed and questionable suspicious findings, the authors recommend reviewing the operative report to understand the surgery and the status of surgical margins. For example, if a T3 tumor was resected with a partial glossectomy and all margins were negative, tumor persistence at the 3-month posttreatment baseline scan is unlikely. In that scenario, questionable areas could be downgraded to a NI-RADS 1. Therefore, the best use of the NI-RADS templates includes experience, and knowledge of expected posttreatment findings:

1. Tongue fasciculations after partial glossectomy and flap reconstruction are a common pitfall that result in increased FDG activity (**Fig. 4**)
2. Diffuse smooth mucosal enhancement is more likely mucositis and should be categorized as NI-RADS 1. More focal or mass-like mucosal enhancement may be either tumor or posttreatment change, and should be categorized as NI-RADS 2.
3. The muscular portion of the flap or vascular pedicle will have differential enhancement and should not be confused with tumor.[18–20]

NECK IMAGING REPORTING AND DATA SYSTEM 2: LOW SUSPICION FOR RECURRENCE → SHORT-TERM FOLLOW-UP OR MUCOSAL INSPECTION
Diagnostic Criteria Box

- Ill-defined soft tissue with only mild differential enhancement; no discrete nodule or mass
- Mild FDG uptake
- NI-RADS 2 descriptors: ill-defined, mildly enhancing, and nondiscrete
- Asymmetric mucosal uptake without a discrete nodule or mass
- CECT and PET findings are discordant.

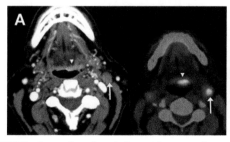
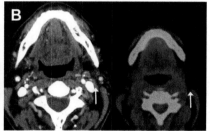

Fig. 1. NI-RADS primary 1 and neck 1: oropharyngeal sqaumous cell carcinoma (SCCA) treated with CRT. (*A*) Staging PET-CECT shows a small left base of tongue (BOT) primary and bilateral FDG avid and morphologically abnormal lymph nodes compatible with T1N2c initial stage. (*B*) 12-week post-CRT, a baseline surveillance PET-CECT shows no residual mucosal enhancement or focal FDG uptake at the primary site and no residual FDG uptake in minimal residual nodal tissue. This was assigned a NI-RADS 1 category and the linked management was routine institutional surveillance of CECT at 6 months.

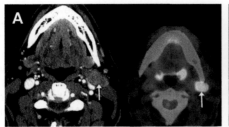
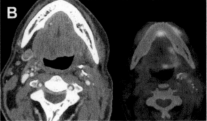

Fig. 2. NI-RADS primary 1 and neck 1: oropharyngeal SCCA treated with transoral robotic surgery (TORS) and neck dissection (ND). (*A*) Staging PET-CECT showed a small left palatine tonsil primary (not as well seen on this CECT axial slice) and FDG avid and morphologically abnormal left level 2A node, compatible with T1NI initial stage. (*B*) 12-week status post-TORS, left selective ND and CRT, a baseline surveillance PET-CECT shows postsurgical distortion at the left glossotonsillar sulcus with no discrete mucosal enhancement or FDG uptake. Postsurgical changes and effacement of fat planes in the left neck are also normal postsurgical findings. Note that the minimal FDG uptake in the primary site and around the postsurgical neck findings was still considered an expected postsurgical finding. This was assigned a NI-RADS 1 category and the linked management was routine institutional surveillance of CECT at 6 months.

Legend with Linked Management

Primary 2
1. 2a (superficial, mucosal surface) → direct visual inspection
2. 2b (deep) → short-interval follow-up (3 months rather than routine 6 months) versus addition of a PET to CECT at 6 months
Neck 2: → short-interval follow-up (3 months rather than routine 6 months) versus addition of a PET to CECT at 6 months.

Neck Imaging Reporting and Data System category 2 has a 17% rate of positive disease
Primary NI-RADS category 2 is subdivided at the primary site to align with practical management recommendations. Mucosal abnormalities are assigned category 2a with the linked management recommendation of direct clinical inspection with biopsy at the discretion of the surgeon. Focal mucosal enhancement or enhancement deep to an ulceration is more concerning than diffuse

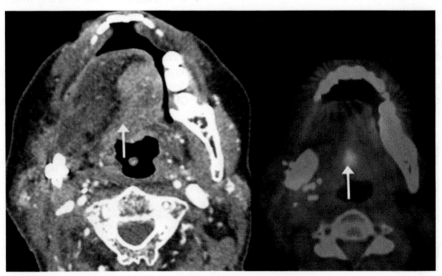

Fig. 3. NI-RADS primary 1: oral cavity SCCA-treated glossectomy (T4aN2b), mandibulectomy, and free fibular flap reconstruction. 12-week status postresection and CRT, a baseline surveillance PET-CECT shows a complicated postsurgical appearance with minimal FDG uptake in the residual oral tongue. This is a common PET pitfall because there are often fasciculations in the residual tongue. In addition, careful review of the record revealed that the surgical margins were negative, so that this was assigned a NI-RADS category 1. Careful examination of the bone and soft tissue components of the flap revealed no nodularity.

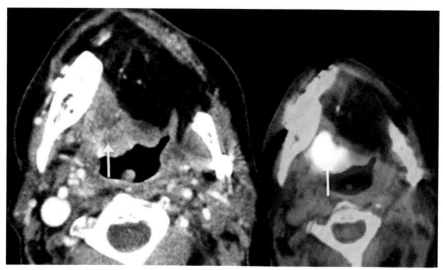

Fig. 4. NI-RADS 1: Fasciculations in residual oral tongue after near total glossectomy. The axial fused PET image demonstrates intense FDG uptake just deep to the flap. However, correlation with the CECT shows this to be residual oral tongue. This is a common PET false-positive and pitfall. A reasonable approach is to review the surgical report for negative margins and confirm that the patient has no pain before assigning this a NI-RADS category 1.

mucosal enhancement (**Fig. 5**). This is assigned a NI-RADS 2a category and should prompt direct clinical inspection as the first management step because this is accessible to clinicians. Some mucosal surfaces, such as the postradiated larynx or hypopharynx, are particularly challenging and PET-CECT often helps direct the clinical examination and biopsies in the posttreatment setting. In the authors' experience, 17% of NI-RADS 2 will turn out to be tumor persistence or recurrence, with the greatest likelihood in category 2a. A deep ill-defined soft tissue abnormality with some differential enhancement or mild FDG uptake would belong in NI-RADS category 2b, with the linked management recommendation for shorter interval follow-up or PET. Most deep ill-defined abnormalities with mild enhancement and mild FDG uptake (NI-RADS 2b) will be posttreatment change (83%) and, therefore, biopsy should be avoided in most circumstances. In rare cases, more immediate management decisions are needed, particularly when trying to start hyperbaric oxygen for presumed radionecrosis if there is a question of coexistent recurrence. Ill-defined mildly enhancing soft tissue that may be initially concerning on CECT can be downgraded

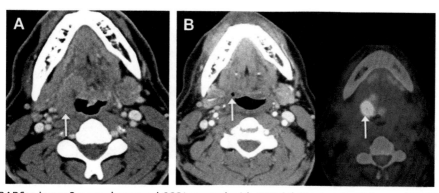

Fig. 5. NI-RADS primary 2a: oropharyngeal SCCA treated with CRT. (*A*) Staging CECT from a PET-CECT shows a large right BOT primary with endophytic growth (invading genioglossus) compatible with T4a initial stage. (*B*) 12-week post-CRT, a baseline surveillance PET-CECT shows a small ulceration along the right base of tongue without deep enhancement or other concerning features on the CECT. However, the PET shows intense focal uptake in this region. The anatomic appearance on CECT is reassuring but this was still assigned a NI-RADS category 2a so that the surgeon would look specifically at this area. On direct inspection, this seemed consistent with radiation injury and a follow-up PET was negative.

to NI-RADS 1 in most cases if there is no FDG up-take on subsequent PET. Likewise, small areas of mild FDG uptake are less concerning if there is no abnormality on the CECT. If a patient receives a category 2b on a CECT only, the recommendation may be PET or short-term follow-up. After the PET, the NI-RADS 2b could either be down-graded to a 1 or upgraded to a 3, depending on FDG uptake.

Neck Lymph nodes that are considered NI-RADS 2 include mild residual FDG uptake in nodes after definitive chemoradiation (**Fig. 6**) or mildly enlarging lymph node without specific morpholog-ically abnormal features (new necrosis or extrac-apsular spread). Importantly, posttreatment pathologic nodes often have central low-density, thin rim enhancement, or necrosis, which are ex-pected posttreatment changes and can still be scored a NI-RADS 1 if there is no FDG uptake, or NI-RADS 2 if there is mild FDG activity. This is different from a newly enlarging node that de-velops new low-density or irregularity, which is a NI-RADS 3. A newly enlarging node on a CECT alone, without definite abnormal features, could be given a NI-RADS 2 with a recommendation for PET. Then, PET would downgrade or upgrade depending on the FDG uptake (**Fig. 7**).

Pearls and pitfalls

1. When deciding between a NI-RADS 2 versus 3, it is helpful to work backwards, considering whether to biopsy now or if it is prudent to wait 3 months and re-image. Often, the choice will become clear because NI-RADS 2 lesions should be ill-defined and, therefore, difficult bi-opsy targets.

2. In most cases, waiting for 3 months will not change the ultimate plan, even if it is proven to represent recurrence. The only exception to this rule is if osteoradionecrosis or soft tissue necrosis is the alternate consideration. Therefore, there may be rare requests to biopsy a NI-RADS 2 lesion because a more immediate pathologic diagnosis is needed to move forward with treatment (hyperbaric oxygen is contraindicated with residual tumor).

3. NI-RADS category 2a is a special category for superficial mucosal abnormalities. Tradition-ally, radiologists have not considered them-selves mucosal doctors; however, it is not uncommon for PET or CECT to show more focal FDG uptake or enhancement along the mucosal surfaces. Instead of expending effort on trying to characterize and then decide on follow-up, radiologists need to communi-cate the location of concern to their surgical colleagues who can easily look at that location and biopsy if there is a worrisome finding.

4. Mucosal lesions in the larynx are often harder for referring clinicians to assess accurately, so PET is very helpful in a postradiated larynx to direct clinical inspection and biopsy. The authors almost always include a PET with CECT for laryngeal SCC treated with CRT.

NECK IMAGING REPORTING AND DATA SYSTEM 3: HIGH SUSPICION FOR RECURRENCE → BIOPSY
Diagnostic Criteria Box

- New or enlarging discrete nodule or mass with significant differential enhancement from sur-rounding soft tissues

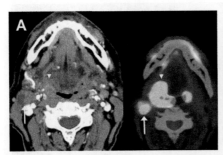
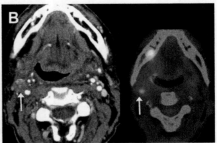

Fig. 6. NI-RADS neck 2: oropharyngeal SCCA treated with CRT. (*A*) Initial staging PET-CECT shows a heterogeneous right level 2A lymph node with focal FDG uptake. The primary right BOT tumor is also well seen on the fused axial PET and partially visualized on the CECT. (*B*) 12-week post-CRT, a baseline surveillance PET-CECT shows interval decrease size and FDG avidity of right level 2A node, but there is 1.2 cm heterogeneous nodal tissue and mild FDG uptake remaining. This was assigned a NI-RADS category 2 because the FDG uptake was very mild. In the authors' past clinical experience, many of these cases with only mild residual FDG uptake were negative at salvage ND. Interestingly, this patient underwent fine needle aspiration (FNA), which was positive, but final path-ologic assessment after salvage ND was negative. It would also be a reasonable approach to offer the patient a short-term follow-up at 3 months.

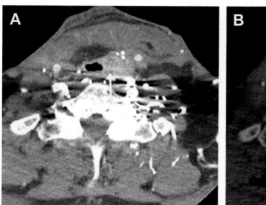
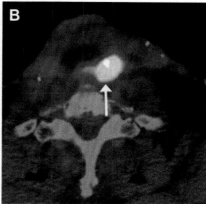

Fig. 7. NI-RADS neck 2 on CECT alone and upgrade to NI-RADS 3 with PET: recurrent laryngeal SCCA, status post total laryngectomy, and pectoralis flap. (A) 12-week postoperative baseline axial CECT alone shows a 1.2-cm discrete enhancing nodule to the left of the neopharynx beneath the pectoralis flap. However, because this was an initial posttreatment baseline and the left ND had been negative, this was assigned a NI-RADS 2 with the recommendation for immediate PET (in large part because the surgeons were confident that this could not be residual disease). Otherwise, the discrete nature of this abnormality and differential enhancement would meet criteria for NI-RADS 3, which would have meant sending the patient for biopsy without a PET. (B) Axial fused PET images from the following week confirmed focal intense FDG uptake and the lesion was upgraded to NI-RADS 3, with the linked management recommendation for biopsy. CT-guided biopsy confirmed residual SCCA.

- Avid focal FDG uptake
- CECT and PET matched suspicion.

Legend with Linked Management

Primary or neck 3 → biopsy
Neck Imaging Reporting and Data System category 3 has a 59% rate of positive disease
Primary NI-RADS category 3 should be assigned to lesions that are high-suspicion and warrant biopsy. Primary site recurrences are either mucosal or submucosal (deep). Most mucosal abnormalities are assigned a NI-RADS 2a category because surgeons can best assess the mucosal surfaces. However, more discrete mucosal abnormalities can be upgraded to a NI-RADS 3, especially if they develop after the posttreatment baseline study. However, the ultimate recommendation and management is often the same because the surgeons will directly inspect and decide on biopsy based on their clinical examination. On the other hand, the decision to biopsy deep abnormalities is primarily based on the imaging appearance, so that the designation of NI-RADS 3 should be reserved for lesions that the radiologist is willing to biopsy by ultrasound or

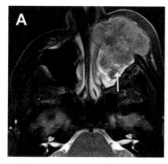
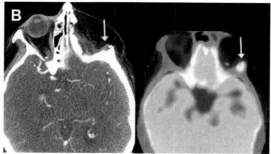

Fig. 8. NI-RADS primary 3: maxillary sinus SCCA status post maxillectomy and orbital exenteration. (A) Axial T2-weighted MR imaging shows large heterogeneous mass centered in the left maxillary sinus with obvious erosion through the anterior and superior walls (seen on other images) of the maxillary sinus. (B) Surveillance PET-CECT showed a very small area of bone irregularity along the residual lateral orbital wall with a subcentimeter discrete enhancing nodule with focal FDG uptake. This was assigned a NI-RADS category 3 and CT biopsy confirmed recurrence.

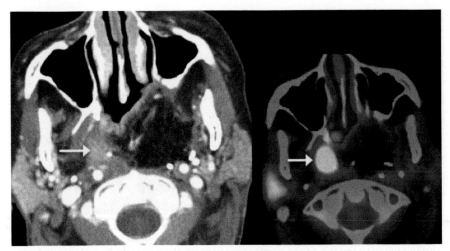

Fig. 9. NI-RADS primary 3: recurrent T4bN0 L soft palate SCC after definitive CRT status post subsequent extensive resection and reconstruction. 12-week postsurgical salvage and reconstruction, a baseline surveillance PET-CECT shows a discrete enhancing nodule deep to the flap reconstruction, posterior to the right medial pterygoid plate with focal intense FDG uptake. This qualifies as a NI-RADS category 3 and biopsy confirmed recurrence.

CT guidance. NI-RADS 3 is not based on size but rather on morphologic appearance and FDG avidity. A subcentimeter discrete lesion with focal intense FDG uptake can be a NI-RADS 3 (**Fig. 8**). Often, deep recurrences of the primary site occur along the margins of the flap (**Fig. 9**). The most common cause of a false-positive in this category is radiation injury to the soft tissue and/or bone, which can have tumefactive appearance on anatomic images and PET with marked FDG uptake (**Fig. 10**).

Assigning a NI-RADS 3 to the primary site, other than the mucosal surface, necessitates that the interpreting radiologist decide if the biopsy can be done with image guidance. When the authors know that we will be responsible for confirming or disproving persistent or recurrent malignancy, equivocal dictations are uncommon.

Neck NI-RADS category 3 in the neck should be assigned for a new lymph node, definite enlargement of a lymph node with focal FDG uptake, or enlargement of a lymph node with new morphologically abnormal features (**Fig. 11**). Although NI-RADS 3 is the high-suspicion category, false-positives do occur and are more commonly seen with PET-CECT than CECT alone.[3]

Pearls and pitfalls

1. Radiation injury in soft tissue or bone can be mass-like and enhance robustly, and are, therefore, tumefactive and difficult to

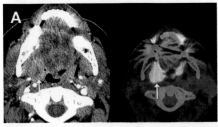
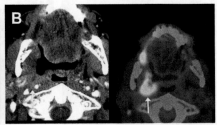

Fig. 10. NI-RADS primary 3: T4aN1 SCCA right tonsil status post CRT. (*A*) Staging PET-CECT shows a large right palatine tonsil primary with extension to the medial pterygoid compatible with T4a initial stage. (*B*) 12-week post-CRT, a baseline surveillance PET-CECT shows a large ulceration in the right tonsillar fossa with mild deep enhancement posteriorly. The fused axial PET images show intense FDG uptake along the margins and deep to this ulceration. The CECT and PET were concordant and were assigned a NI-RADS category 3. Biopsy and subsequent follow-up proved this to be a false-positive from soft tissue radiation injury mimicking residual tumor.

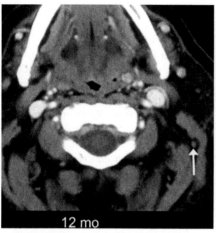
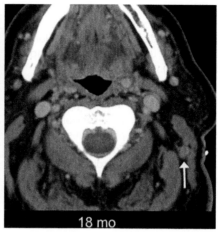

Fig. 11. NI-RADS neck 3: angiosarcoma of the scalp. CECT at 12 months showed no suspicious findings. The CECT at 18 months showed a new small 8-mm left level 2b lymph node. On close inspection, this new node had central necrosis. A new node with definite morphologically abnormal features makes this a NI-RADS 3. Biopsy confirmed recurrence.

distinguish from residual or recurrent tumor. Osteonecrosis has a characteristic appearance on CECT and will have intense FDG uptake. Soft tissue radiation injury will often be a false-positive in this category.

2. If a lesion is borderline between a NI-RADS 3 and 4, an approach is to talk to the clinician to determine if he or she will require a biopsy to prove recurrence before the next stage of treatment. If it is considered definitive by imaging and clinical examination, then it can be assigned a NI-RADS 4.

NECK IMAGING REPORTING AND DATA SYSTEM 4: DEFINITE RECURRENCE
Diagnostic Criteria Box

- Pathologic confirmation
- Definite clinical or radiographic progression
- Unequivocal radiographic appearance.

Primary and neck
Initially, the NI-RADS 4 category was described as biopsy-proven residual or recurrent disease, often in patients on palliation or undergoing

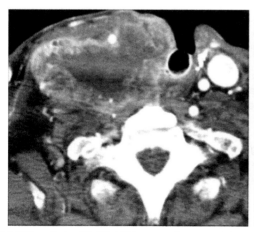
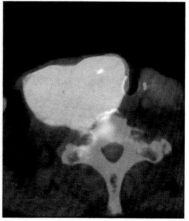

Fig. 12. NI-RADS neck 4: pT4aN2cM0 laryngeal cancer status post total laryngectomy and bilateral ND with clinical examination concerning for recurrence at the stoma. CECT shows large fungating mass in the lower right neck, lateral to the stoma with corresponding intense FDG uptake. This is unequivocal recurrence even at this single time point. The clinicians did not need a biopsy to plan subsequent management. This would qualify for NI-RADS 4 even without pathologic confirmation.

routine imaging as part of a clinical trial. The category has expanded to include cases with definite clinical or radiographic progression or single time point unequivocal radiographic appearance (**Fig. 12**).

SUMMARY

NI-RADS is a practical and clinically useful imaging surveillance template designed to guide appropriate imaging follow-up and next-management steps. The standardization of linked management recommendations and correlation with patient outcomes has the potential to validate performance of the template and highlight the radiologists' significant value in patient care.

REFERENCES

1. Aiken AH, Farley A, Baugnon KL, et al. Implementation of a novel surveillance template for head and neck cancer: neck imaging reporting and data system (NI-RADS). J Am Coll Radiol 2016;13(6):743–6.e1.
2. Dodd GD 3rd, Allen B Jr, Birzniek D, et al. Reengineering the radiology enterprise: a summary of the 2014 Intersociety Committee Summer Conference. J Am Coll Radiol 2015;12(3):228–34.
3. Krieger DA, Hudgins PA, Nayak GK, et al. Initial performance of NI-RADS to predict residual or recurrent head and neck squamous cell carcinoma. AJNR Am J Neuroradiol 2017;38(6):1193–9.
4. Bourhis J, Sire C, Graff P, et al. Concomitant chemoradiotherapy versus acceleration of radiotherapy with or without concomitant chemotherapy in locally advanced head and neck carcinoma (GORTEC 99-02): an open-label phase 3 randomised trial. Lancet Oncol 2012;13(2):145–53.
5. Beswick DM, Gooding WE, Johnson JT. Branstetter BFt. Temporal patterns of head and neck squamous cell carcinoma recurrence with positron-emission tomography/computed tomography monitoring. Laryngoscope 2012;122(7):1512–7.
6. Leung AS, Rath TJ, Hughes MA, et al. Optimal timing of first posttreatment FDG PET/CT in head and neck squamous cell carcinoma. Head Neck 2016;38(Suppl 1):E853–8.
7. Gilbert MR, Branstetter BF, Kim S. Utility of positron-emission tomography/computed tomography imaging in the management of the neck in recurrent laryngeal cancer. Laryngoscope 2012; 122(4):821–5.
8. Koshkareva Y, Branstetter BF, Gaughan JP, et al. Predictive accuracy of first post-treatment PET/CT in HPV-related oropharyngeal squamous cell carcinoma. Laryngoscope 2014;124(8):1843–7.
9. Ong SC, Schoder H, Lee NY, et al. Clinical utility of 18F-FDG PET/CT in assessing the neck after concurrent chemoradiotherapy for Locoregional advanced head and neck cancer. J Nucl Med 2008; 49(4):532–40.
10. Pfister DG, Spencer S, Brizel DM, et al. Head and neck cancers, Version 2.2014. Clinical practice guidelines in oncology. J Natl Compr Canc Netw 2014;12(10):1454–87.
11. Roman BR, Patel SG, Wang MB, et al. Guideline familiarity predicts variation in self-reported use of routine surveillance PET/CT by physicians who treat head and neck cancer. J Natl Compr Canc Netw 2015;13(1):69–77.
12. Roman BR, Goldenberg D, Givi B, Education Committee of American Head and Neck Society (AHNS). AHNS Series–Do you know your guidelines? Guideline recommended follow-up and surveillance of head and neck cancer survivors. Head Neck 2016;38(2):168–74.
13. Hudgins PA, Burson JG, Gussack GS, et al. CT and MR appearance of recurrent malignant head and neck neoplasms after resection and flap reconstruction. AJNR Am J Neuroradiol 1994; 15(9):1689–94.
14. Wray R, Sheikhbahaei S, Marcus C, et al. Therapy response assessment and patient outcomes in head and neck squamous cell carcinoma: FDG PET Hopkins criteria versus residual neck node size and morphologic features. AJR Am J Roentgenol 2016;207(3):641–7.
15. Porceddu SV, Pryor DI, Burmeister E, et al. Results of a prospective study of positron emission tomography-directed management of residual nodal abnormalities in node-positive head and neck cancer after definitive radiotherapy with or without systemic therapy. Head Neck 2011;33(12):1675–82.
16. Sherriff JM, Ogunremi B, Colley S, et al. The role of positron emission tomography/CT imaging in head and neck cancer patients after radical chemoradiotherapy. Br J Radiol 2012;85(1019):e1120–1126.
17. Marcus C, Ciarallo A, Tahari AK, et al. Head and neck PET/CT: therapy response interpretation criteria (Hopkins Criteria)-interreader reliability, accuracy, and survival outcomes. J Nucl Med 2014; 55(9):1411–6.
18. Naidich MJ, Weissman JL. Reconstructive myofascial skull-base flaps: normal appearance on CT and MR imaging studies. AJR Am J Roentgenol 1996;167(3):611–4.
19. Gladish GW, Rice DC, Sabloff BS, et al. Pedicle muscle flaps in intrathoracic cancer resection: imaging appearance and evolution. Radiographics 2007; 27(4):975–87.
20. Theodorou DJ, Theodorou SJ, Kakitsubata Y. Skeletal muscle disease: patterns of MRI appearances. Br J Radiol 2012;85(1020):e1298–1308.

Computed Tomography Versus Magnetic Resonance in Head and Neck Cancer
When to Use What and Image Optimization Strategies

Amy Juliano, MD[a],*, Gul Moonis, MD[b]

KEYWORDS

- Head and neck cancer • AJCC TNM • Anatomic landmarks

KEY POINTS

- CT is a good initial assessment modality when the primary tumor is adjacent to fat, vessels, air-filled aerodigestive tract lumen, and bone/cartilage, such as oropharyngeal cancer, hypopharyngeal cancer, and laryngeal cancer.
- MR imaging offers superior soft tissue contrast, and is preferred when tumor has to be differentiated from adjacent soft tissue structures and bone marrow. This is especially applicable for assessment of nasopharyngeal carcinoma and oral tongue cancer. MR is also useful for problem solving after an initial CT, for example in evaluating for cartilage invasion by a larynx cancer.
- Non–fat-saturated unenhanced T1-weighted MR imaging is a very important sequence for assessing primary tumor and perineural invasion, due to the natural contrast provided by the high signal intensity of fat against tumor, both at the primary site and particularly at the tiny skull base foramina through which cranial nerve branches course through fat.

NASOPHARYNGEAL CARCINOMA

The nasopharynx is an epithelial-lined cavity composed of both stratified squamous and columnar epithelium, located at the upper end of the aerodigestive tract. Its boundaries are: anteriorly, the nasal choana; posteriorly and superiorly, the inferior aspect of the basisphenoid and the entire basiocciput (clivus), anterior arch of C1, a portion of C2, and the overlying prevertebral muscles; inferiorly, continuous with the oropharynx (separated from it by an imaginary line drawn at the level of the hard palate and the Passavant muscle); and laterally, outlined by the fossa of Rosenmüller, the eustachian tube orifice, and torus tubarius.

Squamous cell carcinoma of the nasopharynx (nasopharyngeal carcinoma [NPC]) accounts for 70% of all nasopharyngeal neoplasms and is the most common malignancy of the nasopharynx. The remaining 30% consist of lymphomas, salivary gland tumors, melanomas, and some rare varieties of sarcoma.[1] Some factors thought to be associated with NPC include genetic predisposition linked to human leukocyte antigen loci; latent Epstein-Barr virus (EBV) infection; and environmental exposures, such as nitrosamines in

Disclosure: The authors have nothing to disclose.
[a] Department of Radiology, Massachusetts Eye and Ear Infirmary, Harvard Medical School, 243 Charles Street, Boston, MA 02114, USA; [b] Department of Radiology, Columbia University Medical Center, 622 West 168th Street, New York, NY 10032, USA
* Corresponding author.
E-mail address: amy_juliano@meei.harvard.edu

preserved salted foods, polycyclic hydrocarbons, and chronic nasal inflammation.[2] Patients typically present with a focal neck mass related to metastatic adenopathy because NPC is associated with early lymphatic spread to retropharyngeal nodes (nodes of Rouvière) and nodes along the jugular and spinal accessory chains (**Fig. 1**). The incidence of nodal involvement at presentation has been reported to range from 60% to as high as

96%. Less often, patients present with serous otitis media caused by eustachian tube obstruction (**Fig. 2**), epistaxis, or nasopharyngeal obstruction related to the primary tumor.

Imaging is a key component in the clinical staging of NPC. Recognition of key staging landmarks in the American Joint Committee on Cancer (AJCC) tumor, node, metastasis (TNM) criteria[3] is important for understanding the relative utility of

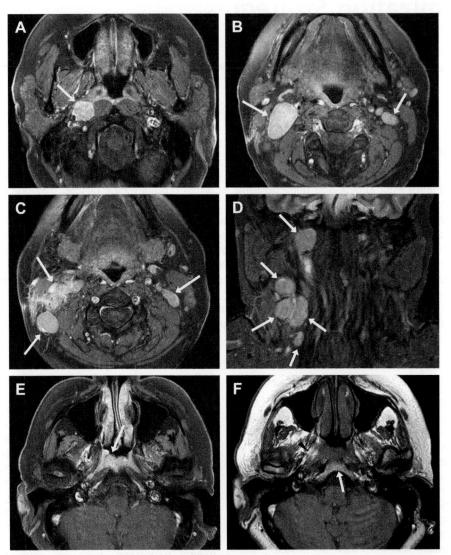

Fig. 1. A 48-year-old woman with EBV and NPC. She initially presented to her primary care physician with a right neck mass, and magnetic resonance (MR) imaging of the nasopharynx and neck was performed. (*A–C*) Axial postcontrast T1-weighted images show avidly enhancing nodes in the lateral retropharyngeal region (node of Rouvière) (*arrow* in *A*) and bilateral level II nodes (*arrows* in *B* and *C*). (*D*) Coronal short-tau inversion recovery image shows the T2-hyperintense nodes (*arrows*). (*E*) Axial postcontrast fat-saturated T1-weighted sequence at the level of the nasopharynx shows nodular soft tissue thickening in the nasopharynx representing the primary tumor, which is small relative to the nodes. Mass effect causes effacement of the fossae of Rosenmüller, more on the right than the left (*arrows*). (*F*) Axial noncontrast T1-weighted sequence helps to assess marrow signal in the clivus (*arrow*) and the parapharyngeal fat (*arrowhead*); in this case, both are uninvolved. The patient subsequently underwent nodal biopsy, which revealed EBV and metastatic carcinoma.

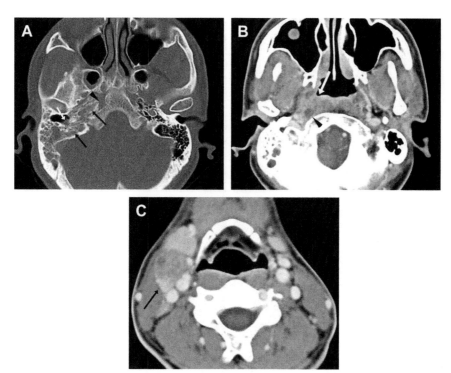

Fig. 2. A 36-year-old man with EBV and NPC. The patient received a course of antibiotics for ear congestion without relief. A cervical node became palpable and neck CT was performed. (*A*) Axial CT image in bone algorithm shows opacification of the right middle ear (*white arrow*), mastoid air cells, and petrous apex air cells without erosion of the bony septations (*black arrows*), presumably representing an effusion. However, close inspection of the skull base reveals abnormal widening of the right foramen lacerum with mild sclerosis of the adjacent bone (*arrowhead*). (*B*) Axial CT image in soft tissue algorithm at the level of the nasopharynx shows enhancing thickened soft tissue effacing the right fossa of Rosenmüller (*arrow*) and a necrotic right node of Rouvière (*arrowhead*). Involvement of the right longus colli muscle is possible but not definitive on CT. (*C*) Axial CT image in soft tissue algorithm further inferiorly shows an abnormal right level II/III node with necrotic components (*arrow*).

computed tomography (CT) versus magnetic resonance (MR) imaging. The imaging modality should be selected to optimize visualization of these landmark structures. For establishing the T category, structures (other than the primary tumor mass) that have to be identified on imaging include:

- Nasopharynx
- Oropharynx
- Nasal cavity
- Parapharyngeal space
- Medial pterygoid muscle
- Lateral pterygoid muscle
- Prevertebral muscles
- Bony structures at the skull base (including skull base foramina such as foramen lacerum)
- Cervical vertebrae
- Bony pterygoid (pterygoid process, pterygoid plates)
- Paranasal sinuses
- Intracranial structures (dura, leptomeninges, brain parenchyma, cavernous sinus, Meckel cave)

- Cranial nerves
- Hypopharynx
- Orbit
- Parotid gland
- Structures lateral to the lateral pterygoid muscle

CT is able to offer excellent bony delineation, especially of cortical margins, and is helpful in assessment of the bony skull base (including the clivus, bony pterygoids, and skull base foramina) (see **Fig. 2**), vertebral body margins, bony margins of sinonasal cavities and nasal septum, and orbital margins. Otherwise, soft tissue structures predominate the T criteria, and visualization of these soft tissue structures (such as muscles, fat, fascial compartments, and head and neck spaces) and delineation of tumor from these structures is crucial. Therefore, MR imaging is considered the preferred modality because of its ability to offer superior soft tissue contrast (**Fig. 3**).[3] Intracranial involvement and perineural tumor spread are also best assessed by MR imaging.[4] As well, MR

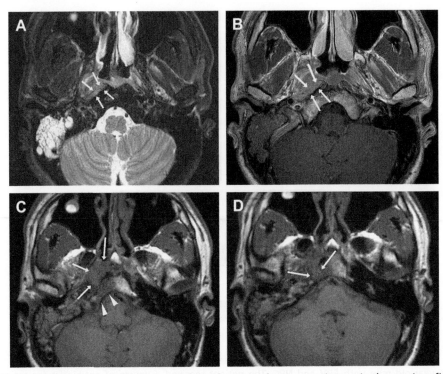

Fig. 3. NPC. MR imaging was performed 1 week from the CT on the same patient as in the previous figure. Axial T2-weighted image (*A*) and postcontrast T1-weighted image (*B*) show increased T2 signal and enhancement of the anterior portion of the right longus colli muscle (*arrows*), confirming tumor involvement. (*C*) Axial noncontrast T1-weighted image shows the primary tumor (*arrows*) extending superoposteriorly toward the skull base. There is infiltration of the clivus, as shown by the loss in normal T1-hyperintense fatty marrow signal (*arrowheads*). (*D*) Axial noncontrast T1-weighted image slightly more rostral shows tumor extending through and widening the right foramen lacerum (*arrows*).

imaging is able to detect marrow involvement; this is especially important when assessing the clivus, which is not as well evaluated by CT (see **Figs. 2** and **3**). If MR does not show frank marrow infiltration but tumor can be seen to abut bone, CT can be a good complementary second modality to exclude bone involvement.

Assessment of nodal status may be accomplished by either CT or MR imaging, with attention paid not only to the size of the nodes (greatest dimension in any direction) but also laterality, location, and the most caudal extent of nodal involvement. Nodal necrosis and extranodal extension of tumor are important features to note (**Fig. 4**).

The most common sites of distant metastases are lung, bone, liver, and distant nodes (defined as all nodes inferior to the clavicle). Distant metastasis can be detected by whole-body 18F-fluorodeoxyglucose PET/CT. However, a CT scan of the chest and upper abdomen is commonly performed for initial staging and surveillance, especially because it may not be logistically or financially feasible for the patient to undergo repeated staging PET/CT studies.

NPC is typically treated by radiation therapy. Posttreatment imaging surveillance of the primary site is well accomplished by MR imaging, with CT of the chest and upper abdomen helpful to monitor for distant metastases.

MR imaging of the nasopharynx should be performed using large-field-of-view, high-resolution, thin (3 mm) imaging slices. Noncontrast T1-weighted imaging can be extremely helpful, because of the high signal contrast between fat (normal, whether in tissue planes or within marrow) and tumor, especially when evaluating skull base foramina for tumor involvement. Nerves should always be surrounded by fat, and, when normal fat signal is absent or infiltrated (eg, in foramen ovale, vidian canal, pterygopalatine fossa, inferior alveolar foramen, infraorbital canal, or foramen in the premaxillary region), then tumor involvement should be suspected. On contrast-enhanced T1-weighted sequences, tumor is typically intermediate in T2 signal intensity and enhancement (**Fig. 5**), and, if so, can be distinguished from adjacent normal fat and muscle.

CT should likewise be performed with thin (2 mm) imaging slices and presented in both soft

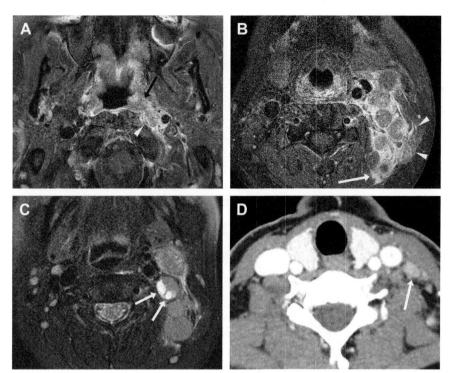

Fig. 4. A 40-year-old woman with NPC. (*A*) Axial contrast-enhanced T1-weighted image shows the primary tumor (*arrow*) and an abnormal left node of Rouvière (*arrowhead*). The node has surrounding enhancing infiltrating tissue, suggestive of extracapsular/extranodal extension (ENE) of disease. (*B*) Axial contrast-enhanced T1-weighted image more inferiorly shows multiple bulky left neck nodes with ill-defined irregular margins and surrounding infiltrative enhancement extending to the adjacent paraspinal musculature (*arrow*) and sternocleidomastoid muscle (*arrowheads*), features compatible with extracapsular extension. (*C*) Axial T2-weighted image shows T2-hyperintense areas within some of the nodes, indicating necrosis (*arrows*). (*D*) Axial CT image in soft tissue algorithm shows metastatic nodes continuing below the level of the cricoid (*arrow*), which portends a worse prognosis.

tissue and bone algorithms. Contrast administration can help increase tumor visibility to a certain extent but is especially helpful for highlighting the vessels in the skull base, to determine whether there is carotid artery invasion or encasement. Assessment of nodal status in the neck by CT is vastly improved with the presence of intravenous contrast as well, helping to differentiate nodes of Rouvière from the adjacent internal carotid artery and longus colli muscle, jugular chain nodes from muscles (see **Fig. 4**D) and vessels, and also in helping to discern any necrotic components within the nodes (see **Fig. 2**B, C).

ORAL CAVITY CARCINOMA

The oral cavity is the most ventral portion of the aerodigestive tract. It is separated from the oropharynx by a ring of structures consisting of the circumvallate papillae of the tongue, the soft palate, and the anterior tonsillar pillars. The oral cavity is divided into a central part, the oral cavity proper, and a lateral part, the vestibule.

The vestibule is a cleft lined by the buccal mucosa laterally; superiorly and inferiorly by reflections of the buccal mucosa onto the mandible and maxilla, respectively, referred to as the upper and lower gingivobuccal sulci (GBS); the gingival mucosa medially; the lips anteriorly; and leads to the retromolar trigone posteriorly.[5] The anatomic subsites of the oral cavity are (1) the lips, (2) the floor of the mouth, (3) the oral tongue (ie, the anterior two-thirds of the tongue), (4) the buccal mucosa, (5) the upper and lower gingivae, (6) the hard palate, and (7) the retromolar trigone.

Oral cavity squamous cell carcinoma (OCC) is the most common malignancy of the head and neck (excluding nonmelanoma skin cancer)[6] and is the sixth most common cancer worldwide. Most cases are related to consumption of alcohol and tobacco.[7] In the Western world, the most common site for OCC is the tongue, which accounts for approximately 40% to 50% of all cases.[6] Almost all tongue lesions occur on the lateral and ventrolateral aspects. The second

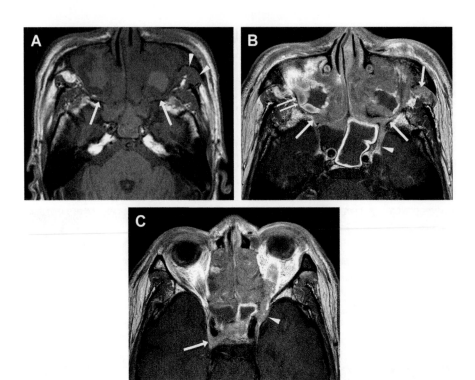

Fig. 5. Aggressive recurrent NPC. A 71-year-old man with EBV and NPC after chemotherapy and radiation; 1 year later, the patient had recurrent disease in the neck and underwent salvage neck dissection. Another year after that, this MR imaging was performed because of new epistaxis and cheek paresthesias. (*A*) Axial noncontrast T1-weighted image shows obliteration of the fat in bilateral pterygopalatine fossae by infiltrative recurrent tumor (*arrows*), extending laterally on the left along the retromaxillary fissure toward the temporalis muscle (*arrowheads*). Soft tissue in the paranasal sinuses is nonspecific on this sequence. (*B*) Axial contrast-enhanced T1-weighted image shows recurrent tumor showing intermediate signal intensity/enhancement in bilateral pterygopalatine fossae; laterally along the retromaxillary fissure to the temporalis muscle (*arrows*); along the left foramen rotundum (*arrowhead*); and invading into the right sphenoid sinus, nasal cavity, and maxillary sinuses (left > right). Peripheral soft tissue at the lateral portion of the right maxillary sinus has MR appearance compatible with inflammatory mucosal enhancement and submucosal edema rather than tumor involvement (*small double arrows*). (*C*) Axial contrast-enhanced T1-weighted image slightly rostrally shows tumor involvement of the cavernous sinus (*arrow*) and left superior orbital fissure (*arrowhead*).

most common oral cavity site is the floor of the mouth. However, in India, where betel nut chewing is a risk factor, the tongue and buccal mucosa are the most common sites for OCC.

Imaging aids in determining the extent of the primary tumor, regional lymph node spread, and distant metastasis in patients with OCC. The eighth edition of the AJCC Cancer Staging Manual describes the TNM staging criteria for OCC.[3] There is a revised T staging for OCC. Depth of invasion has been recognized as a better predictive parameter for tumor aggressiveness than tumor thickness in oral tongue lesions. Depth of invasion has replaced extrinsic muscle infiltration for T4 designation in oral tongue lesions. Less invasive (depth <5 mm) carcinomas should be distinguished from moderately invasive (depth 5–10 mm) and deeply invasive (depth >10 mm) carcinomas. The oral cavity T staging is the same for all subsites, except the criteria for moderately advanced local disease (T4a) for lip is a separate entity.

The factors that influence treatment options are size of tumor, location, bony involvement, status of nodes, and histology (type, grade and depth of invasion).

The anatomic landmarks that are important for staging in OCC and need to be examined specifically on imaging include:

- Maxilla and mandible
- Maxillary sinus
- Floor of mouth
- Pterygopalatine fossa
- Masticator space
- Pterygoid plates
- Skull base
- Internal carotid artery

Overall evaluation of OCC can be limited on CT scans because of dental amalgam. The puffed-check technique may be helpful to detect buccal cancers on CT (**Fig. 6**). MR imaging offers better soft tissue characterization and anatomic detail,[5] although some investigators have found good correlation between CT-based tumor thickness and measurements on pathologic specimens.[8] However, superficial mucosal tumors can be entirely missed on both CT and MR imaging. MR imaging should be performed using high-resolution small-field-of-view imaging. In addition to fat-saturated T2-weighted and postgadolinium fat-saturated T1-weighted images, it is important to obtain thin-section (3 mm) non–fat-saturated T1-weighted images to take advantage of the natural contrast provided by the high signal intensity of fat.[9] MR imaging is considered an accurate method to detect depth of invasion of oral tongue cancers and has predictive value for nodal metastasis.[10–13] Alsaffar and colleagues[14] found strong correlation between pathologic, MR imaging, and clinical measurements in deep tumors (≥5 mm). In superficial tumors (<5 mm), clinical and MR imaging examination had low correlation with pathologic thickness. Extension of the tumor from its primary site to adjacent areas should be sought in each case because it is important in staging. Evaluation of the neurovascular bundle (NVB) or midline septum involvement is important for preoperative planning. Hemiglossectomy is precluded if the contralateral NVB is involved and if the midline is transgressed. In general, a good-quality CT scan is adequate to answer this question.

T4a lesions (moderately advanced local disease) include maxillary or mandibular bony involvement or extension into the maxillary sinus (**Fig. 7**). For lip cancers, T4a cancers extend to the bone, inferior alveolar nerve, floor of mouth, or skin of face. Of note, superficial erosion of

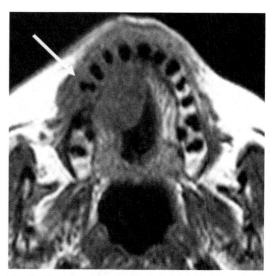

Fig. 7. Alveolar ridge carcinoma (*arrow*). There is an oral cavity lesion along the labial and buccal surfaces of the right upper alveolar ridge with resorption of the intervening cortices and the trabecular elements surrounding the lateral incisor, canine, and first premolar teeth.

bone or tooth socket alone by a gingival primary is not sufficient to classify a tumor as T4.

Very advanced (T4b) disease is defined as involvement of the masticator space, pterygoid plates, or skull base, or encasement of the internal carotid artery (**Fig. 8**). Extrinsic tongue muscle infiltration is no longer a staging criterion for T4 disease.

Mandibular involvement in OCC occurs by direct infiltration of the tumor through the alveolar ridge or lingual cortical plate at the point of abutment with the lesion.[15] The treatment options are either segmental (full thickness) or marginal (partial thickness in height or width) mandibulectomy. Marginal surgery is less morbid and is indicated if there is limited cortical involvement clinically or by imaging.[16] If there is extensive involvement of the marrow, then segmental surgery should be performed. Some investigators advocate clinical examination, intraoperative periosteal stripping, and at least 2 imaging techniques that complement each other in terms of specificity and sensitivity as the basis for deciding whether and what type of mandibular resection should be performed.[17]

The literature is still divided on the best imaging modality to evaluate for mandibular invasion.[15] Plain films, orthopantomograms, CT scans, MR imaging, and bone scans have been used with varying degrees of accuracy. With axial, coronal, and sagittal reconstructions on CT scan, even subtle tumor invasion of the mandible can be

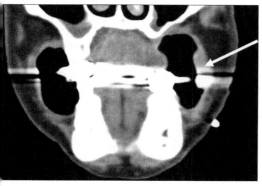

Fig. 6. Left buccal cancer (*arrow*) seen on puffed cheek technique on a coronal CT scan.

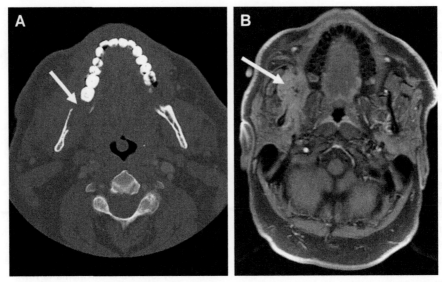

Fig. 8. T4b carcinoma of the mandible. (*A*) Axial CT image shows erosion of the right posterior mandibular body (*arrow*). (*B*) Post-gadolinium T1-weighted axial MR image shows involvement of the right masticator space (*arrow*).

detected, and 3D reconstructions can be helpful for assessment. Cone-beam CT shows promising results in identification of mandibular invasion by OCC with a much higher sensitivity for cortical bone invasion and a better negative predictive value.[18]

In our experience, cortical erosion of mandible or maxilla is best performed with CT. On MR imaging, cortical bone might not be well seen. Bone marrow involvement may be seen on unenhanced T1-weighted images as replacement of the fatty signal and enhancement on postgadolinium T1-weighted images with fat saturation. However, these findings are not very specific, and mimics include infection, recent tooth extraction, and osteoradionecrosis. Chemical shift artifact on MR imaging induced by bone marrow fat can also result in false-positive results. Bone scintigraphy can be very sensitive but not very specific and is not routinely used in our practice.

Incidence of perineural invasion (PNI) or perineural spread (PNS) in OCC is as high as 40%.[19] PNI may be evident on CT as enlarged or irregular foramina but, in our opinion, high-resolution MR imaging (including axial thin-section non–fat-saturated T1-weighted images) is more sensitive to map out the course of the nerve in its entirety from the oral cavity to the brain. MR imaging should be performed even if the CT is positive for PNS because skip lesions may occur. The nerves that are usually involved in OCC include branches of V3 (inferior alveolar nerve, mental nerve, lingual nerve, buccal branches) or V2 (greater or lesser palatine nerves, or infraorbital nerve). Perineural spread is manifested on MR imaging as loss of foraminal fat, and enlargement and enhancement of the involved nerve (**Fig. 9**). Denervation changes in the muscles of mastication can also be seen.[20]

Nodal involvement is the single most important prognostic indicator in OCC and oropharyngeal carcinoma (OPC).[21] The first nodal stations to be involved in OCC are levels I and II. RMT, floor of the mouth, and oral tongue cancers are more likely to present with adenopathy than other oral cavity subsites.[21] CT scan with contrast performed with 2 mm slices is adequate for nodal staging and MR imaging is not needed for this evaluation. Attention should be paid to the size of the nodes (greatest dimension in any direction), laterality, location, nodal necrosis and extra nodal extension.

OROPHARYNGEAL CARCINOMA

The oropharynx consists of the soft palate, base (or posterior one-third) of tongue (BOT), palatine tonsils, palatoglossal folds, valleculae, and posterior pharyngeal wall. The junction of the hard and soft palate from above and the circumvallate papillae from below separate it from the oral cavity. In addition to traditional modifiable risk factors like tobacco and alcohol, human papillomavirus (HPV) has emerged as a major causal factor for OPC.

HPV types 16 and 18 are the most commonly detected transcriptionally active HPV types in head and neck cancer.[22] HPV-associated OPC occurs in younger, healthier individuals with no significant tobacco exposure, is highly responsive to therapy, and carries an excellent prognosis.

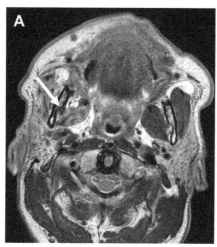
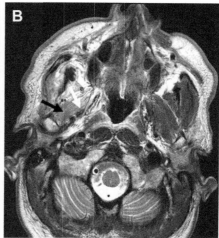

Fig. 9. Perineural spread from a right buccal cancer. Axial T2-weighted MR images show enlargement of the right inferior alveolar nerve (*white arrow* in *A*) and V3 (*white arrow* in *B*), and denervation changes within the right muscles of mastication (*black arrow* in *B*).

Immunohistochemistry for overexpression of tumor suppressor protein p16 is a robust surrogate marker for HPV-mediated carcinogenesis. Approximately 60% of OPCs present with nodal metastases, of which 30% are bilateral. BOT is associated with the highest frequency of nodal disease followed by tonsillar fossa, oropharyngeal wall, and soft palate.[21] Cystic adenopathy is seen with HPV-positive OCC and may mimic a branchial cleft cyst (**Fig. 10**).

The recently released eighth edition of the AJCC Staging Manual introduces some modifications in the TNM staging of OPC.[3] In HPV-associated OPC, clinically or radiologically affected nodes whether single or multiple as long as they are less than 6 cm and remain ipsilateral are included in the same N category (N1). Clinically or radiologically evident bilateral or contralateral nodes less than 6 cm are in N2 category. Nodes greater than 6 cm are designated N3.

T4b category has been removed from p-16 positive OPC. Extranodal extension (ENE) has been added as an additional criterion for N3 designation for non–HPV-associated OPC. On imaging, ENE is suspected when the node shows indistinct, shaggy margins with nodal capsular enhancement and infiltration into adjacent fat or soft tissue planes.[23] CT and MR imaging have been found to be comparable for detection of ENE.[24] However, overall imaging is still not considered to have high enough sensitivity and specificity to detect ENE. Therefore, for diagnosis of ENE, both radiological and clinical evidence are needed (skin invasion, infiltration of muscle, dysfunction of subjacent nerve). ENE has no effect on the staging of HPV-positive OPC.

Important imaging landmarks for T staging of OPC include:

- Extrinsic muscles of tongue
- Lingual surface of the epiglottis
- Larynx
- Pterygoid muscles
- Pterygoid plate

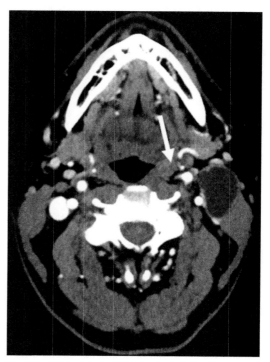

Fig. 10. HPV-related OPC. Cystic left level II lymph node on axial CT in this patient with a subtle left oropharyngeal tumor (*arrow*).

- Hard palate
- Mandible
- Lateral nasopharynx
- Skull base
- Internal carotid artery encasement

Of note, mucosal extension to the lingual surface of the epiglottis from primary tumors of the BOT does not constitute involvement of the larynx. Laryngeal involvement precludes partial glossectomy and preepiglottic space invasion correlates with increased nodal metastasis. Preepiglottic invasion is discussed in more detail later.

CT is the modality of choice for initial staging because of its speed and ease of acquisition, although MR imaging provides superior evaluation of soft tissue involvement. Extension into the intrinsic muscles should be sought (best seen on T1-weighted non–fat-saturated sagittal images). Like oral tongue and floor of the mouth carcinoma, evaluation of the neurovascular bundle and midline septum involvement are important factors to assess for preoperative planning. Hemiglossectomy is precluded if contralateral NVB is involved and if the midline is transgressed. Tonsillar cancers can have substantial submucosal involvement that may be occult on clinical examination. Extension to the pterygoid muscles, nasopharynx, or skull base (along the pterygomandibular raphe) should also be assessed and is adequate with a good-quality CT scan (**Fig. 11**). Osseous involvement of the pterygoid plates is better seen on CT.

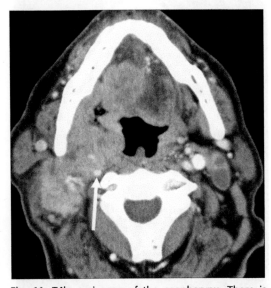

Fig. 11. T4b carcinoma of the oropharynx. There is very locally advanced disease on an axial CT scan with encasement of the right internal carotid artery (*arrow*) and invasion of the lateral pterygoid muscle. Bilateral level II nodes are noted, right matted with ENE and left necrotic.

HYPOPHARYNGEAL CARCINOMA

The hypopharynx extends from lateral pharyngoepiglottic folds superiorly to the upper esophageal segment inferiorly and includes the postcricoid segment, the pyriform sinuses, and the posterior hypopharyngeal walls. The aryepiglottic folds (a supraglottic structure) forms the anteromedial margin of the piriform sinus.

Most hypopharyngeal cancers arise in the pyriform sinus, with the postcricoid region the least common site of involvement. Hypopharyngeal cancers are generally clinically occult until a late stage and the disease is frequently advanced at presentation. Nodal metastasis is present in 50% to 70% of cases at presentation. Submucosal extension of tumor on imaging may be greater than expected on laryngoscopy. Both CT and MR imaging are accurate methods to detect the primary tumor[25] but CT scan is easier and faster to perform and is the preferred modality for tumor detection and staging.

The structures that are important for the imaging checklist in hypopharyngeal cancers according to the AJCC TNM criteria[3] for hypopharyngeal cancer are:

- Pyriform sinus
- Posterior hypopharyngeal wall
- Postcricoid region
- Thyroid cartilage/other laryngeal cartilages
- Thyrohyoid membrane
- Esophagus
- Carotid artery
- Prevertebral fascia/muscles

Images should be assessed for involvement of different hypopharyngeal subsites, the paraglottic space, thyroid cartilage, and extrapharyngeal spread via the thyrohyoid membrane along the superior laryngeal neurovascular bundle (**Fig. 12**). When lateral spread occurs, involvement of the carotid artery should be assessed. The best imaging option for detection of laryngeal cartilage, carotid artery, and paravertebral fascia/muscle involvement is discussed later, because these features are common to both extensive laryngeal and hypopharyngeal cancers.

LARYNGEAL CARCINOMA

Imaging of the neck at initial presentation aids in the determination of laryngeal tumor subsite (supraglottic, glottic, or subglottic), local extent of the primary tumor, and nodal status. Knowledge of laryngeal anatomy and staging criteria is essential.

The larynx is marginated superolaterally by the epiglottis and laryngeal (anterior) aspect of the

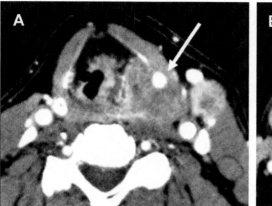
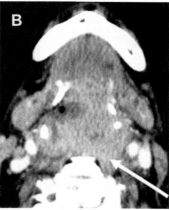

Fig. 12. Hypopharyngeal cancers. (A) Axial contrast-enhanced CT image shows a T4a (moderately advanced local disease) hypopharyngeal carcinoma with extension through the thyrohyoid membrane and invasion of the strap muscle (*arrow*). (B) Axial contrast-enhanced CT image in a different patient shows a T4b (advanced local disease) hypopharyngeal carcinoma with tumor invasion of the prevertebral fascia (*arrow*).

aryepiglottic folds. Posteriorly, it is delimited by the arytenoid cartilages, interarytenoid space, and posterior surface of the cricoid cartilage. Anteriorly, it is marginated by the lingual (anterior) surface of the epiglottis, thyrohyoid membrane, anterior commissure, anterior thyroid cartilage, cricothyroid membrane, and anterior cricoid cartilage. The inferior margin is formed by a horizontal plane along the inferior border of the cricoid ring.

A supraglottic carcinoma involves the epiglottis, laryngeal aspect of the aryepiglottic folds, arytenoids, and false vocal cords/folds (**Fig. 13**). A tumor is considered glottic if it involves the true cords, including the anterior and posterior commissures, and structures within a 1-cm thickness starting from a horizontal plane along the inferolateral margin of the laryngeal ventricles (**Fig. 14**). A subglottic tumor involves structures between the inferior margin of the glottis and the inferior margin of the cricoid cartilage (**Fig. 15**).

Laryngeal cancers are staged by the TNM system, with the latest AJCC guidelines published in 2017.[3] Supraglottic, glottic, and subglottic tumors each have their own T staging criteria, but, for all 3, the structures important for radiologists to identify include:

- Base of tongue
- Vallecula
- Medial wall of pyriform sinus
- Postcricoid pharynx
- Preepiglottic space
- Paraglottic space
- Thyroid cartilage (inner cortex, outer cortex)
- Extralaryngeal soft tissues of the neck
  - Deep extrinsic muscles of the tongue
  - Strap muscles

- Thyroid gland
- Trachea
- Esophagus
- Prevertebral space
- Carotid artery
- Mediastinal structures

Determination of tumor subsite is readily accomplished by CT (in combination with endoscopy to determine vocal cord mobility). CT offers high spatial resolution, and image acquisition can be

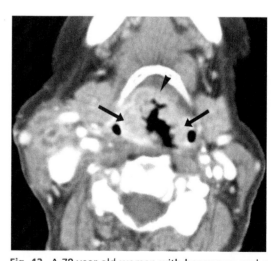

Fig. 13. A 78-year-old woman with hoarseness and a new right neck mass. She underwent direct laryngoscopy and biopsy, confirming invasive squamous cell carcinoma of the supraglottic larynx. Axial contrast-enhanced CT image in soft tissue algorithm shows heterogeneously enhancing mass with ulcerated margins involving the root of the epiglottis (petiole) and bilateral aryepiglottic folds (*arrows*), with infiltration into the preepiglottic space (*arrowhead*).

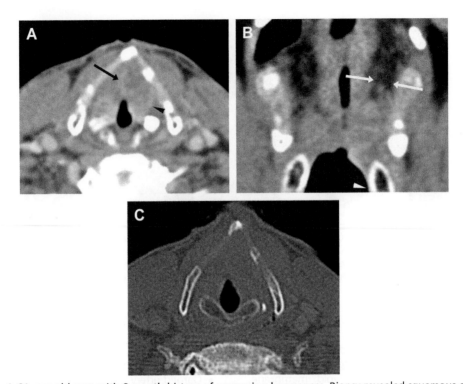

Fig. 14. A 64-year-old man with 8-month history of worsening hoarseness. Biopsy revealed squamous cell carcinoma of the anterior commissure and the entirety of the left true cord. (*A*) Axial contrast-enhanced CT image in soft tissue algorithm shows soft tissue thickening at the anterior commissure (*arrow*), extending to the left true cord, which is asymmetrically bulkier than the right (*arrowhead*). (*B*) Coronal reformatted image confirms involvement of the left true cord with expansile bulging margins, but without frank extension into the supraglottic paraglottic fat (*arrows*) or subglottis (*arrowhead*). (*C*) Axial CT image in bone algorithm shows heterogeneous ossification of the thyroid cartilage lamina without erosive changes or soft tissue extension beyond the outer surface of the cartilage.

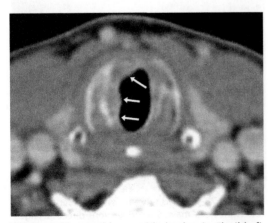

Fig. 15. A 60-year-old man with dysphonia. Flexible fiberoptic laryngoscopy revealed subglottic tissue irregularity that extended up to the right true cord. Biopsy confirmed squamous cell carcinoma. Axial contrast-enhanced CT image shows irregular soft tissue thickening at the right subglottis abutting the inner surface of the cricoid cartilage (*arrows*).

accomplished within seconds, avoiding motion artifact that may be an issue for MR imaging, especially in the region of the larynx where swallowing or even quiet breathing or subtle phonation may lead to substantial degradation of image quality (**Fig. 16**). Contrast is routinely administered, and soft tissue and bone algorithms are produced. Reformatted axial images with small-field-of-view, thin (1.5 or 2 mm) image slice thickness in a plane parallel to the plane of the true cords in combination with coronal reformats allow radiologists to distinguish between supraglottic, glottic, and subglottic larynx. For the supraglottic subsite, the epiglottis and aryepiglottic folds are clearly contrasted with the adjacent air-filled valleculae, laryngeal lumen, and pyriform sinuses, whereas the false cords are recognized by the presence of fat lateral to them (**Fig. 17A**). Continuing caudally on axial images, once the fat disappears and 3 sets of cartilages can be seen on a single image (vocal process of the arytenoids, cricoid cartilage, and thyroid cartilage), this indicates the level of the true cord (see **Fig. 17B**), and the glottic subsite continues from

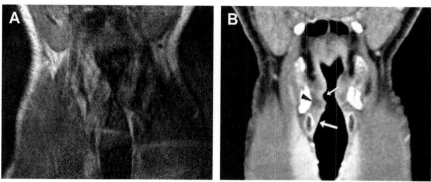

Fig. 16. A 66-year-old man with hoarseness, found to have right vocal fold paresis on fiberoptic laryngoscopy. CT was performed to assess for a potential lesion along the right vagus or recurrent laryngeal nerve, which revealed subglottic soft tissue thickening suspicious for tumor. MR imaging was subsequently performed for further evaluation. (A) Coronal postcontrast T1-weighted MR image shows significant motion artifact, perhaps from breathing or swallowing and vascular pulsations, degrading quality and compromising diagnostic capability. (B) Coronal reformatted contrast-enhanced CT image has no motion artifact, and clearly shows enlargement of the right laryngeal ventricle (*arrow*) and atrophy of the right thyroarytenoid muscle (*arrowhead*), compatible with right true cord paresis. There is also soft tissue thickening along the right subglottic larynx (*large arrow*), which on biopsy proved to represent squamous cell carcinoma.

that point caudally for 1 cm. On coronal images, the glottis is outlined by the lower border of the air-filled laryngeal ventricles (**Fig. 17C**), continuing inferiorly for 1 cm. The subglottis begins 1 cm caudal to the top of the true cords and continues down to the inferior border of the cricoid cartilage, both easily identifiable on coronal CT images (see **Fig. 17C**), whereas on axial images the complete cricoid ring

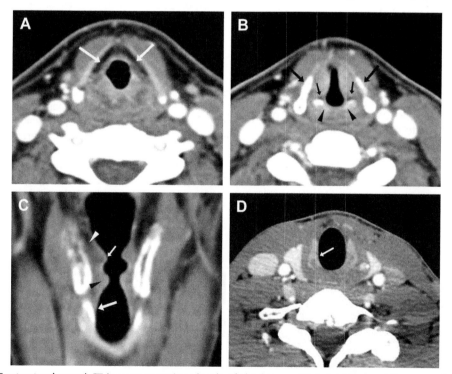

Fig. 17. Contrast-enhanced CT images at various levels of the larynx. (A) Axial image at the supraglottic level shows supraglottic paraglottic fat bilaterally (*arrows*). (B) Axial image at the glottic level, where the arytenoid (*small arrows*), cricoid (*arrowheads*), and thyroid (*large arrows*) cartilages are seen at the same time. (C) Coronal image shows the false cords (*small arrow*) and supraglottic paraglottic fat (*white arrowhead*) at the supraglottic larynx, the true cords and thyroarytenoid muscles (*black arrowhead*) at the glottic larynx, and the subglottis starting 1 cm inferior to the top of the true cords (*large arrow*). (D) Axial images shows the subglottis, where luminal air abuts the cricoid ring (*arrow*).

should be seen without any intervening tissue between the cricoid cartilage and the air-filled lumen (**Fig. 17D**).

It is important to be able to recognize a higher-stage tumor (T3 and T4) from a T1 or T2 primary, and to be able to distinguish between T3 and T4 tumors, because their management approaches differ.

T3

A T3 tumor invades the preepiglottic space (fat) (**Fig. 18A**), paraglottic space (fat) (**Fig. 18B**), and/or inner cortex of the thyroid cartilage (calcification). Fat and calcification are both well seen by CT, and therefore CT remains the routine first imaging modality of choice.[26] Infiltration of fat by soft tissue can be readily appreciated on CT, and sagittal images in soft tissue algorithm are helpful for identifying preepiglottic space involvement. Involvement of the inner cortex of the thyroid cartilage should theoretically be detectable by CT as an area of erosion or inhomogeneity that abuts abnormal tumoral soft tissue in the larynx. However, in situations in which the thyroid cartilage is irregularly ossified or nonossified, it may be difficult to differentiate between uneven ossification (physiologic) and regional cortical erosion (pathologic, from malignancy), unless there is frank soft tissue extension through the thickness of the cartilage to the extralaryngeal side of the cartilage[27] (in this case the tumor would be upstaged from T3 to T4a). In those scenarios, MR may be helpful to assess the marrow space of the ossified portion of the cartilage, to determine whether there is tumor infiltration that would support involvement of the inner cortex (discussed later) (**Fig. 19**).

T4

Invasion through the outer cortex of the thyroid cartilage is one of the staging criteria for a T4a tumor. Note that tumor tends to invade ossified

cartilage; nonossified cartilage is generally resistant to tumor invasion.[28] CT findings that would raise the suspicion for cartilage invasion by tumor includes erosion/lysis, sclerosis of the arytenoid and cricoid cartilages, and cartilage penetration with tumor seen on the outer aspect of the cartilage.[28] However, erosion of ossified cartilage can resemble normal irregularly ossified cartilage (**Fig. 20A**) or nonossified cartilage (**Fig. 20B**). Asymmetric sclerosis (see **Fig. 20A**) is a nonspecific finding and can be seen in the arytenoids in more than 12% of normal individuals.[29] Through-and-through cartilage penetration is the most specific sign (**Fig. 21**), but is not always evident.

In those cases in which cartilage invasion is indeterminate on CT, MR imaging should be performed (**Fig. 22**).[30] On T1-weighted sequences, hyperintense areas represent fatty marrow within ossified cartilage and are therefore normal; intermediate or hypointense areas are indeterminate. On T2-weighted sequences, hypointense areas represent nonossified cartilage and are therefore normal because those areas resist tumor invasion. Intermediate T2 signal is suspicious for tumor invasion, and this may be confirmed by enhancement seen on postgadolinium T1-weighted sequences; radiologists can be even more confident of cartilage invasion if the area is isointense to tumor on all sequences. Fat-suppressed sequences are helpful for distinguishing tumor from fatty marrow. If T2 signal is hyperintense, reactive edema or inflammation is probably more likely. MR imaging is more sensitive than CT but less specific,[30] and tends to overestimate cartilage invasion by tumor, whereas CT underestimates cartilage invasion.[31,32] Of note, at the level of the anterior commissure, where the vocal ligaments attach to the thyroid cartilage via Broyles ligament, there is a focal absence of perichondrium. As such, even a small anterior commissure tumor can have associated early local cartilage invasion, and careful scrutiny of this area is warranted on imaging. MR

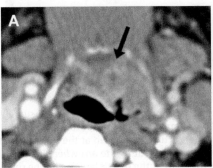
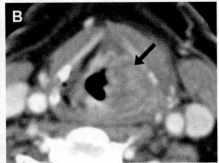

Fig. 18. Axial contrast-enhanced CT images show a T3 supraglottic tumor invading the preepiglottic fat (*arrow* in A) and left supraglottic paraglottic fat (*arrow* in B).

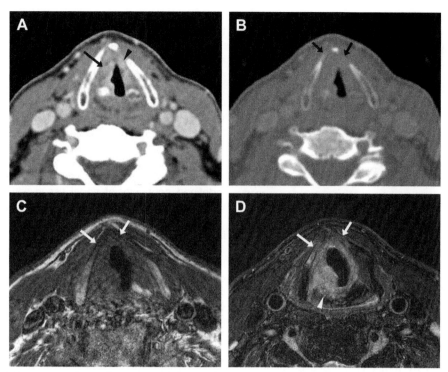

Fig. 19. Axial contrast-enhanced CT images show a right glottic tumor (*arrow* in *A*) extending across the anterior commissure toward the anterior left true cord (*arrowhead* in *A*). Tumor abuts the anterior thyroid cartilage lamina bilaterally where there is focal thinning (*arrows* in *B*). However, it is difficult to determine whether this is physiologic or caused by tumor involvement. Axial T1-weighted MR images obtained before (*C*) and following (*D*) contrast administration show intermediate signal in those areas of the thyroid cartilage (*arrows* in *C*) and associated enhancement (*arrows* in *D*), isointense to tumor, compatible with cartilage invasion. Note that tumor also invades the right posterior cricoid cartilage (*arrowhead* in *D*).

imaging may be a useful early adjunct to CT evaluation in this situation.[33] In recent years, dual-energy CT has been explored as an alternate imaging technique to diagnose cartilage invasion, although its use is as yet not widespread.[28,34] Another staging criterion for a T4a tumor is extralaryngeal spread of disease: up toward the tongue or inferiorly involving the strap muscles, thyroid

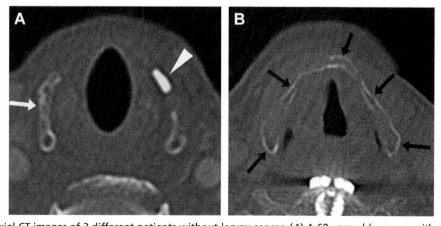

Fig. 20. Axial CT images of 2 different patients without larynx cancer. (*A*) A 68-year-old woman with some areas of the thyroid cartilage ossified, including a region that appears irregular (*arrow*). Another area is densely sclerotic (*arrowhead*). (*B*) A 63-year-old man with noncontiguous areas of ossified cartilage (*arrows*) separated by nonossified cartilage.

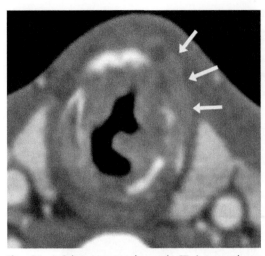

Fig. 21. Axial contrast-enhanced CT image shows abnormal soft tissue beyond the outer surface of the laryngeal cartilages (*arrows*), which unequivocally confirms cartilage invasion on CT and T4 status of the tumor.

gland, trachea, and esophagus. Invasion of the thyroid gland by tumor is obvious on contrast-enhanced CT, because the thyroid gland is normally much denser than tumor (**Fig. 23**). As for the tongue/floor of mouth, strap muscles, trachea, and esophagus, if the tumor is bulky, expansile, and infiltrative, then invasion can be diagnosed by CT (**Fig. 24**). However, in some cases it is difficult to determine whether the outward expanding margin of the tumor encroaches on these structures; in these situations, MR imaging can again be very useful for its ability to distinguish between various normal soft tissue structures and tumor.

A T4b tumor invades the prevertebral space, encases the carotid artery, or invades mediastinal structures (**Fig. 25**). Encasement of the carotid artery and mediastinal extension can usually be well shown by CT, but prevertebral involvement may be difficult to appreciate by CT, and MR imaging can be crucial for accurate staging in these CT-equivocal cases. In a recent study, MR imaging had higher negative predictive value and higher specificity in predicting the absence of prevertebral fascia invasion compared with CT, and preservation of the retropharyngeal fat plane on MR imaging was thought to reliably predict the absence of prevertebral space fixation.[35]

Cervical nodes are well assessed by contrast-enhanced CT.[36] Size (measurement in greatest dimension), number, and laterality are important, as expected. In addition, if nodes appear round, lack fatty hila, enhance heterogeneously, and have necrotic elements (**Fig. 26**), they should be viewed with suspicion, although these features

are not part of the N staging criteria. In the eighth edition of the AJCC staging criteria, ENE of tumor is especially emphasized. ENE has a profound effect on the prognosis of non–HPV-related head and neck cancers, and this is reflected in the latest N criteria. The presence of ENE in any node of any size upstages the disease to N3. Imaging findings suspicious for ENE include loss of a smooth, well-defined margin between the node and adjacent fat; infiltrative soft tissue extending from the node to surrounding fat or normal soft tissue structures (**Fig. 27**); and most definitively if there is ill-defined contiguity of nodal tissue with adjacent musculature, vessel wall, and/or skin, suggesting invasion and tethering.[3]

The true cords have a paucity of lymphatic drainage, and nodal extension from a purely glottic tumor is unusual, especially if the primary tumor is small. However, when advanced, a large glottic tumor can lead to surrounding direct tissue invasion, breaching the conus elasticus, as well as nodal metastases to regional nodes and nodes along the jugular chains. The supraglottic region has an extensive lymphatic network, and supraglottic tumors tend to be associated with adenopathy, often bilateral, and usually along the upper jugular and midjugular chains (levels II and III); level I involvement is less common. Subglottis is the least common subsite, and, as a subglottic tumor grows, it shows direct surrounding tissue invasion, as well as nodal metastases to regional nodes and nodes along the midjugular and lower jugular chains (levels III and IV). Level VII nodes (in the suprasternal notch) are considered regional metastases (N status), whereas mediastinal nodes inferior to the level of the innominate artery are considered distant metastases, and upstage the M status of disease.

Other than mediastinal nodes, other sites of distant metastases include lungs, and less frequently liver or bone. Chest CT is a practical and effective imaging tool primarily for detection of metastatic pulmonary nodules. PET/CT offers a comprehensive whole-body assessment, but is not currently reimbursable for routine repeated restaging purposes. Overall, distant metastasis is uncommon unless there is bulky regional adenopathy.[3]

UNKNOWN PRIMARY TUMORS OF THE HEAD AND NECK

Head and neck cancers of unknown primary are uncommon, constituting 1% to 4% of all head and neck cancers.[37,38] Patients present with metastatic neck nodes without a clear primary origin even after extensive clinical and imaging

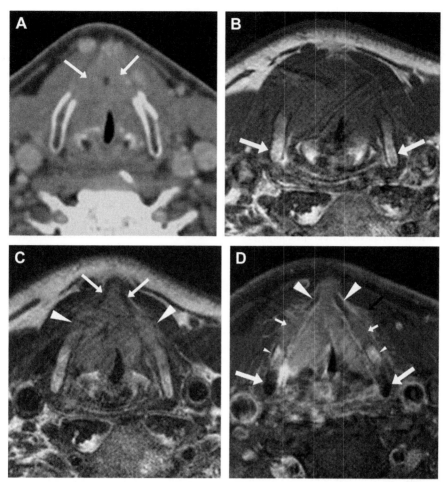

Fig. 22. A 60-year-old man with T4a squamous cell carcinoma of larynx. (*A*) Axial contrast-enhanced CT image shows tumor abutting the thyroid cartilage (*arrows*), but it is difficult to determine whether there is cartilage invasion by tumor. (*B*) Axial non–contrast-enhanced T1-weighted MR image shows hyperintense signal in the posterior portions of the cartilage, compatible with fatty marrow in normal ossified cartilage (*arrows*). The remainder of the cartilage remains indeterminate. (*C*) Axial T2-weighted MR image shows hypointense signal in the anterior-most portion of the cartilage (*arrows*), compatible with normal nonossified cartilage. The areas of intermediate signal intensity (*arrowheads*) are indeterminate. (*D*) Axial fat-suppressed contrast-enhanced T1-weighted MR image shows normal ossified cartilage (*large white arrows*, hypointense because of suppressed signal in fat), normal nonossified cartilage (*large white arrowheads*, hypointense because of cartilage), tumor invasion (*small white arrows*, intermediate signal, isointense to tumor), and probable inflammatory reaction (*small white arrowheads*, avid enhancement and more hyperintense T2 signal). There is tumor penetration beyond the thyroid cartilage toward the strap muscles, worse on the left (*black arrow*).

investigation.[39] Theories as to why the primary tumor might remain occult include small size, location not easily accessible by clinical examination and biopsy, early metastatic phenotype, and inherent limitations of diagnostic techniques.[40] More than two-thirds of these cases are squamous cell carcinomas,[41–43] and the abnormal nodes are typically located in the upper neck and midneck. When abnormal nodes are in the lower neck, the primary site is more likely to be infraclavicular; when they are in the parotid glands, the primary tumor is usually a cutaneous malignancy

rather than a squamous cell carcinoma of the head and neck.[40,41]

The typical presentation is a painless neck mass not responsive to antibiotic therapy.[44] The task then includes determination of the histology of the node, localization of the primary tumor, and assessment of additional pathologic nodes in the neck bilaterally. Work-up typically starts with fine-needle aspiration (FNA) biopsy, which may be performed under ultrasonography guidance as warranted. Ultrasonography guidance is especially helpful if the node is deep, is in close

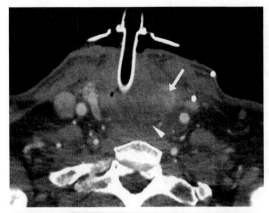

Fig. 23. A 54-year-old heavy smoker with a 6-month history of hoarseness underwent fiberoptic laryngoscopy and biopsy that confirmed necrotic and poorly differentiated squamous cell carcinoma of the larynx, subsequently developing airway obstruction and respiratory distress necessitating emergent tracheostomy. Axial contrast-enhanced CT image shows invasion of the left lobe of the thyroid gland (*arrow*) and the esophagus (*arrowhead*). The laryngeal lumen is completely obliterated by tumor, necessitating a tracheostomy tube.

proximity to the carotid, or if there are cystic/ necrotic elements that should be avoided to minimize the risk of a nondiagnostic sample. If the FNA results are inconclusive or negative (discordant with clinical findings), patients might proceed to core needle biopsy. Open biopsy is an option, but in recent years has been discouraged because of the risks of tumor spillage, disruption of fascial planes that serve as protective barriers to tumor

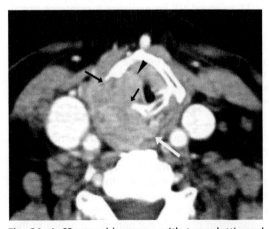

Fig. 24. A 62-year-old woman with transglottic and hypopharyngeal T4a squamous cell carcinoma. Axial contrast-enhanced CT image shows tumor involving the right true cord (*black arrowhead*) with cartilage invasion (*black arrows*), extralaryngeal spread, and esophageal invasion (*large white arrow*).

spread, and changes to the lymphatic drainage system. A preferred next step could be planned excisional biopsy with immediate frozen section analysis followed by a neck dissection if the node is positive for squamous cell carcinoma.[45,46] Once metastatic squamous cell carcinoma is confirmed in the node and no cutaneous source is evident, the primary site is sought via a combination of physical examination, CT, MR imaging, PET/CT, panendoscopy (endoscopic examination under anesthesia – [EUA]) with biopsies, and/or direct laryngoscopy (DL) with biopsies.[40,45] A recent study suggests that testing for biomarkers such as HPV, p16, and EBV when sampling the metastatic node via FNA offers additional guidance in the search for the occult primary and increases the detection rate of occult primary tumors not evident on physical examination, EUA/DL, and imaging studies, including CT, MR imaging, and PET/CT, knowing that HPV and p16 positivity are associated with oropharyngeal cancers, whereas EBV positivity is associated with NPCs.[47] When no clear primary is evident after exhaustive investigation using these tools, many investigators advocate ipsilateral or bilateral tonsillectomy as the next step because the palatine tonsil is the most common site to harbor an occult primary, followed by the base of tongue.[40,45,48] In multiple studies, the rate of detection of a tonsillar primary after tonsillectomy ranged from 26% to 39%.[49–54] In some cases, the tonsillar primary was contralateral to the metastatic node.[49] In one study of 23 cases, only 13% of tonsillar biopsies were positive for carcinoma, whereas tonsillectomy yielded a diagnosis of cancer in 39% of cases.[52] These investigators concluded that routine bilateral tonsillectomy (not tonsil biopsy) should be performed as part of the work-up for patients with an unknown primary. In recent years, transoral robotic surgery–assisted endoscopy/ tongue base mucosectomy has been described to improve diagnostic yield.[48,55]

In terms of imaging investigation, one series found that more patients had suspicious findings on CT and/or MR imaging than on physical examination, and CT more often revealed suspicious findings compared with MR imaging.[40] On CT, radiologists should carefully scrutinize for any subtle asymmetry in size, contour, and internal density/ enhancement pattern within the palatine tonsils and along the base of tongue. Additional areas to examine include the nasopharynx (particularly among the endemic population), circumferentially around the oropharynx (particularly if the pathologic neck node is cystic, raising the suspicion for an HPV and primary tumor), the hypopharynx, as well as the larynx. The location of the pathologic

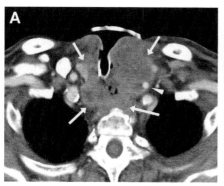
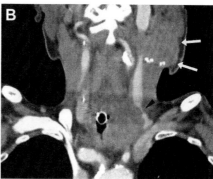

Fig. 25. A 72-year-old man with T4b transglottic tumor. Axial and coronal contrast-enhanced CT images show extensive bulky necrotic mass invading the esophagus, thyroid gland, trachea, prevertebral soft tissues, and mediastinum (*arrows* in *A*). It surrounds the left common carotid artery (*arrowhead* in *A*), invades the left internal jugular vein (*black arrowhead* in *B*), and there is necrotic nodal mass with extracapsular extension in the left upper neck to midneck (*white arrows* in *B*).

nodes and knowledge of any biomarker positivity in the FNA nodal sample is useful for guiding the search pattern as well. When there are bilateral nodal metastases, the more likely candidates are the nasopharynx, base of tongue, hypopharynx, and other midline areas.[45] MR imaging offers excellent soft tissue contrast delineation but is best used in detecting a small occult primary if there is a specific area prescribed for focused interrogation, such that the imaging protocol can be tailored for small-field-of-view, high-resolution imaging of that particular area using thin imaging slices. An MR imaging examination using a generic neck protocol leads to thick imaging slices and generally more technique and motion artifact

compared with a neck CT of comparable craniocaudal excursion, and is therefore less desirable than a neck CT or a targeted (eg, oropharynx, nasopharynx, base of skull) MR imaging.

Not only can the CT or MR imaging help to identify a potentially occult primary, it can also provide comprehensive assessment of cervical nodal disease. As with N staging for other head and neck malignancies, the size, laterality, and number of nodes are important to note.[3] Features suspicious for nodal involvement include enlarged size, round contour with loss of fatty hilum, and heterogeneous density suggestive of cystic or

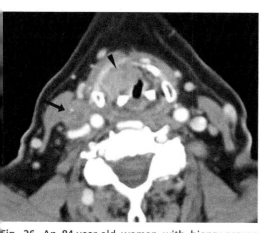

Fig. 26. An 84-year-old woman with biopsy-proven right supraglottic and glottic tumor with ipsilateral metastatic level III node. Axial contrast-enhanced CT images show the primary tumor effacing the right supraglottic paraglottic fat (*arrowhead*), and a right level III node that is round, lacks a fatty hilum, and has necrotic components (*arrow*).

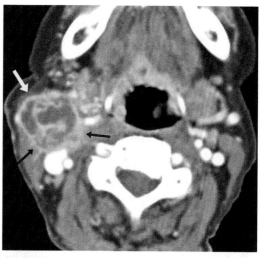

Fig. 27. A 77-year-old woman with supraglottic cancer and bilateral metastatic nodes. Axial contrast-enhanced CT image shows a large necrotic right level II node with ill-defined irregular margins suggestive of ENE of tumor. Note infiltrative appearance at the rim bordering on adjacent fat (*white arrow*) and musculature (*black arrows*).

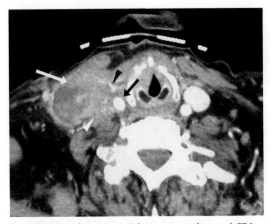

Fig. 28. ENE of tumor. Axial contrast-enhanced CT image shows a right level III/IV nodal mass with necrotic components and ill-defined infiltrative border, inseparable from the sternocleidomastoid muscle (*white arrow*) and scalene muscle (*white arrowhead*), and infiltrating the fat around the carotid sheath (*black arrow*). The internal jugular vein is compressed (*black arrowhead*).

necrotic components. In addition, findings that indicate ENE, such as indistinct nodal margins, irregular nodal capsular enhancement, and infiltration of the surrounding fat or soft tissue structures, are particularly ominous, and alter the clinical N stage up to N3b (**Figs. 28** and **29**).[3]

Although PET/CT is able to image the whole body and detect areas of hypermetabolic activity, and may increase sensitivity and specificity compared with cross-sectional imaging alone, there are risks of false-negatives in small nodes or cystic/necrotic nodes, and false-positives in reactive nodes, and it must be interpreted with

caution. For investigation of a primary site, PET/CT has shown a high false-positive rate in the base of tongue and tonsils in multiple studies,[40,56,57] and these are also the most likely locations of the occult primary. The reliability of PET/CT can be improved when the attenuation-correction non-contrast CT is followed by contrast-enhanced diagnostic CT, and the two are interpreted in conjunction.

REFERENCES

1. Som PM, Curtin HD. Head and neck imaging. St Louis (MO): Elsevier Mosby; 2011.
2. Tsao SW, Yip YL, Tsang CM, et al. Etiological factors of nasopharyngeal carcinoma. Oral Oncol 2014;50: 330–8.
3. Amin MB, Greene FL, Edge SB, et al. The Eighth Edition AJCC Cancer Staging Manual: Continuing to build a bridge from a population-based to a more "personalized" approach to cancer staging. CA Cancer J Clin 2017;67:93–9.
4. Landry D, Glastonbury CM. Squamous cell carcinoma of the upper aerodigestive tract: a review. Radiol Clin North Am 2015;53:81–97.
5. Arya S, Chaukar D, Pai P. Imaging in oral cancers. Indian J Radiol Imaging 2012;22:195–208.
6. Chi AC, Day TA, Neville BW. Oral cavity and oropharyngeal squamous cell carcinoma–an update. CA Cancer J Clin 2015;65:401–21.
7. Shah JP, Gil Z. Current concepts in management of oral cancer–surgery. Oral Oncol 2009;45:394–401.
8. Madana J, Laliberté F, Morand GB, et al. Computerized tomography based tumor-thickness measurement is useful to predict postoperative pathological tumor thickness in oral tongue squamous cell carcinoma. J Otolaryngol Head Neck Surg 2015;44:49.
9. Curtin HD. Detection of perineural spread: fat is a friend. AJNR Am J Neuroradiol 1998;19:1385–6.
10. Park JO, Jung SL, Joo YH, et al. Diagnostic accuracy of magnetic resonance imaging (MRI) in the assessment of tumor invasion depth in oral/oropharyngeal cancer. Oral Oncol 2011;47:381–6.
11. Goel V, Parihar PS, Parihar A, et al. Accuracy of MRI in prediction of tumour thickness and nodal stage in oral tongue and gingivobuccal cancer with clinical correlation and staging. J Clin Diagn Res 2016;10: TC01–05.
12. Lam P, Au-Yeung KM, Cheng PW, et al. Correlating MRI and histologic tumor thickness in the assessment of oral tongue cancer. AJR Am J Roentgenol 2004;182:803–8.
13. Preda L, Chiesa F, Calabrese L, et al. Relationship between histologic thickness of tongue carcinoma and thickness estimated from preoperative MRI. Eur Radiol 2006;16:2242–8.

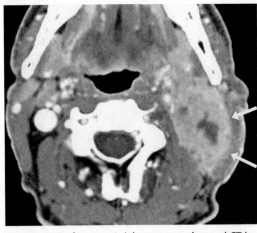

Fig. 29. ENE of tumor. Axial contrast-enhanced CT image shows a large left level II node with necrotic components and ill-defined margins infiltrating the sternocleidomastoid muscle (*arrows*).

14. Alsaffar HA, Goldstein DP, King EV, et al. Correlation between clinical and MRI assessment of depth of invasion in oral tongue squamous cell carcinoma. J Otolaryngol Head Neck Surg 2016;45:61.

15. Rao LP, Shukla M, Sharma V, et al. Mandibular conservation in oral cancer. Surg Oncol 2012;21:109–18.

16. Chen YL, Kuo SW, Fang KH, et al. Prognostic impact of marginal mandibulectomy in the presence of superficial bone invasion and the nononcologic outcome. Head Neck 2011;33:708–13.

17. Brown JS, Lewis-Jones H. Evidence for imaging the mandible in the management of oral squamous cell carcinoma: a review. Br J Oral Maxillofac Surg 2001; 39:411–8.

18. Hakim SG, Wieker H, Trenkle T, et al. Imaging of mandible invasion by oral squamous cell carcinoma using computed tomography, cone-beam computed tomography and bone scintigraphy with SPECT. Clin Oral Investig 2014;18:961–7.

19. Varsha BK, Radhika MB, Makarla S, et al. Perineural invasion in oral squamous cell carcinoma: Case series and review of literature. J Oral Maxillofac Pathol 2015;19:335–41.

20. Moonis G, Cunnane MB, Emerick K, et al. Patterns of perineural tumor spread in head and neck cancer. Magn Reson Imaging Clin North Am 2012;20: 435–46.

21. Trotta BM, Pease CS, Rasamny JJ, et al. Oral cavity and oropharyngeal squamous cell cancer: key imaging findings for staging and treatment planning. Radiographics 2011;31:339–54.

22. Lydiatt WM, Patel SG, O'Sullivan B, et al. Head and neck cancers–major changes in the American Joint Committee on Cancer Eighth Edition Cancer Staging Manual. CA Cancer J Clin 2017;67:122–37.

23. Kimura Y, Sumi M, Sakihama N, et al. MR imaging criteria for the prediction of extranodal spread of metastatic cancer in the neck. AJNR Am J Neuroradiol 2008;29:1355–9.

24. King AD, Tse GM, Yuen EH, et al. Comparison of CT and MR imaging for the detection of extranodal neoplastic spread in metastatic neck nodes. Eur J Radiol 2004;52:264–70.

25. Daisne JF, Duprez T, Weynand B, et al. Tumor volume in pharyngolaryngeal squamous cell carcinoma: comparison at CT, MR imaging, and FDG PET and validation with surgical specimen. Radiology 2004;233:93–100.

26. Koopmann M, Weiss D, Steiger M, et al. Thyroid cartilage invasion in laryngeal and hypopharyngeal squamous cell carcinoma treated with total laryngectomy. Eur Arch Otorhinolaryngol 2016;273: 3789–94.

27. Becker M, Zbären P, Delavelle J, et al. Neoplastic invasion of the laryngeal cartilage: reassessment of criteria for diagnosis at CT. Radiology 1997;203: 521–32.

28. Dadfar N, Seyyedi M, Forghani R, et al. Computed tomography appearance of normal nonossified thyroid cartilage: implication for tumor invasion diagnosis. J Comput Assist Tomogr 2015;39:240–3.

29. Zan E, Yousem DM, Aygun N. Asymmetric mineralization of the arytenoid cartilages in patients without laryngeal cancer. AJNR Am J Neuroradiol 2011;32: 1113–8.

30. Castelijns JA, Gerritsen GJ, Kaiser MC, et al. Invasion of laryngeal cartilage by cancer: comparison of CT and MR imaging. Radiology 1988;167: 199–206.

31. Zbaren P, Becker M, Lang H. Staging of laryngeal cancer: endoscopy, computed tomography and magnetic resonance versus histopathology. Eur Arch Otorhinolaryngol 1997;254(Suppl 1):S117–22.

32. Allegra E, Ferrise P, Trapasso S, et al. Early glottic cancer: role of MRI in the preoperative staging. Biomed Res Int 2014;2014:890385.

33. Wu JH, Zhao J, Li ZH, et al. Comparison of CT and MRI in diagnosis of laryngeal carcinoma with anterior vocal commissure involvement. Sci Rep 2016; 6:30353.

34. Kuno H, Onaya H, Fujii S, et al. Primary staging of laryngeal and hypopharyngeal cancer: CT, MR imaging and dual-energy CT. Eur J Radiol 2014;83: e23–35.

35. Imre A, Pinar E, Erdoğan N, et al. Prevertebral space invasion in head and neck cancer: negative predictive value of imaging techniques. Ann Otol Rhinol Laryngol 2015;124:378–83.

36. Tibbetts KM, Tan M. Role of advanced laryngeal imaging in glottic cancer: early detection and evaluation of glottic neoplasms. Otolaryngol Clin North Am 2015;48:565–84.

37. Rodel RM, Matthias C, Blomeyer BD, et al. Impact of distant metastasis in patients with cervical lymph node metastases from cancer of an unknown primary site. Ann Otol Rhinol Laryngol 2009;118:662–9.

38. Grau C, Johansen LV, Jakobsen J, et al. Cervical lymph node metastases from unknown primary tumours. Results from a national survey by the Danish Society for Head and Neck Oncology. Radiother Oncol 2000;55:121–9.

39. Pavlidis N, Pentheroudakis G. Cancer of unknown primary site. Lancet 2012;379:1428–35.

40. Cianchetti M, Mancuso AA, Amdur RJ, et al. Diagnostic evaluation of squamous cell carcinoma metastatic to cervical lymph nodes from an unknown head and neck primary site. Laryngoscope 2009; 119:2348–54.

41. Al Kadah B, Papaspyrou G, Linxweiler M, et al. Cancer of unknown primary (CUP) of the head and neck: retrospective analysis of 81 patients. Eur Arch Otorhinolaryngol 2017. http://dx.doi.org/10.1007/s00405-017-4525-8.

42. Galer CE, Kies MS. Evaluation and management of the unknown primary carcinoma of the head and neck. J Natl Compr Cancer Netw 2008;6:1068–75.

43. Koivunen P, Laranne J, Virtaniemi J, et al. Cervical metastasis of unknown origin: a series of 72 patients. Acta Otolaryngol 2002;122:569–74.

44. Strojan P, Ferlito A, Langendijk JA, et al. Contemporary management of lymph node metastases from an unknown primary to the neck: II. a review of therapeutic options. Head Neck 2013;35:286–93.

45. Arosio AD, Pignataro L, Gaini RM, et al. Neck lymph node metastases from unknown primary. Cancer Treat Rev 2017;53:1–9.

46. Martin HE, Morfit HM. Cervical lymph node metastasis as the first symptom of cancer. Surg Gynecol Obstet 1944;78:133–59.

47. Cheol Park G, Roh JL, Cho KJ, et al. 18 F-FDG PET/CT vs. human papillomavirus, p16 and Epstein-Barr virus detection in cervical metastatic lymph nodes for identifying primary tumors. Int J Cancer 2017;140:1405–12.

48. Hatten KM, O'Malley BW Jr, Bur AM, et al. Transoral robotic surgery-assisted endoscopy with primary site detection and treatment in occult mucosal primaries. JAMA Otolaryngol Head Neck Surg 2017;143:267–73.

49. Koch WM, Bhatti N, Williams MF, et al. Oncologic rationale for bilateral tonsillectomy in head and neck squamous cell carcinoma of unknown primary source. Otolaryngol Head Neck Surg 2001;124:331–3.

50. Kothari P, Randhawa PS, Farrell R. Role of tonsillectomy in the search for a squamous cell carcinoma from an unknown primary in the head and neck. Br J Oral Maxillofac Surg 2008;46:283–7.

51. Lapeyre M, Malissard L, Peiffert D, et al. Cervical lymph node metastasis from an unknown primary: is a tonsillectomy necessary? Int J Radiat Oncol Biol Phys 1997;39:291–6.

52. McQuone SJ, Eisele DW, Lee DJ, et al. Occult tonsillar carcinoma in the unknown primary. Laryngoscope 1998;108:1605–10.

53. Randall DA, Johnstone PA, Foss RD, et al. Tonsillectomy in diagnosis of the unknown primary tumor of the head and neck. Otolaryngol Head Neck Surg 2000;122:52–5.

54. Righi PD, Sofferman RA. Screening unilateral tonsillectomy in the unknown primary. Laryngoscope 1995;105:548–50.

55. Winter SC, Ofo E, Meikle D, et al. Trans-oral robotic assisted tongue base mucosectomy for investigation of cancer of unknown primary in the head and neck region. the UK experience. Clin Otolaryngol 2017. http://dx.doi.org/10.1111/coa.12860.

56. Dong MJ, Zhao K, Lin XT, et al. Role of fluorodeoxyglucose-PET versus fluorodeoxyglucose-PET/computed tomography in detection of unknown primary tumor: a meta-analysis of the literature. Nucl Med Commun 2008;29:791–802.

57. Rusthoven KE, Koshy M, Paulino AC. The role of fluorodeoxyglucose positron emission tomography in cervical lymph node metastases from an unknown primary tumor. Cancer 2004;101:2641–9.

Practical Tips for MR Imaging of Perineural Tumor Spread

Claudia F.E. Kirsch, MD[a],*, Ilona M. Schmalfuss, MD[b]

KEYWORDS

- Perineural tumor spread • Perineural invasion • Perineural involvement • Adenoid cystic carcinoma
- Trigeminal nerve • Facial nerve • Auriculotemporal nerve • Greater superficial petrosal nerve
- MR imaging

KEY POINTS

- Any cranial nerve can be affected by perineural tumor spread even in asymptomatic patients.
- Perineural tumor spread may not be continuous on imaging and can occur in antegrade or retrograde direction, requiring the radiologist to map the entire nerve from its origin to all distal branches.
- Radiologists need to be aware of preexisting connections between different nerves to appropriately map the extent of perineural tumor spread.

INTRODUCTION

More than 500,000 new head and neck cancers are diagnosed worldwide annually, accounting for approximately 300,000 deaths annually.[1] Major prognostic factors of head and neck cancer include locoregional metastases, lymphatic or vascular invasion, positive surgical margins, extracapsular metastatic lymphadenopathy, and perineural invasion (PNI) or perineural tumor spread (PNS).[2–8]

Perineural involvement by head and neck cancer was first noted in the literature in the 1800s.[9,10] However, it was not until 1963 that clinicians began to realize that this occurred more often than previously thought. They noted that there was a relation between clinical symptoms and tumor recurrence.[11] Currently, PNI is defined as tumor cells within any of the 3 layers of the nerve sheath (epineurium, perineurium, and endoneurium) or tumor cells surrounding at least 33% of the nerve.[5,6,8,12,13] PNI is inconsistently visualized

radiographically. In contrast, PNS, defined as dissemination of the main tumor along the cranial nerve (CN), is often radiographically detectable, even before patients become symptomatic.[4] Although it is mandated by the United Kingdom's Royal College of Pathologists[14] and the American College of Pathologists to report the histopathological presence or absence of PNI or PNS for head and neck malignancies,[15] there is no universally accepted definition.[16] Lack of a universal standard means that the reported histopathologic detection rates of PNI and PNS may vary depending on the specimen, immunohistochemistry staining, relation to resection margins, and pathologist's expertise.[17]

The importance of determining PNI and PNS cannot be understated because the extent of PNS and its relation to the tumor margin correlates with decreased disease-free survival, regardless of the type or size of the involved nerve.[6] The mechanism allowing cancer to spread along nerves remains unknown. Recent research of

Disclosures: C.F.E. Kirsch is a consultant for Primal Pictures 3D Anatomy, Informa; RTOG, grant 3504. I.M. Schmalfuss has nothing to disclose.
a Division of Neuroradiology Imaging Service Line, Department of Radiology, Northwell Health, Donald and Barbara Zucker School of Medicine at Hofstra/Northwell, 300 Community Drive, Manhasset, NY 11030, USA;
b Department of Radiology, University of Florida, Veterans Administration Medical Center, 1601 Southwest Archer Road, Gainesville, FL 32608, USA
* Corresponding author.
E-mail address: ckirsch@northwell.edu

cutaneous squamous cell cancers, revealed differentially expressed genes between tumors with PNI versus tumors without PNI.[12,13] However, why certain tumors, such as adenoid cystic carcinoma (ACC), have a propensity for PNI or PNS remains unknown. Because PNI and PNS cannot be differentiated on imaging, the term PNS will be used for both types of neural involvement in the subsequent sections of this article.

ACC of the minor or major salivary glands is the tumor most likely to develop PNS, with a prevalence of up to 56%. However, because ACC is a rare tumor, representing 1% to 3% of all head and neck cancers, it accounts only for a small number of patients reported with PNS.[18,19] The highest number of PNS is diagnosed in patients with squamous cell carcinoma because it is the most common head and neck cancer even though it has lower propensity for neural involvement than ACC with reported incidence of 2% to 34%.[19–22] Additional tumors that may develop PNS include mucoepidermoid and basal cell carcinomas, as well as desmoplastic melanomas, sarcomas, and lymphomas.[23,24]

Because PNS is associated with increased risk of tumor recurrence and higher morbidity and mortality, accurate radiographic determination of PNS is imperative for early initiation of appropriate treatment.[24,25] Delineation of PNS requires detailed knowledge of the neural anatomic pathways that the primary tumor may take and of pertinent juxtaforaminal fat planes that may be effaced. The trigeminal nerve (CN V) and facial nerve (CN VII) are most commonly involved by PNS with the highest prevalence seen along the maxillary division of CN V.[25–27] Although CN V and CN VII are frequently affected by PNS, the radiologist must be aware that any CN and/or preexisting connections between different nerves may be involved by PNS, leading to variable pathways of neuronal involvement.[26,27]

This article provides practical tips for perineural spread using MR imaging and, for the sake of ease of understanding, focuses on 6 major Ps: CN Pathways, fat Pads, CN V and CN VII Points of connection, and MR imaging Protocols with radiographic Pathologic assessment and Pearls for diagnosing PNS.

NORMAL ANATOMY AND IMAGING TECHNIQUES

As previously mentioned, CN V and CN VII are the 2 nerves most commonly affected by PNS. To adequately map PNS, the radiologist must be familiar with the course of each nerve from the brainstem to its distal innervation, juxtaforaminal fat pads and connecting points between CN V and CN VII that may allow tumor to spread between these 2 nerves (**Figs. 1 and 2**).[25,28]

Trigeminal Nerve

The trigeminal nerve, CN V, provides sensory innervation for touch, pain and temperature of the skin and/or mucous membranes of the face, scalp, intracranial dura, orbit, sinonasal region, oral cavity, teeth, and palate via the paired ophthalmic (V1), maxillary (V2) and mandibular

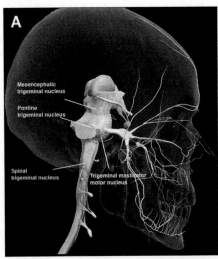
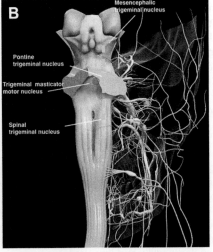

Fig. 1. CN V (*A, B*): Sensory nuclei (*dashed green line*). The mesencephalic nucleus for proprioceptive fibers from muscles of mastication is in the midbrain. The dominant pontine trigeminal nucleus for facial pressure and touch is anterolateral to the fourth ventricle in the pons, the spinal trigeminal nucleus is located inferiorly in medulla to and extends inferiorly to approximately the C2 cervical vertebral level for deep touch, pain, and pain temperature.

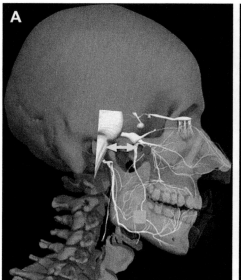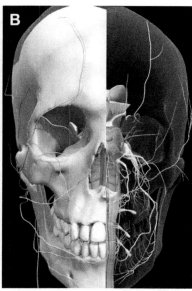

Fig. 2. The key interconnections between CN V and CN VII (*A*): Aqua blue double sided arrow is in the region of the auriculotemporal nerve between the neck of the mandible and sphenomandibular ligament. The auriculo-temporal nerve arises as 2 roots from V3 that encircle the middle meningeal artery and connect with CN VII branches in the parotid gland. The red dot marks the pterygopalatine ganglion where V2 and vidian nerve meet. Brown square represents the submandibular ganglion extending inferiorly from V3 lingual nerve to receive branches from CN VII chorda tympani nerve. (*B*) Distal fibers of CN VII zygomatic branches are in continuity with distal V1 sensory branches.

(V3) divisions.[29] In addition, V3 carries motor fibers to the muscles of mastication (masseter, temporalis, and pterygoid muscles) and to the tensor veli palatini, tensor tympani, mylohyoid, and anterior belly of the digastric muscles.[30–32]

V1 is the smallest branch formed by coalescence of the frontal, lacrimal, nasociliary, and dural branches. The nerve courses in the orbital roof fat pad located superior to the levator palpebrae superioris and superior rectus muscles with the frontal branch extending superiorly within the forehead fat pad (**Fig. 3**). The V1 nerve exits posteriorly from the orbit via the superior orbital fissure into the lateral cavernous sinus wall (see **Fig. 3**).[31–33]

As previously mentioned, V2 is most commonly involved by PNS. Its infraorbital nerve branch forms in the preantral fat pad (**Figs. 4** and **5**), and extends posteriorly within the infraorbital canal along the orbital floor, where it merges with the superior alveolar branches. It extends through the retroantral fat pad into the pterygopalatine fossa. The greater and lesser palatine nerves from the soft and hard palate course superiorly within the same named canals to merge with the infraorbital nerve within the pterygopalatine fossa. A small fat pad is identified at the greater palatine canal opening and within the pterygopalatine fossa (**Fig. 6**). V2 continues posteriorly through

the foramen rotundum and subsequently within the lateral wall of the cavernous sinus below V1 (**Fig. 5D–F**).

V3 is the largest division of CN V and contains both sensory and motor components previously mentioned. The inferior alveolar nerve is the largest branch of V3, giving rise to the mental nerve anterior to the mandible. The mental nerve extends through a small fat pad along the mental foramen (**Fig. 7A,B**) into the inferior alveolar canal within the mandible, where it coalesces with inferior dental nerves. The inferior alveolar nerve exits the mandible through the mandibular foramen that also contains a small fat pad (see **Fig. 7C**) to course superiorly through the infratemporal fossa to the skull base. The lingual nerve forms within the floor of the mouth to course posteriorly between the hyoglossus and mylohyoid muscles. It continues superiorly medial to the mandibular ramus to join the inferior alveolar nerve and the motor branches of V3 just below the skull base. V3 traverses the skull base through the foramen ovale and subsequently along the lateral wall of the cavernous sinus below V2 to reach the trigeminal ganglion (see **Fig. 7D**).[32,33]

The sensory fibers of V1, V2, and V3 unite to form the semilunar or trigeminal ganglion located in the inferolateral Meckel cave. CN V extends

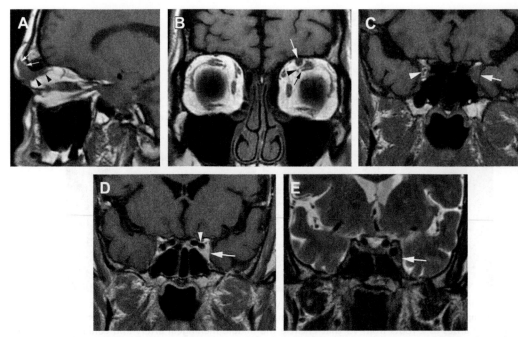

Fig. 3. Sagittal T1 image (*A*) shows obliteration of the left forehead fat pad (*arrows* in A) extending along the anterior orbital roof (*arrowheads* in A), concerning for PNS along V1. The coronal T1 images (*B, C*) confirm PNS reflected as markedly enlarged V1 (*white arrow* in B) superior to the levator palpebrae superioris (*arrowhead* in B) and superior rectus (*black arrow* in B) muscles that manifests posteriorly as near complete obliteration of the fat pad within the orbital apex (*arrow* in C) compared with the normal orbital apex fat pad on the right (*arrowhead* in C). The PNS continues posteriorly to the cavernous sinus with subtle widening and enhancement (*arrow* in D) inferior to the internal carotid artery (*arrowhead* in D) on coronal postcontrast T1 image (*D*), corresponding to a markedly enlarged V1 (*arrow* in E) on the coronal T2 image (*E*).

posteriorly through the Meckel cave as separate rootlets and as a main trunk on each side within the prepontine cistern. CN V enters the lateral pons to reach its 4 nuclei: the 3 sensory nuclei consisting of the principal pontine sensory

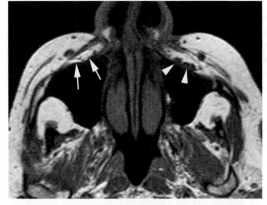

Fig. 4. Axial T1 image demonstrates normal preantral fat pad on the right (*arrows*) and partial obliteration on the left caused by noticeable enlargement of the infraorbital nerve branches (*arrowheads*) within the preantral fat pad.

nucleus, the mesencephalic nucleus, and the spinal trigeminal nucleus; as well as the single motor nucleus (see **Fig. 1**).[31–34]

Facial Nerve

The facial nucleus within the posterior pons gives rise to CN VII. Their fibers drape around the abducens nucleus on each side to form the facial colliculi along the anterior wall of the fourth ventricle. The fibers then travel through the lateral pons to exit at the lateral pontomedullary junction. The nerve courses through the cerebellopontine angle into internal auditory canal to enter the temporal bone and to continue as the labyrinthine segment through the anterior otic capsule, anterior genu and tympanic segment through the middle ear cavity, posterior genu, and mastoid segment within the mastoid portion of the temporal bone. CN VII exits the temporal bone through the stylomastoid foramen that contains a small fat pad (**Fig. 8**) to course through the parotid gland. Within the parotid gland, it gives rise to its peripheral branches: posterior auricular, temporal, zygomatic, buccal, marginal mandibular, and cervical nerves. These split up into numerous little

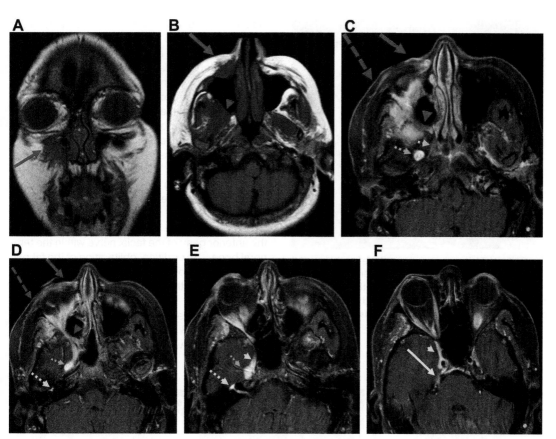

Fig. 5. A 57-year-old woman with progressive CN palsies from lymphoma. Coronal (*A*) and axial (*B*) T1 images, show loss of fat planes in the right preantral region (*red arrows* in *A* and *B*) and in the right pterygopalatine fossa (*red arrowhead* in *B*) on the right. Axial, postcontrast T1 images with fat saturation (*C–F*) reveal enhancing tumor in preantral soft tissues (*red arrow* in *C* and *D*), infratemporal fossa, and masticator space with involvement of the muscles of mastication (*red dashed arrows* in *C* and *D*). Notice the PNS of V2 via infraorbital nerve to pterygopalatine fossa (*red arrowhead* in *C* and *D*), vidian nerve in vidian canal (*yellow dashed arrow* in *C*), V2 in foramen rotundum to cavernous sinus (*green arrowhead* in E-F), and V3 in the foramen ovale (*pink dashed arrow* in *C–E*). There is also extension of PNS from vidian nerve to greater superficial petrosal nerve to right CN VII geniculate ganglion (*light peach dashed arrow* in *D* and *E*) with PNS extension into the intracanalicular segment of CN VII. Notice also the PNS of the cisternal segment of CN V (*light blue arrow* in *F*).

branches to provide motor innervation to muscles of facial expression. In addition, CN VII provides motor innervation to the stylohyoid, stapedius, and posterior belly of the digastric muscles, as well as special sensory and parasympathetic innervation to the glandular tissue in the head and neck.[31,35]

Neuronal Connections Between Cranial Nerves V and VII

The vidian nerve, also referred to as the nerve of the pterygoid canal, is formed by the confluence of the greater superficial petrosal nerve (GSPN), a branch of the facial nerve, and the deep petrosal nerve, a branch of the carotid plexus. The fibers for the GSPN arise from the CN VII lower pontine

superior salivatory nucleus and leave the brain stem as the nervus intermedius with the CN VII motor root and CN VIII to course together through the internal auditory canal. The parasympathetic fibers of the nervus intermedius give rise to the GSPN at the anterior genu of CN VII without synapsing at the CN VII geniculate ganglion. These preganglionic parasympathetic fibers of the GSPN extend under the dura in the sphenopetrosal groove to the anterior aspect of the foramen lacerum. The deep petrosal nerve carries the postganglionic sympathetic fibers of the sympathetic plexus of the internal carotid artery and joins the GSPN at the foramen lacerum to form the vidian nerve. The vidian nerve extends anteriorly within the vidian canal, where it is joined by an ascending sphenoidal branch from the otic ganglion. The

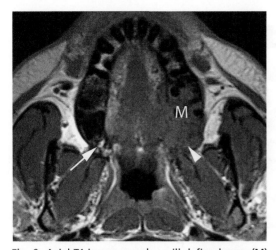

Fig. 6. Axial T1 image reveals an ill-defined mass (M) in the left posterolateral maxilla. On the right, a normal fat pad (*arrow*) is visualized within the greater palatine foramen, whereas this fat pad (*arrowhead*) is obliterated by tumor on the left consistent with PNS.

vidian canal is located inferomedial to foramen rotundum along the floor of the sphenoid sinus. It forms a connection between the foramen lacerum and the pterygopalatine fossa. The vidian nerve synapses in the pterygopalatine ganglion and provides vasoconstrictor and secretomotor postganglionic fibers to the nasal mucosa and lacrimal gland.[31] The pterygopalatine ganglion is an important neuronal connection between V2 within the pterygopalatine fossa and CN VII via the vidian nerve and GSPN. Therefore, PNS along these nerves manifests as enhancement and or enlargement of the vidian nerve within the vidian canal and of the GSPN along the posterolateral wall of the petrous canal of the internal carotid artery to reach the anterior genu of the facial nerve within the temporal bone.[35] In addition, obliteration of the fat pad within the anterior vidian canal is usually observed with PNS along the vidian nerve (see **Figs. 2**A and 5D,E; **Fig. 9**).

The auriculotemporal nerve forms a connection between V3 and CN VII (see **Fig. 2**A). It originates from V3 within the infratemporal fossa to

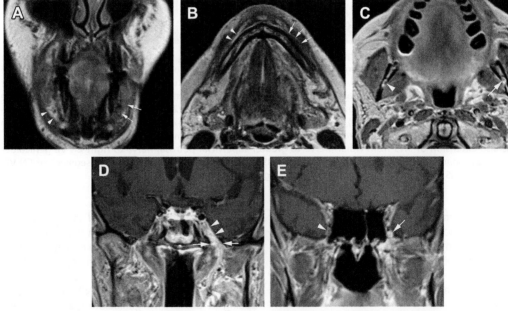

Fig. 7. A 75-year-old man with history of left lower lip cancer underwent MR imaging examination for work-up of left lower face numbness. The coronal T1 (*A*) and axial T2 (*B*) images reveal obliteration of the left fat pad anterior to the mental foramen (*arrows* in A and B) compared with the normal appearance on the right (*arrowheads* in A and B). Axial, postcontrast T1 through the ramus of the mandible (*C*) demonstrates symmetric fat pads and inferior alveolar nerves within the mandibular foramina; however, the left inferior alveolar nerve (*arrow* in C) shows subtle enhancement compared with the normal right side (*arrowhead* in C), concerning for persistent PNS. Coronal, postcontrast T1 images (*D, E*) reveal pronounced PNS at the left foramen ovale manifesting as significant enhancement and enlargement of the left V3 (between *arrows* in D) and involvement of the left cavernous sinus (*arrowheads* in D). Notice the marked enhancement of V2 in the left foramen rotundum (*arrow* in E) compared with the normal right side (*arrowhead* in E), indicating antegrade PNS, illustrating the need to map PNS along each branch of V2.

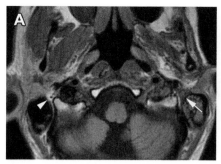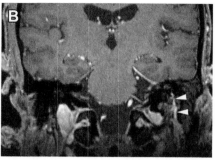

Fig. 8. A 65-year-old man woman status post left parotidectomy for adenoid cystic carcinoma underwent MR imaging for work-up of facial nerve palsy. Axial T1 (*A*) images shows a normal fat pad within the stylomastoid foramen on the right (*arrowhead* in *A*), whereas it is obliterated on the left (*arrow* in *A*) consistent with PNS along the main trunk of CN VII. The coronal, postcontrast 3D isotropic T1 image confirms the PNS manifesting as marked enhancement and thickening of the descending segment of the left CN VII (*arrowheads* in *B*).

course laterally around the middle meningeal artery just below the foramen spinosum and continues laterally posterior to the ramus of the mandible to reach CN VII within the parotid gland (**Figs. 10** and **11**). The auriculotemporal nerve supplies the temporomandibular joint and usually presents with temporomandibular joint dysfunction when affected by a pathologic condition.[36,37]

Additional connections between CN V and CN VII include (see **Fig. 2**)

- The lacrimal nerve, a V1 branch arising from the supraorbital nerve, connects with the zygomatic branch of V2 and the temporal branches of CN VII
- The mental nerve, a V3 branch, connects with the marginal mandibular branch of CN VII
- The buccinator nerve, a V3 branch, connects with the zygomatic, buccal, and/or marginal mandibular branches of CN VII

- The cutaneous connections of the distal zygomatic branches of CN VII connect with the distal sensory branches of V1.[36–38]

Additional studies have reported on PNS along other CNs, the scope of which is beyond this article. Radiologists, however, need to keep in mind that any CN with Schwann cells, including CN III, IV, VI, and VIII to XII, in the region of a primary tumor has the capacity to be a conduit in which PNS may occur.[39–41]

Imaging Techniques

MR imaging is considered the study of first choice in work-up of patients with risk for PNS with scanners of 1.5 or 3 T being preferred. The imaging volume should span the entire course of the nerve at risk and include the nerve nuclei in the brainstem, the main nerve branches, and all distal branches because these represent blind spots

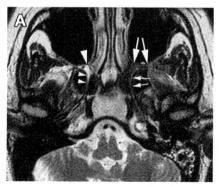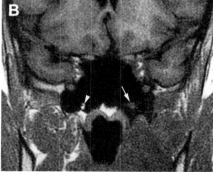

Fig. 9. Axial T2 (*A*) and coronal T1 (*B*) images show a normal fat pad in the anterior vidian canal on the right (*small arrowheads*). This fat pad is infiltrated by tumor on the left (*small arrows*) consistent with PNS along the vidian nerve. Notice the associated obliteration of the fat pad within the left pterygopalatine fossa (*large arrows*) compared with its normal appearance on the right (*large arrowhead*).

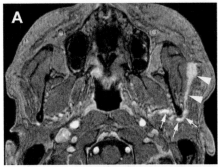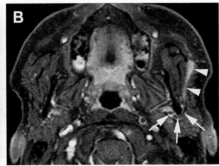

Fig. 10. Axial, postcontrast 3D isotropic T1 image (*A*) reveals marked, linear enhancement along the lateral masseter muscle (*arrowheads*) draping around the ramus of the mandible (*small arrows*). The appearance is concerning for PNS along the buccal branch of CN V (*arrowheads*) and the auriculotemporal nerve (*small arrows*). The axial, postcontrast T1 image with fat suppression (*B*) confirms PNS involvement along the buccal branch (*arrowheads*) with a flow void in the retromandibular region (*large arrows*), illustrating how asymmetric venous structures may mimic PNS, requiring correlation to all available sequences to avoid such a mistake.

for radiologist, in particular at the skin and subcutaneous levels (see **Fig. 10**; **Fig. 12**).[42,43] Demonstration of PNS along large nerve branches may require only 1.5 T; however, 3T has been shown to be superior in evaluation of PNS along smaller nerve branches within the preauricular, periparotid, parotid, and temporal regions (see **Fig. 12**).[44,45] In addition, 3-T MR imaging has the advantage of shorter scan times, resulting in less motion; however, it is prone to susceptibility artifacts from air tissue interface, such as in patients with marked pneumatization of the skull base. In these situations, 1.5 T may be preferable to evaluate for PNS.[46]

Although there are scanner and institutional preferences on how to work up a patient at risk for PNS, certain general imaging techniques need to be considered:

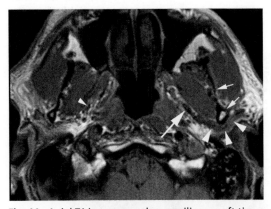

Fig. 11. Axial T1 image reveals a curvilinear soft tissue lesion (*large arrowheads*) draping posterior to the ramus of the mandible (*small arrows*) and extending to an enlarged V3 (*large arrow*) compared with the normal size on the right (*small arrowhead*), consistent with PNS along the auriculotemporal nerve and V3.

Slice thickness and field of view

To best demonstrate the small CNs, high-resolution imaging is required with thin sections and a small field of view. The image slice thickness should be less than or equal to 3 mm with many radiologists routinely using 3-dimensional (D) isotropic sequences for workup of patients at risk for PNS. 3D isotropic imaging allows reformations in standard planes (axial, coronal, and sagittal) and along the course of an affected nerve, which might increase a radiologist's confidence in mapping the extent of PNS (see **Figs. 8B and 10A**). The main disadvantage of 3D isotropic imaging is the longer acquisition time compared with standard imaging, which might lead to motion degradation and potentially nondiagnostic images in some patients. Therefore, a combination of standard and 3D isotropic imaging is the most optimal. A field of view of less than or equal to 16 cm is often applied; however, in some patients, a more targeted view to the area of concern using smaller field of view might be necessary to increase the sensitivity to delineate the PNS, such as in patients with involvement of peripheral branches of the facial nerve.[40,44–47]

Sequences

The noncontrast T1 sequence, typically acquired in the axial and coronal planes, is among the most important sequences in the workup of patients with potential PNS. It best delineates the normal hyperintense appearance of the juxtaarticular fat pads from the lower signal intensity of PNS (see **Fig. 3A–C, 4, 5A, 6, 7A, 8A, and 9**). Therefore, it is particularly important in evaluation of the extracranial segments of CNs.[40,46–48]

The T2 sequences are superior in detection of edema and, therefore, helpful in diagnosing acute denervation of muscles supplied by the affected nerve (**Fig. 13**). This is particularly

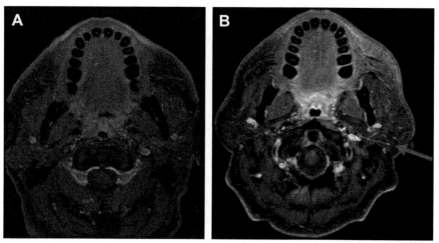

Fig. 12. A 53-year-old man with history of left preauricular squamous cell carcinoma presents with difficulty of blinking the left eye. (A) Axial, postcontrast T1 images with fat suppression performed on a 1.5-T MR imaging scanner shows a normal left parotid gland. Immediately after completion of the study, the patient underwent additional scanning (B) on a 3-T MR imaging scanner that revealed a thin, linear horizontal Y-shaped enhancement in left parotid gland (red arrow) with surgery and histopathology confirming PNS along extracranial intraparotid branches of CN VII.

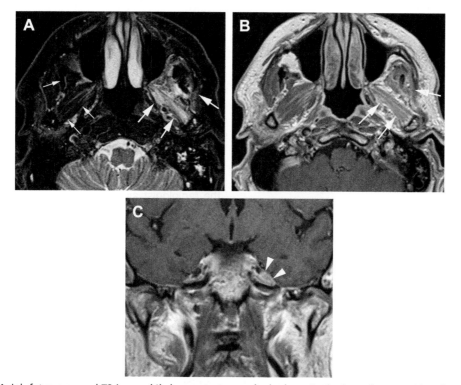

Fig. 13. Axial, fat-suppressed T2 image (A) demonstrates marked edema in the lateral pterygoid and temporalis (large arrows) muscles on the left compared with normal signal on the right (small arrows). This is associated with marked enhancement (arrows in B) on the axial, postcontrast T1 image (B). Such findings are consistent with acute denervation atrophy of the muscle of mastication concerning for PNS along V3. The coronal, postcontrast T1 image (C) confirms this finding because the left Meckel cave is partially obliterated by tumor (arrowheads).

true when combined with a fat suppression technique. In addition, T2-weighted images better delineate vascular flow voids that occasionally lead to enlarged neural foramina and mimic PNS.

Fat suppression techniques are typically used in combination with T2 and postcontrast T1 imaging. These have the advantages to suppress the bright signal of fat and enhance the visibility of edema and enhancement, respectively (see **Fig. 13**). However, they may be compromised by inadequate fat suppression that often occurs in areas of air bone interface. In addition, dental filling artifacts or other metallic implants cause more profound artifacts on the fat-suppressed images than on standard T1 and T2 images.[40,46–49] Such areas of inadequate fat suppression may mimic areas of enhancement, leading to the incorrect diagnosis of PNS. Therefore, it is always recommended to correlate the findings on fat-suppressed images with the other obtained sequences. Postcontrast T1-weighted scans without fat suppression are less likely to be degraded by artifacts; however, the differentiation between affected nerve and the adjacent fat is often difficult because the PNS enhances and assumes only slightly greyer appearance relative to the adjacent bright fat.[48]

MR neurography uses special sequences, such as 3D double-echo steady-state with water excitation to enhance the nerve conspicuity.[45] It has shown to have high sensitivity for detection of neuronal pathologic condition, including PNS with reported sensitivities of 95% to 100%.[49–51] Utilization of dedicated MR imaging techniques and a heightened awareness to look for PNS along the entire nerve is required to prevent missing this critical finding.[40,52]

Gadolinium administration
Gadolinium-enhanced T1-weighted images should be performed in all patients unless the risk of contrast administration outweighs the benefits. Contrast administration is particularly important for mapping of intracranial involvement because PNS might manifest as enhancement-only without nerve enlargement (see **Fig. 7C,E**).

Imaging planes
The imaging planes selected depend on the nerve at risk. Axial and coronal planes are usually used for imaging of CN V and CN VII, the most commonly involved CNs by PNS. In the coronal plane, it is easier to assess V3, foramen ovale and rotundum, Meckel cave, greater and lesser palatine nerves, trigeminal nerve main trunk, and

the infraorbital nerve (see **Fig. 7D-E and 13C**). The axial plane best demonstrates the fat pad in the preantral and retroantral region, as well as within the pterygopalatine fossa, orbital apex, and mandibular foramen (see **Figs. 4, 5B,** and **7C**). In addition, it lays out V2 within the foramen rotundum and the vidian canal (see **Fig. 5D–F** and **9A**). The need for selection of an imaging plane is obviated when 3D imaging techniques are used.[40]

IMAGING PROTOCOLS

Examples of imaging protocols for the workup of patients with PNS along the CN V and CN VII are provided in **Tables 1** and **2**.

IMAGING FINDINGS AND PATHOLOGIC ASSESSMENT

A spectrum of imaging findings can indicate the presence of PNS.

Enlargement and/or Enhancement of a Nerve

PNS typically manifests as enhancement of the involved nerve. Often this is associated with enlargement of the affected nerve (see **Fig. 3B-E, 5C–F, 7D–E, 8B,** and **10**); however, sometimes, the nerve remains normal in size (see **Fig. 7C**), making it harder for the radiologist to detect PNS.

Enlargement and/or Erosion of Neural Foramina or Canals

Enlargement of the nerve affected by PNS may lead to expansion of the neural foramen or canal that it passes through. This is typically noticed by the radiologist as asymmetry from side to side. Such foraminal enlargement is nonspecific and might be related to benign disease processes or anatomic variation. Additional erosions of the foramen and/or canal are greater indicators of a malignant etiologic factors such as PNS.

Obliteration of Fat Planes

Fat planes are considered a radiologist's friend in head and neck imaging.[46,48] They occur along the course of different nerves. When obliterated, fat planes provide an important clue to the presence of a pathologic condition along a nerve.[48] The different fat planes pertinent to CN V and VII were previously discussed in the anatomy section and are summarized in **Table 3**.

Thickening and/or Enhancement of the Superior Muscular Aponeurotic System

Most CN VII peripheral branches spread throughout the face along the superior muscular aponeurotic system (SMAS). Therefore, it is not surprising that PNS along peripheral branches of CN VII manifests as thickening and/or enhancement of the SMAS on cross-sectional imaging (see **Fig. 10**). Thickening of SMAS is often overlooked and has been reported as among the radiologist's blind spots.[42,43] Only careful, direct comparison from side to side on each image might help the radiologist detect early PNS along a peripheral branch of CN V or CN VII.[44,54,55]

Muscular Denervation

PNS can lead to denervation of the muscles supplied by the involved nerve. In the acute phase, this manifests as edema and marked enhancement that is easiest visualized on fat-suppressed T2 and postcontrast, fat-suppressed T1-weighted images, respectively (see **Fig. 13**).[25] In the chronic phase, the denervated muscles atrophy and undergo fatty replacement, which is best seen on T1-weighted and T2-weighted images without fat suppression. In fact, the radiologist might miss the fatty muscular replacement if fat suppression techniques are applied.

DIAGNOSTIC CRITERIA

Almost all of the previously listed imaging findings are not specific for PNS and may be related to other disease entities (see later discussion of differential diagnosis). In most patients, these imaging findings provide an important hint for some type of pathologic condition, often in combination with patient's history and clinical symptoms, that leads to the correct diagnosis. Erosions of a neural foramen and/or canal are more specific for a malignant process such as PNS; however, they can be difficult to detect with MR imaging in the early stages.

DIFFERENTIAL DIAGNOSIS

Benign nerve tumors and neuritis are the 2 major differential diagnostic considerations to PNS. Benign nerve tumors, such as schwannomas or neurofibromas, can affect any portion of the nerve. They are rare in patients without neurofibromatosis and usually manifest as bulky enlargement of the involved nerve segment at the time of symptoms. In contrast, neuritis usually manifests as marked enhancement of portion or of the entire nerve without significant enlargement of the nerve. Neuritis can have various infectious causes, such as different viruses; Lyme disease; and, more rarely, poliomyelitis or syphilis, accounting for most cases.[56] Occasionally, neuritis is caused by trauma, postradiation changes, or autoimmune disorders such as sarcoidosis and amyloidosis.[57]

In many patients, correlation to clinical history and examination leads to the correct diagnosis. However, in cases in which it may be difficult to resolve the nature of the disease, repeat short-term follow-up imaging is often helpful: neuritis usually improves, whereas PNS tends to progress and benign neural tumors remain stable in appearance.

PEARLS, PITFALLS, AND VARIANTS

When interpreting MR imaging studies of patients at risk for PNS, comparison to the contralateral, unaffected side can serve as a control for easier detection of obliterated fat planes, presence of enhancement, thickening of SMAS, or enlargement of neural foramina or canals. However, the radiologist must be aware of possible anatomic variations that can lead to asymmetric appearance of these structures that include the following.

Physiologic Enhancement of Facial Nerve

The facial nerve typically shows physiologic enhancement, with the geniculate ganglion (97%) and the tympanic segment (88%) being most commonly involved. Occasionally, such enhancement can be asymmetric and, therefore, can be mistaken for pathologic nerve involvement. Correlation with clinical history can be helpful in such cases. However, enhancement of the labyrinthine or mastoid segments of the facial nerve, of the facial nerve outside of the facial canal, or associated enhancement of the vestibulocochlear nerve are greater indications of pathologic enhancement, such as that related to PNS.[57]

Variations in Venous Structures

Variations in size and course of venous structures are very common throughout the body. In the head and neck region, variation of the venous pterygoid plexus is most frequently encountered, leading to asymmetric enhancement in the infratemporal fossa and parapharyngeal space. Occasionally, this may be mistaken for PNS along the auriculotemporal nerve. Noticing flow voids in the regions of asymmetric enhancement, best seen

Table 1
Comparison of variable MR imaging sequences and variability in use of postgadolinium with fat saturation in the literature

Author Reference, Year	Magnet Strength Tesla (T)	Field of View (FOV)	Slice Thickness	Matrix	Precontrast	Postcontrast Plane with or without Fat Suppression	T2-Weighted	3D FT T1 0.6–1 mm VIBE Postgadolinium or Other Sequence
Moraldi et al,[21] 2008	—	Small FOV	High spatial resolution T1	—	—	High spatial resolution T1 with fat suppression	High resolution axial SE T2	Isotropic high-spatial resolution VIBE voxel size 0.5–0.7 mm, started 2 min after contrast administration
Borges & Casselman,[53] 2010	—	230 mm	<3 mm without interslice gap	160 × 256	Axial T1, T2	Axial and coronal T1 with fat saturation	Axial FSE T2	Multiplanar gradient echo, GRASS, or MPRAGE with reconstructions
Morani et al,[40] 2011	1.5-T synergy coils with standard head coils 3T do not use synergy coils, Microscopic coils for small superficial branches	Sequence-dependent (see Table 2)	Sequence-dependent (see Table 2)	Sequence-dependent (see Table 2)	Assess fat, especially in coronal plane for loss of fat planes	Fat-suppressed T1 useful if lesion in fat-containing area that is, orbits; however, may cause artifacts in skull base; use parallel imaging, or alternative, including a short-tau inversion recovery (STIR) sequence, especially if metal hardware	T2 images without fat saturation may provide better contrast for lesions in cavernous sinus	For peripheral nerve segments high-resolution T1 SPIN echo, or turbo SPIN-echo

						2D T1 with contrast and fat saturation	Coronal T2 fat-suppressed for muscle denervation	3D isotropic T1 postgadolinium, with sagittal and coronal reformations
Gandhi et al,[45] 2011	3 T	Small FOV, axial orbital roof-mandible, coronal globes posterior temporal bones	2 mm with 0.4–1 mm spacing	240 × 320	Axial and coronal T1	2D T1 with contrast and fat saturation	Coronal T2 fat-suppressed for muscle denervation	3D isotropic T1 postgadolinium, with sagittal and coronal reformations
Moonis et al,[23] 2012	—	—	3 mm	—	Axial T1 thin section	Axial and coronal T1 with gadolinium and without fat saturation	—	—
Stambuk,[41] 2013	Depends on skull base aeration if increased 1.5 T preferred	18 cm	3 mm	320 × 192	Axial T1	3-mm axial and coronal T1 postgadolinium without fat saturation	Yes, for muscle denervation	—

Abbreviations: FSE, fast spin-echo; FT, fourier transform; GRASS, gradient recalled acquisition in the steady state; MP-RAGE, Magnetisation Prepared RApid Gradient Echo; SE, spin-echo; VIBE, volumetric interpolated breath-hold examination.

Table 2
Detailed MR imaging sequences for assessment of cranial nerves V to XII

Slice Orientation	Sagittal T1 Head	DWI Head	Axial Flair Head	Axial T2	Axial T1	Postaxial T1	Axial T1 Fat-Saturated	Coronal T1	Axial T1 Head
FOV (mm)	240	230	230	160	160	160	160	160	240
Matrix	304/512	128/256	320/512	336/400	224/288	224/288	224/288	224/288	256/512
Number of slices/location	21	28	25	34	34	34	34	38	25
Slice thickness/gap	5/1 mm	4/1 mm	5/1 mm	4/1 mm	4/1 mm	4/1 mm	4/1 mm	3/default	5/1 mm
Contrast	Pre	Pre	Pre	Pre	Pre	Post	Post	Post	Post
TE	10	59	125	90	9.1	8	8	10.5	10
TR	Shortest	Shortest	11,000	Shortest	500	590	545	500	500
Flip Angle	—	90	—	90	75	90	90	90	90
Number of excitation	1	1	1	1	1	3	2	4	1

Axial from frontal sinus to the mid C3 cervical vertebral level, mandible to spinous process.
Coronal from frontal sinus to posterior pons.
Abbreviations: DWI, diffusion weighted imaging; TE, echo time.
Adapted from Morani AC, Ramani NS, Wesolowski JR. Skull base, orbits, temporal bone, and cranial nerves: anatomy on MR imaging. Magn Reson Imaging Clin N Am 2011;19(3): 439–56; with permission.

on T2-weighted images, usually leads to the correct diagnosis (see **Fig. 10**).

Occasionally, accessory or aberrant vessels, usually venous in nature, course through the neural foramina, causing asymmetric size and/or enhancement that might be overcalled as PNS. The foramen ovale is most commonly affected by such an anatomic variation. This has been attributed to an aberrant course of the sphenoid emissary vein through the foramen ovale in the absence of foramen Vesalius.[58]

WHAT THE REFERRING PHYSICIAN NEEDS TO KNOW

The referring physician needs to know if and to what extent PNS is present because it substantially alters patient prognosis and treatment plan. Limited involvement of nerve by PNS might be resectable, whereas more advanced PNS requires radiation therapy. For both scenarios, detailed mapping of each nerve at risk and their possible neuronal connections is required to

Table 3
Location of fat pads along the course of cranial nerves V and VII

Nerve	Fat Pad Location	Imaging Plane in Which Best Visualized	Examples
V1	Forehead, anterior to frontal sinus	Sagittal	Fig. 3A
	Along orbital roof	Sagittal	Fig. 3A
	Orbital apex	Coronal and axial	Fig. 3C
V2	Preantral	Axial	Figs. 4 and 5B
	Postantral	Axial	Fig. 5B
	Greater palatine foramen	Axial and coronal	Fig. 5B
	Pterygopalatine fossa	Axial and coronal	Fig. 6
V3	Premental	Axial and coronal	Fig. 7A,B
	Mandibular foramen	Axial and coronal	Fig. 7C
Vidian nerve	Anterior vidian canal	Axial and coronal	Fig. 9
CN VII	Stylomastoid foramen	Axial and coronal	Fig. 8

allow complete surgical resection or full radiation coverage of the PNS.[59]

SUMMARY

Over the past decade, both the knowledge and awareness of the prognostic implications of PNS have increased in the fields of pathology, oncology, surgery, radiation oncology, and radiology. Goethe famously once said, "We only see what we know"; however, there is still much we do not see radiographically and do not know regarding PNS, including why this occurs in certain tumors and not others, and how best to identify PNS as early as possible to improve patient outcomes. Continuous technological enhancements help us to better delineate PNS, particularly along smaller neural branches, and more advancements are anticipated with the use of MR neurography in the near future.

REFERENCES

1. Torre LA, Siegel RL, Ward EM, et al. Global cancer incidence and mortality rates and trends an update. Cancer Epidemiol Biomarkers Prev 2016; 25(1):16–27.
2. Simard EP, Torre LA, Jemal A. International trends in head and neck cancer incidence rates: differences by country, sex and anatomic site. Oral Oncol 2014;50(5):387–403.
3. Available at: https://www.cancer.org/cancer/oral-cavity-and-oropharyngeal-cancer/about/key-statistics.html. Accessed May 2017.
4. Rahima B, Shingaki S, Nagata M, et al. Prognostic significance of perineural invasion in oral and oropharyngeal carcinoma. Oral Surg Oral Med Oral Pathol Oral Radiol Endod 2004;97(4):423–31.
5. Woolgar JA. Histopathological prognosticators in oral and oropharyngeal squamous cell carcinoma. Oral Oncol 2006;42(3):229–39.
6. Miller ME, Palla B, Chen Q, et al. A novel classification system for perineural invasion in noncutaneous head and neck squamous cell carcinoma: histologic subcategories and patient outcomes. Am J Otolaryngol 2012;33(2):212–5.
7. O'brien CJ, Lahr CJ, Soong SJ, et al. Surgical treatment of early-stage carcinoma of the oral tongue—would adjuvant treatment be beneficial? Head Neck Surg 1986;8(6):401–8.
8. Liebig C, Ayala G, Wilks JA, et al. Perineural invasion in cancer. Cancer 2009;115(15):3379–91.
9. Cruveilheir J. Maladies des nerfs anatomie pathologique du corps Humain. 2nd edition. Paris: JB Bailliere; 1835.
10. Neumann E. Secundäre Cancroidinfiltration des Nervus mentalis bei einem Fall von Lippencancroid.

Archiv für pathologische Anatomie und Physiologie und für klinische Medizin 1862;24(1–2):201–2.
11. Ballantyne AJ, McCarten AB, Ibanez ML. The extension of cancer of the head and neck through peripheral nerves. Am J Surg 1963;106(4):651–67.
12. Mays AC, Chou J, Craddock AL, et al. Gene variability between perineural-positive and perineural-negative squamous cell skin cancers. J Clin Med Genomics 2015;3(133):2.
13. Doumas S, Paterson JC, Norris PM, et al. Fractalkine (CX3CL1) and fractalkine receptor (CX3CR1) in squamous cell carcinoma of the tongue: markers of nerve invasion? Oral Maxillofac Surg 2015;19(1):61–4.
14. Available at: http://www.rcpath.org. Accessed May 2017; see: Head and Neck Datasets, Section A.
15. Available at: http://www.cap.org/web/home/resources/cancer-reporting-tools/cancer-protocol-templates? Accessed May 2017.
16. Chatzistefanou I, Lubek J, Markou K, et al. The role of perineural invasion in treatment decisions for oral cancer patients: a review of the literature. J Craniomaxillofac Surg 2017;45(6):821–5.
17. Kurtz KA, Hoffman HT, Zimmerman MB, et al. Perineural and vascular invasion in oral cavity squamous carcinoma: increased incidence on re-review of slides and by using immunohistochemical enhancement. Arch Pathol Lab Med 2005;129(3): 354–9.
18. Barrett AW, Speight PM. Perineural invasion in adenoid cystic carcinoma of the salivary glands: a valid prognostic indicator? Oral Oncol 2009;45(11): 936–40.
19. Amit M, Binenbaum Y, Trejo–Leider L, et al. International collaborative validation of intraneural invasion as a prognostic marker in adenoid cystic carcinoma of the head and neck. Head Neck 2015;37(7):1038–45.
20. Roh J, Muelleman T, Tawfik O, et al. Perineural growth in head and neck squamous cell carcinoma: a review. Oral Oncol 2015;51(1):16–23.
21. Maroldi R, Farina D, Borghesi A, et al. Perineural tumor spread. Neuroimaging Clin N Am 2008;18(2): 413–29.
22. Fagan JJ, Collins B, Barnes L, et al. Perineural invasion in squamous cell carcinoma of the head and neck. Arch Otolaryngol Head Neck Surg 1998; 124(6):637–40.
23. Moonis G, Cunnane MB, Emerick K, et al. Patterns of perineural tumor spread in head and neck cancer. Magn Reson Imaging Clin N Am 2012;20(3):435–46.
24. Binmadi NO, Basile JR. Perineural invasion in oral squamous cell carcinoma: a discussion of significance and review of the literature. Oral Oncol 2011;47(11):1005–10.
25. Badger D, Aygun N. Imaging of perineural spread in head and neck cancer. Radiol Clin North Am 2017; 55(1):139–49.

26. Johnston M, Yu E, Kim J. Perineural invasion and spread in head and neck cancer. Expert Rev Anticancer Ther 2012;12(3):359–71.

27. Caldemeyer KS, Mathews VP, Righi PD, et al. Imaging features and clinical significance of perineural spread or extension of head and neck tumors. Radiographics 1998;18(1):97–110.

28. Curtin HD. Detection of perineural spread: fat is a friend. AJNR Am J Neuroradiol 1998;19(8):1385–6.

29. Gil Z, Carlson DL, Gupta A, et al. Patterns and incidence of neural invasion in patients with cancers of the paranasal sinuses. Arch Otolaryngol Head Neck Surg 2009;135(2):173–9.

30. Davidson JR, Mack J, Gutnikova A, et al. Developmental changes in human dural innervation. Childs Nerv Syst 2012;28(5):665–71.

31. Monkhouse S. Cranial nerves: functional anatomy. Cambridge (UK): Cambridge University Press; 2005.

32. Williams LS, Schmalfuss IM, Sistrom CL, et al. MR imaging of the trigeminal ganglion, nerve, and the perineural vascular plexus: normal appearance and variants with correlation to cadaver specimens. AJNR Am J Neuroradiol 2003;24(7):1317–23.

33. Bathla G, Hegde AN. The trigeminal nerve: an illustrated review of its imaging anatomy and pathology. Clin Radiol 2013;68(2):203–13.

34. Gonella MC, Fischbein NJ, So YT. Disorders of the trigeminal system. Semin Neurol 2009;29(1):36–044.

35. Phillips CD, Bubash LA. The facial nerve: anatomy and common pathology. Semin Ultrasound CT MR 2002;23(3):202–17.

36. Diamond M, Wartmann CT, Tubbs RS, et al. Peripheral facial nerve communications and their clinical implications. Clin Anat 2011;24(1):10–8.

37. Schmalfuss IM, Tart RP, Mukherji S, et al. Perineural tumor spread along the auriculotemporal nerve. AJNR Am J Neuroradiol 2002;23(2):303–11.

38. Li C, Jiang XZ, Zhao YF. Connection of trigeminal nerve and facial nerve branches and its clinical significance. Shanghai Journal of Stomatology 2009; 18(5):545–50 [in Chinese].

39. Kumar VA, Shah KB, Ginsberg LE. Perineural Tumor Spread to the oculomotor (CN III) nerve. J Comput Assist Tomogr 2013;37(4):525–7.

40. Morani AC, Ramani NS, Wesolowski JR. Skull base, orbits, temporal bone, and cranial nerves: anatomy on MR imaging. Magn Reson Imaging Clin N Am 2011;19(3):439–56.

41. Stambuk HE. Perineural tumor spread involving the central skull base region. Semin Ultrasound CT MR 2013;34(5):445–58.

42. Panizza BJ. An overview of head and neck malignancy with perineural spread. J Neurol Surg B Skull Base 2016;77(02):081–5.

43. Balamucki CJ, Mancuso AA, Amdur RJ, et al. Skin carcinoma of the head and neck with perineural invasion. Am J Otolaryngol 2012;33(4):447–54.

44. Penn R, Abemayor E, Nabili V, et al. Perineural invasion detected by high-field 3.0-T magnetic resonance imaging. Am J Otolaryngol 2010;31(6):482–4.

45. Gandhi MR, Panizza B, Kennedy D. Detecting and defining the anatomic extent of large nerve perineural spread of malignancy: comparing "targeted" MRI with the histologic findings following surgery. Head Neck 2011;33(4):469–75.

46. Kirsch CF. Advances in magnetic resonance imaging of the skull base. Int Arch Otorhinolaryngol 2014;18(S 02):S127–35.

47. Ong CK, Chong VF. Imaging of perineural spread in head and neck tumors. Cancer Imaging 2010; 10(1A):S92–8.

48. Curtin HD. Detection of perineural spread: fat suppression versus no fat suppression. AJNR Am J Neuroradiol 2004;25(1):1–3.

49. Gandhi M, Sommerville J. The imaging of large nerve perineural spread. J Neurol Surg B Skull Base 2016;77(02):113–23.

50. Baulch J, Gandhi M, Sommerville J, et al. 3T MRI evaluation of large nerve perineural spread of head and neck cancers. J Med Imaging Radiat Oncol 2015;59(5):578–85.

51. Álvarez BB, Gómez MT. Perineural spread in head and neck tumors. Radiologia 2014;56(5):400–12.

52. Lee KJ, Abemayor E, Sayre J, et al. Determination of perineural invasion preoperatively on radiographic images. Otolaryngol Head Neck Surg 2008;139(2): 275–80.

53. Borges A, Casselman J. Imaging the trigeminal nerve. Eur J Radiol 2010;74(2):323–40.

54. Ginsberg LE, De Monte F, Gillenwater AM. Greater superficial petrosal nerve: anatomy and MR findings in perineural tumor spread. AJNR Am J Neuroradiol 1996;17(2):389–93.

55. Fujii H, Fujita A, Yang H, et al. Visualization of the peripheral branches of the mandibular division of the trigeminal nerve on 3D double-echo steady-state with water excitation sequence. AJNR Am J Neuroradiol 2015;36(7):1333–7.

56. Jain V, Deshmukh A, Gollomp S. Bilateral Facial paralysis case presentation and discussion of differential diagnosis. J Gen Intern Med 2006;21(7): C7–10.

57. Martin-Duverneuil N, Sola-Martinex MT, Miaux Y, et al. Contrast enhancement of the facial nerve on MRI: normal or pathological? Neuroradiology 1997; 39(3):207–12.

58. Ginsberg LE, Pruett SW, Chen MYM, et al. Skull-Base foramina of the middle cranial fossa: reassessment of normal variations with high-resolution CT. AJNR Am J Neuroradiol 1994;15:283–91.

59. Galloway TJ, Morris CG, Mancuso AA, et al. Impact of radiographic findings on prognosis for skin carcinoma with clinical perineural invasion. Cancer 2005; 103(6):1254–7.

High-Resolution Isotropic Three-Dimensional MR Imaging of the Extraforaminal Segments of the Cranial Nerves

CrossMark

Jessica Wen, MD[a], Naman S. Desai, MD[b],
Dean Jeffery, MD[b], Nafi Aygun, MD[b],*, Ari Blitz, MD[b]

KEYWORDS

- High-resolution MR imaging • Cranial nerves • Segmental classification
- Extraforaminal cranial nerves

KEY POINTS

- High-resolution isotropic 3-dimensional (D) MR imaging with and without contrast is now routinely used for imaging evaluation of cranial nerve anatomy and pathologic abnormality.
- Previous work has highlighted the utility of sequences, including constructive interference in steady-state without and with intravenous contrast, in such cases.
- The extraforaminal segments are well-visualized on these techniques, especially in the setting of contrast against varying tissue types.
- The extraforaminal segments are affected by a wide range of pathologic entities, which may cause enhancement or displacement of the nerve; in such pathologic conditions, the relevant findings are also visible to an extent not available on standard 2D imaging.

INTRODUCTION

For the purposes of imaging, the cranial nerves (CNs) may be divided into 7 segments based on anatomic context (**Fig. 1**),[1] designated as segments a through g. Each of the CNs, with the exception of the vestibulocochlear nerve (CN VIII), is partly found outside of the head, passing beyond a line drawn between the margins of the outer table of the skull at each side of the skull base foramina; that is, in the extraforaminal segment, which may be designated as CN #.g for rapid reference. More specifically, segments a and b remain within the central nervous system and are designated the nuclear and parenchymal fascicular segments, respectively. The cisternal segment, c, is that portion that lies within the cistern having exited the brainstem until it reaches the entrance of the dural cave segment, d. More distally, the CN courses beyond the inner dural layer, is no longer surrounded by cerebrospinal fluid (CSF), becomes associated with a venous plexus, and is considered as the interdural segment, e. After piercing the outer layer of dura, the CN is foraminal, f. The final extraforaminal segment, g, is reached when the nerve exits the skull base.

Disclosure: Dr A. Blitz has been on the medical advisory board for Guerbet. He is also partially funded by R21 NS096497 and FAIN U01DC013778 grants.
[a] The Russell H. Morgan Department of Radiology and Radiologic Science, The Johns Hopkins Hospital, 600 North Wolfe Street, Baltimore, MD 21287, USA; [b] Division of Neuroradiology, The Russell H. Morgan Department of Radiology and Radiologic Science, The Johns Hopkins Hospital, Phipps B-100, 600 North Wolfe Street, Baltimore, MD 21287, USA
* Corresponding author.
E-mail address: naygun1@jhmi.edu

mri.theclinics.com

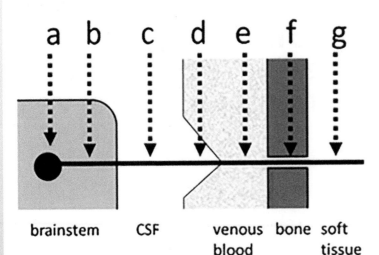

Fig. 1. The different anatomic segments of the cranial nerves. CSF, cerebrospinal fluid. (*From* Blitz AM, Aygun N, Herzka DA, et al. "High resolution three-dimensional MR imaging of the skull base: compartments, boundaries, and critical structures." Radiol Clin North Am 2017;55(1):21; with permission.)

CNs serve various functions, including but not limited to vision, movements of extraocular and facial muscles, and hearing. It is in the extraforaminal segments that the CNs may be seen extending through surrounding soft tissue to (in the case of motor innervation) or from (in the case of sensory innervation) the organs they innervate. Clinical suspicion of an extraforaminal location of disease affecting the CNs is sometimes possible due to the branching pattern of the CNs, proximity with other CNs with interrupted function, and/or a known abnormality such as dermatologic malignancy in the region of suspected CN dysfunction. Currently, MR imaging is the gold standard for visualization of various pathologic abnormalities associated with CNs. However, imaging of the extraforaminal segments of the CNs presents a particular challenge due to their small size, complex course, and varying anatomic context as they course adjacent to a variety of soft tissue structures. High-resolution 3-dimensional (D) MR imaging allows for visualization of a greater extent of the normal and abnormal extraforaminal segments of the CNs than was previously possible, although substantial challenges remain. Differential diagnosis of lesions is based on the location and gross anatomic features evident on imaging.

Cranial neuropathy may arise from disease affecting fiber bundles at any anatomic segment, from the nuclear segment (CN #.a) to the innervated end organs in the extraforaminal segments (CN #.g). Segmental classification of the CNs has been described elsewhere and is summarized in **Fig. 1.**[1] Readers interested in imaging of the CNs from their nuclear to the foraminal segments with their associated pathologic conditions can refer to review articles written elsewhere.[1–3] The extraforaminal segment, g, begins at the level of the

outer cortex of the appropriate foramen. This article focuses on the normal high-resolution anatomy and appearance of several featured CNs, with specific emphasis on the extraforaminal segment, along with selected pathologic conditions affecting those segments.

IMAGING APPROACHES

At the authors' institution, high-resolution isotropic 3D MR imaging protocol consists of the following sequences: precontrast and postcontrast 3D constructive interference in steady-state (CISS), 3D T2-weighted short-tau inversion recovery (STIR) SPACE (Sampling Perfection with Application optimized Contrasts using different flip angle Evolution), precontrast volumetric interpolated breath-hold examination (VIBE), and postcontrast VIBE with fat saturation (**Table 1**).[4] In addition, standard precontrast imaging through the head is typically performed before the high-resolution imaging and standard postcontrast imaging is generally performed following the high-resolution sequences listed.

CISS sequences acquire high-signal, high-resolution isotropic 3D images, which can be reconstructed in multiple planes to visualize complex skull base and CN anatomy. The use of CISS imaging with and without contrast has been described for evaluation of the course of the CNs from the cisternal through extraforaminal segments.[1] Even though it is a gradient echo technique, CISS sequence includes both T1-weighting and T2-weighting, which enables postcontrast evaluation of structures, such as small regions of pathologic enhancement encountered in perineural spread of malignancies.[5] Additionally, nonpathologic postcontrast enhancement enables exquisite

Table 1
Parameters of high-resolution skull base MR imaging protocol at the authors' institution[a]

	TR (ms)	TE (ms)	TI (ms)	Flip Angle (degree)	Field of View (mm)	Slices	Voxel Size (mm)[b]	Averages	Time of Acquisition
STIR SPACE	3000	256	220	—	256	88	1.0 × 1.0 × 1.0	1.4	5:23
VIBE	4.93	2.46	—	9	210	112	0.78 × 0.78 × 0.8	3	4:38
CISS[c]	5.46	2.43	—	42	152	112	0.6 × 0.6 × 0.6	1	5:17
Intravenous contrast									
CISS	5.46	2.43	—	42	152	112	0.6 × 0.6 × 0.6	1	5:17
VIBE with SPAIR FS	11.6	4.3	—	10.5	210	112	0.73 × 0.73 × 0.8	1	4:16

MR imaging protocol for high-resolution skull base imaging at the authors' institutions, which includes a precontrast and postcontrast CISS sequence.

[a] Please note that standard precontrast imaging through the head is typically performed before the high-resolution skull base examination and standard postcontrast imaging of the head is generally performed following the high-resolution sequences listed.

[b] Reconstructed voxel size.

[c] Acquired and reconstructed voxel size are identical.

Adapted from Blitz AM, Aygun N, Herzka DA, et al. High resolution three-dimensional MR imaging of the skull base: compartments, boundaries, and critical structures. Radiol Clin North Am 2017;55(1):20; with permission.

visualization of mucosal surfaces and soft tissue planes. Due to both T1-weighting and T2-weighting in CISS sequences, isotropic 3D STIR sequence is performed to analyze T2-weighted signal characteristics of a lesion.

Fat appears hyperintense on both CISS and nonfat-suppressed VIBE sequences. Because many extraforaminal CNs traverse through fat, subtle pathologic contrast enhancement would be difficult to appreciate in the background of hyperintense fat. Therefore, postcontrast VIBE sequences are performed with fat saturation to make pathologic contrast enhancement more apparent (**Fig. 2**).

High-resolution isotropic 3-dimensional MR imaging protocol has several advantages compared with conventional techniques used for CN imaging. CISS imaging can be performed in a clinically acceptable time period, with evaluation of skull base and posterior fossa at 0.6-mm isotropic resolution in less than 6 minutes. Additionally, due to the isotropic nature of the images, often, much of the length of the extraforaminal CNs can be depicted with the aid of multiplanar reconstructions. On conventional T1-weighted and T2-weighted imaging, susceptibility artifacts near air-containing structures limit evaluation of extraforaminal components of CNs in those regions. However, due to reduced T2* (T2 star) sensitivity of balanced stead state free precession (SSFP) sequences, as well as utilization of small voxels, resultant artifacts usually do not

significantly limit such evaluation. Additionally, CISS images are also relatively insensitive to motion.[6]

Several other high-resolution MR imaging techniques have been used for imaging of the extraforaminal course of the CNs. For example, the extraforaminal course of CNs have been visualized using a high-resolution imaging technique of 3D reversed fast imaging with steady-state precession (3D-PSIF) with diffusion-weighted MR sequence. Zhang and colleagues[7] were able to demonstrate extracranial portions of CNs II to XII, except nerves within the cavernous sinuses. However, they concluded that, due to motion artifacts and susceptibility artifacts at the skull base and upper neck, the 3D-PSIF should be used in conjunction with other standard sequences.

Similarly, 3D double-echo steady-state (DESS) with water excitation (WE) has been used in healthy volunteers to depict the intraparotid course of the normal facial nerve, including its relationship to the parotid duct.[8,9] Qin and colleagues[8] demonstrated that, on 3D DESS WE images, facial nerve exhibits high-signal intensity with surrounding tissues demonstrating low-signal intensity. The main trunk and cervicofacial division of the facial nerve, as well as the parotid ducts, were identified with great fidelity. Similarly, the authors' institution has also successfully used DESS sequences to demonstrate lingual nerve and inferior alveolar nerve in the parapharyngeal space.

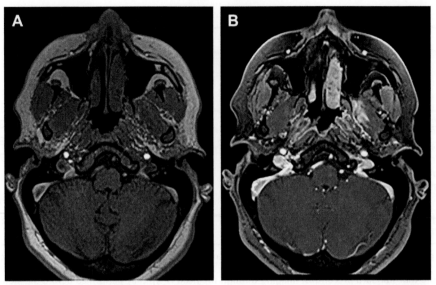

Fig. 2. Axial T1 precontrast nonfat-saturated (*A*) and postcontrast fat-saturated (*B*) images at the level of the torus tubarius. Addition of postcontrast fat-saturated images allows exquisite visualization of mucosal surfaces as evidenced by visualization of anterior (*B, yellow arrow*) and posterior (*B*, red *arrow*) walls of the torus tubarius. Additionally, fossa of Rosenmüller (*B, blue arrow*) is also easily visualized on T1-weighted postcontrast fat-saturated images.

Diffusion tensor tractography has been used to visualize neural fibers of CN VII in the head and neck region at 3 T. However, because neural fibers are often small in diameter than a standard voxel, these techniques are limited by partial volume averaging. In contrast, CISS anisotropic and high spatial resolution sequences can readily detect these branches.

TECHNIQUE (CONSTRUCTIVE INTERFERENCE IN STEADY-STATE)

CISS sequence is a high-spatial resolution, refocused gradient echo sequence that can be obtained with isotropic resolution in a clinically acceptable acquisition time. Images can be reconstructed in any plane. CISS images have the appearance of T2-weighted images, although increased signal is easily recognized after administration of gadolinium-based contrast material in tissues that show contrast enhancement on T1-weighted images. Precontrast and postcontrast CISS sequences can be performed in less than 6 minutes, each with an isotropic resolution of 0.6 mm.

3D T1-weighted sequences before administration of contrast without fat saturation (VIBE) are performed in less than 5 minutes with isotropic resolution of 0.8 mm. It allows for the evaluation of presence or absence of fat as intrinsic T1 hyperintensity within the medullary space, extracranial space, or the lesion itself. Postcontrast 3D T1 sequences with fat saturation (postcontrast VIBE

with fat saturation) are performed similarly in less than 5 minutes with isotropic resolution of 0.8 mm. Fat saturation is used to provide high conspicuity for enhancement, as well as characterization of precontrast T1 hyperintensity secondary to presence of fat.

DISCUSSION

CN dysfunction can occur as a result of pathologic abnormality at any point along the nerve fibers, including the extraforaminal segments. The wide range of pathologic entities affecting CN#.a to CN #.f has been discussed elsewhere.[1-3] This article highlights pathologic abnormality localized to the extraforaminal segment, with characteristic examples featured along with the discussion of normal CN anatomy.

Several entities may affect CNs in a similar manner, leading to the corresponding CN palsy. Congenital absence or atresia can lead symptoms that may be low-grade, vague, intermittent, and chronic for many years before diagnosis. Inflammatory conditions, including sarcoidosis, Wegener granulomatosis, and Tolosa Hunt syndrome, may produce painful symptoms, leading to imaging workup. Infectious agents, including viral infections, can have a tropism for CN involvement.

Malignant lesions may also arise from or directly involve the extraforaminal CNs. The extensive network of innervation within the head and neck, and the wide array of pathologic abnormality that

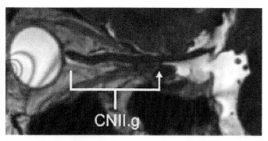

Fig. 3. Sagittal CISS reformat through the orbit clearly depicts the entire course of the optic nerve, including the extraforaminal portion anterior to the optic canal.

can arise from cutaneous, mucosal, and salivary, among other tissue types, allows for many different sources of perineural disease spread. Benign lesions may also arise from the CNs, including schwannomas and neurofibromas, which are more frequently seen involving particular CNs than others (see later discussion).

Each of the extraforaminal CNs are discussed individually, with particular emphasis on CNs III, V, VII, and X, given the complexity of their extraforaminal anatomy and complex innervation of the head and neck.

CRANIAL NERVE II: OPTIC NERVE, ANATOMY

The optic nerve is unique in that it is an extension of the central nerve system and not a CN by strict

definition. It is surrounded entirely by meninges rather than Schwann cells, therefore all segments are considered intradural (segmentation of CN II has been discussed elsewhere), and the extraforaminal portion is located within the orbit after passage through the optic canal. CSF fluid and the optic sheath surround the optic nerve, separating it from the adjacent orbital fat (**Fig. 3**).

Cranial Nerve II.g: Selected Pathologic Abnormalities

Inflammatory conditions and neoplastic lesions are among the many types of pathologic abnormalities involving CN II.g. Optic neuritis is an inflammatory disorder, often times demyelinating, which can cause acute painful visual loss in young patients (**Fig. 4**).

Other inflammatory conditions, including sarcoidosis, may also involve the optic nerve and show varying involvement of the optic sheath and/or nerve, also potentially mimicking the previously described pathologic abnormalities.[10] Optic gliomas, along with other neoplastic processes, including lymphoma and metastases, may mimic optic neuritis.[11] In the diagnosis of mass lesions, the relationship to and involvement or lack thereof of the optic sheath is crucial for image interpretation and surgical planning. With the spatial resolution provided on contrast-enhanced (CE) CISS, detecting these differences is possible. Optic nerve

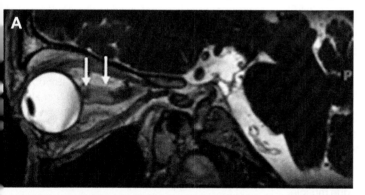

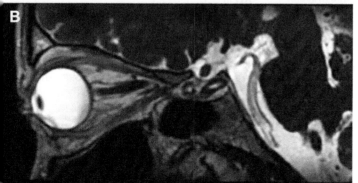

Fig. 4. (A) Sagittal postcontrast CISS demonstrates enhancement and thickening of the intraorbital segment of the left optic nerve (*white arrows*) in this patient with optic neuritis. (B) In the normal contralateral right eye, the optic sheath is well depicted, with normal CSF signal seen surrounding the optic nerve.

sheath meningiomas, for example, will exhibit features compatible with a dural-based mass originating from the optic nerve sheath rather than the optic nerve itself. A tram-track sign has been described with optic nerve sheath meningiomas.

The presence of orbital fat often complicates MR imaging of the optic nerve. CE-CISS sequence, among others, is limited due to lack of fat suppression, which potentially decreases the conspicuity of an enhancing mass surrounded by hyperintense orbital fat. In these cases, high-resolution postcontrast, fat-suppressed, T1-weighted images, such as 3D CE-VIBE sequences, may be a useful complementing sequence.[2]

The extraforaminal ocular motor CNs share a common location within the orbit for the innervation of the extraocular muscular apparatus and are, therefore, discussed together. Particular emphasis is placed on CN III due to its size and neural supply, with brief mention of CNs IV and VI given their similar functions and pathologic abnormalities.

CRANIAL NERVE III.g: OCULOMOTOR NERVE, ANATOMY

The oculomotor nerve enters the orbital apex via the superior orbital fissure. It then branches into superior and inferior divisions. The superior division supplies the superior rectus muscle and levator palpebrae, whereas the inferior division innervates the medial and inferior rectus muscles (**Fig. 5**), as well as supplying parasympathetic innervation to the ciliary ganglia responsible for the pupillary reflex.[2,12]

CRANIAL NERVE IV.g: TROCHLEAR NERVE, ANATOMY

CN IV.g exits the skull in the superolateral portion of the superior orbital fissure, external to the annulus of Zinn, along with the frontal and lacrimal branches of the ophthalmic division of CN V.1.g,[12] eventually innervating the superior oblique muscle.

CRANIAL NERVE VI.g: ABDUCENS NERVE, ANATOMY

CN VI.f travels through the central portion of the superior orbital fissure along with the CN III.f to enter into the orbit and innervates the lateral rectus muscle.[12]

CRANIAL NERVES III.g, IV.g, AND VI.g: SELECTED PATHOLOGIC ABNORMALITIES

A wide range of causes of ocular CN palsies exist, including diabetic neuropathy, trauma,

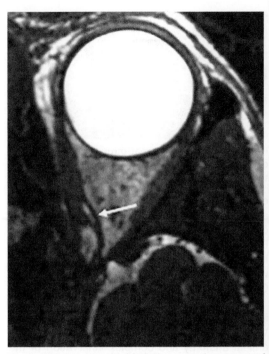

Fig. 5. CISS sequence highlighting normal anatomy of the inferior division of CN III.g (*arrow*) directly innervating the medial rectus muscle.

demyelinating disorders, congenital abnormality or absence,[13] and idiopathic disease.[14–16] Pathologic abnormalities that involve the ocular motor CNs can present with classic symptoms localizing to a specific CN palsy. However, given the close proximity of these nerves within the orbital apex, pathologic abnormalities involving 1 nerve may also masquerade as palsy of another.[2] Symptoms such as proptosis and pain may signify an abnormality within the region of the orbital apex without more localizing clinical clues. Tolosa-Hunt, for example, is a condition producing granulomatous inflammation within the cavernous sinus that can extend into the superior orbital fissure and orbital apex, producing painful opthalmaplegia.[17,18]

CN III palsy is most commonly associated clinically with extrinsic mass effect on the oculomotor nerve from uncal herniation or aneurysm. However, it can also be an indicator of intrinsic pathologic abnormality. The long course of the trochlear nerve through the subarachnoid space makes it vulnerable to injury from trauma, compression, ischemia, and infection, including via the subarachnoid space.[16,19,20]

Mass lesions involving the ocular motor CNs are often slow growing; however, they may cause symptoms at very small sizes due to mass effect. Up to 4% of orbital tumors have been attributed to peripheral nerve sheath tumors, both benign

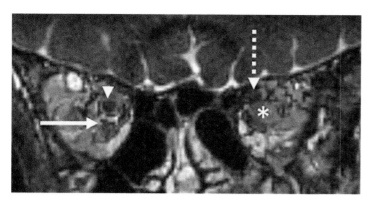

Fig. 6. Coronal postcontrast CISS on a 1.5-T magnet. On the right, there is normal anatomic relationship between the optic nerve (*arrowhead*) and CN III (*solid arrow*). On the left, the optic nerve is displaced superiorly and medially (*dashed arrow*) by an enhancing lesion (*asterisk*) that appears to originate from CN III.g. In the setting of a clinical history of neurofibromatosis, findings are most likely to represent a plexiform neurofibroma originating from the inferior division of CN III.g on the left.

and malignant[21]; 6% of all schwannomas are reported to be orbital in origin.[22,23] These lesions are rare and are usually seen in cases of neurofibromatosis[23–25] (**Fig. 6**). Several cases of oculomotor nerve schwannomas have been reported, with patients presenting with CN III palsy,[22,26,27] proptosis,[28] and even an entity called ophthalmoplegic migraine in which the patient experiences migraine symptoms followed by pupillary abnormalities and diplopia.[24] Schwannomas of the trochlear and abducens nerve have also been reported but are much less common.[29–32]

The reported incidence of a focal lesion as the source for a monocular neuropathy identified on imaging varies.[33,34] Patients with a history of malignancy may be at higher risk for having focal lesions affecting peripheral CNs, including those within the orbit. Adequately visualizing and also determining the relationship of a lesion to the native CN to identify its origin is crucial to accurate diagnosis. The complex anatomy of the orbital apex requires that minute structures be differentiated from each other with high signal-to-noise ratio and high-resolution imaging.[24]

CRANIAL NERVE V: TRIGEMINAL NERVE

The trigeminal nerve is the largest of the CNs, with 3 main divisions supplying sensation to different regions of the face, as well as motor innervation to the muscles of mastication via the third division (CN V.3). The extraforaminal segment of each division and their associated pathologic abnormalities are discussed individually.

Cranial Nerve V.1.g: Ophthalmic Division, Trigeminal Nerve Anatomy

Branches of CN V.1.g begin in the face and become the foraminal segment (CN V.1.f) as it enters the superior orbital fissure. Within the orbit, V1 includes 3 branches: the frontal, lacrimal, and nasociliary nerves (**Fig. 7**). The frontal and lacrimal nerves are located superiorly in the superior orbital fissure and supply sensation to the upper face and the lacrimal gland, respectively. The frontal nerve is the largest of the branches of V1, and gives off supratrochlear and supraorbital branches. The nasociliary branch is located more inferiorly and innervates the globe and nasal cavity. A unique feature of the nasociliary nerve is that it is the only CN V.1 branch, which is intraconal, traveling through the annulus of Zinn.[35] In addition to sensory innervation of the nasal skin and mucosa, the long ciliary nerve branches maintain the corneal blink reflex through noncutaneous sensory innervation of the cornea.[35,36]

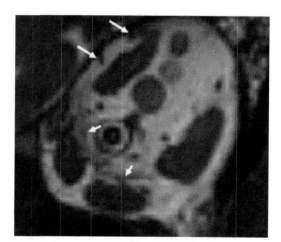

Fig. 7. Coronal CISS image of the left orbit showing multiple branches of the V1 branch of the trigeminal nerve. V1 travels through Meckel cave into the cavernous sinus and through the superior orbital fissure, where it gives off frontal, lacrimal, and nasociliary branches. The supratrochlear (medial) and supraorbital (lateral) branches of the left frontal nerve are well seen in the orbit (*white arrows*).

Cranial Nerve V.1.g: Selected Pathologic Abnormalities

Pathologic abnormality involving branches of the ophthalmic division are less common than those affecting CN V.2 and CN V.3, and are often cutaneous in cause given the large area of sensory innervation supplied by CN V.1.g branches. Squamous cell carcinoma (SCC), basal cell carcinoma (BCC), and melanoma may all result in perineural spread of tumor, particularly along the dominant frontal nerve[35,36] (**Fig. 8**). CE-CISS sequences can also show prominent enhancement due to perineural spread of the lacrimal nerve (**Fig. 9**), which can occur with pathologic abnormality such as adenoid cystic carcinoma.[37,38] Enhancement and enlargement of the extraforaminal branches are findings associated with perineural spread and invasion.

Cranial Nerve V.2.g: Maxillary Division, Trigeminal Nerve Anatomy

The branches of the extraforaminal segment of the maxillary division, CN V.2, of the trigeminal nerve converge on the pterygopalatine fossa (PPF) passing posteriorly to enter the foraminal segment in the foramen rotundum (CN V.2.f) (**Fig. 10**). It is well-

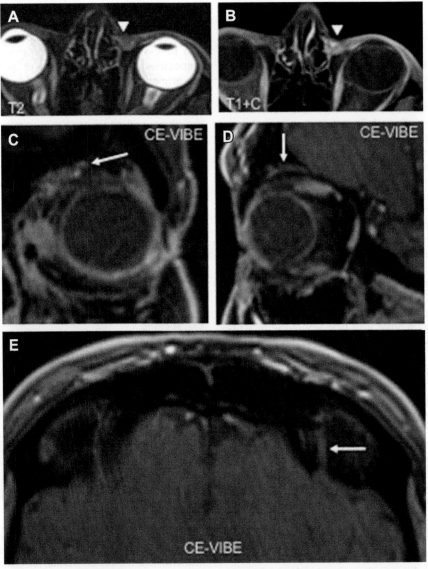

Fig. 8. (*A, B*) Conventional 2D sequences show a T2 hyperintense and enhancing lesion (*arrowheads*) along the left nasal fold compatible with a known BCC. (*C, D, E*) CE-VIBE) in all 3 planar reformations shows enhancement and thickening of the left lacrimal nerve (*arrows*), suspicious for perineural spread of disease.

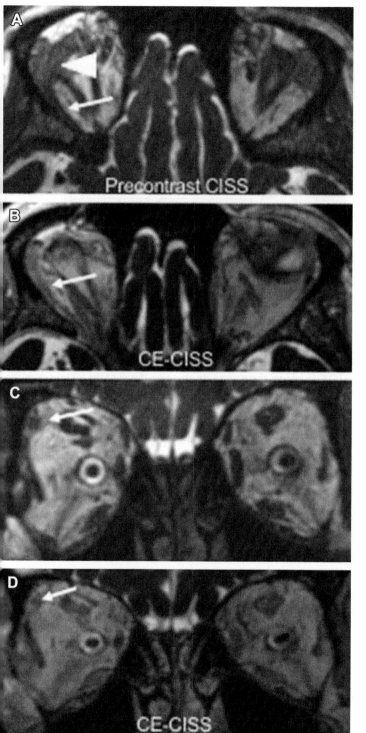

Fig. 9. (*A*) Axial precontrast CISS shows the lacrimal gland (*arrowhead*) innervated by the lacrimal nerve (*arrow*). (*B*) CE-CISS demonstrates enhancement of the nerve (*white arrow*) in this patient with a history of right supraorbital SCC of the skin suspicious for perineural spread. (*C*) Coronal precontrast reformatted image contrasts the lacrimal nerve (*white arrow*) with the surrounding bright orbital fat. (*D*) Contrast-enhancement on CISS makes this contrast less conspicuous; however, it still clearly shows enhancement (*white arrow*) relative to surrounding structures.

depicted on CISS sequences due to enhancement of the surrounding perineural vascular plexus.[39,40] Branches of CN V.2.g include the infraorbital nerve, zygomatic, and superior alveolar nerves that supply sensory innervation to the midface. The PPF houses the pterygopalatine ganglion. The PPF is a central hub of communication between multiple neural pathways, as well as a site of

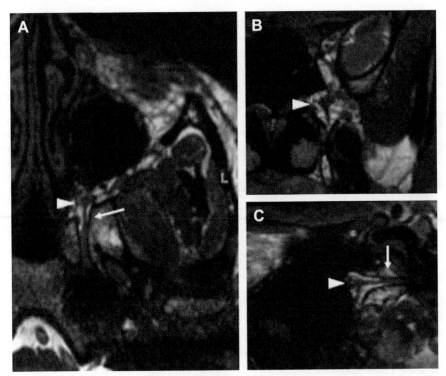

Fig. 10. Axial (*A*), coronal (*B*), and sagittal (*C*) CISS images show exquisite anatomic detail of the V2 branch of the trigeminal nerve (*arrows*) traveling through foramen rotundum into the PPF, which houses the pterygopalatine ganglion (*arrowheads*).

connection with the infratemporal fossa via the pterygomaxillary fissure, the nasopharynx via the palatovaginal canal, the palate through the greater and lesser palatine foramina, the nasal cavity via the sphenopalatine foramen, and the orbits superiorly and face inferiorly via inferior orbital fissure.[36,41]

Cranial Nerve V.2.g: Selected Pathologic Abnormalities

A wide range of benign and malignant pathologic abnormalities can affect the mandibular branch of the trigeminal nerve and present with maxillofacial pain. Rare entities include inflammatory pseudotumor,[42] postinfectious neuralgia,[43] and sinonasal sarcoidosis.[44] Wegener granulomatosis is a rare inflammatory cause of CN palsy, as is seen in the case involving the CN V.2 branch before entering the infraorbital foramen (**Fig. 11**). Given the extensive connections between the PPF and the multiple compartments of the face, various neoplastic processes of the head and neck can also result in perineural spread to the skull base. This includes cutaneous lesions within the midface distribution via the infraorbital nerve; nasopharyngeal carcinoma through the sphenopalatine foramen and palatovaginal canal; and,

finally, oropharyngeal and minor salivary gland tumors derived from the palate.[45] Comparison of non–CE-CISS and CE-CISS, as well as 3D T1-weighted imaging, can demonstrate an abnormal signal in many of these regions, as well as showing thickening and enhancement of distal extra-CN branches within the soft tissues.

Cranial Nerve V. 3.g: Mandibular Division, Trigeminal Nerve, Anatomy

The mandibular division, CN V.3, of the trigeminal nerve exits the foramen ovale, where it is surrounded by a perineural venous plexus and well-visualized on CE-CISS[39] (**Fig. 12**). It extends caudally into the masticator space. The branches of CN V.3.g supply sensory innervation to the lower face, including the jaw, floor of the mouth, and tongue, as well as motor-innervation of the muscles of mastication, tensor tympani, tensor veli palatini, mylohyoid, and anterior belly of the digastric muscles.[46] CN V.3.g then divides into anterior and posterior divisions; the anterior division supplies motor innervation and 1 sensory branch to the cheek (buccal nerve), and the posterior division supplies the auriculotemporal, lingual, and inferior alveolar nerves.[46] The auriculotemporal branch is unique given its extension into the

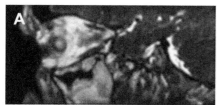
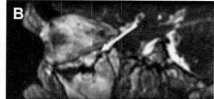

Fig. 11. (A) Sagittal precontrast CISS and (B) sagittal CE-CISS showing a small focus of enhancement (arrow) within a branch of V2 before entering the infraorbital foramen.

parotid gland, where it closely approximates the branches of the CN VII.g, acting as a main route of perineural spread of disease.[47] It is formed by 2 roots encircling the middle meningeal artery that combine and travel through the stylomandibular tunnel, supplying sensation to the nearby temporomandibular joint[45,48] (Fig. 13). The inferior alveolar nerve travels through the mandible via the mandibular foramen, giving off the mental nerve at its terminal branch along the jaw (Fig. 14). The lingual nerve branches off just medial and anterior to the inferior alveolar nerve, traveling along the medial aspect of the mandible to the floor of the mouth.

Cranial Nerve V.3.g: Selected Pathologic Abnormalities

Similar to the CN V.1 and V.2 divisions, a variety of benign and malignant entities can affect CN V.3.g. Cases of nasopharyngeal inflammatory pseudotumor,[48] peripheral metastatic mandibular lesions,[49] and rare solitary fibrous tumor involving foramen ovale[50] have all been reported. More common neurogenic tumors, including neurofibromas, schwannomas, and malignant nerve sheath tumors, may arise in the masticator space along CN V.3.g branches.[51] The presence of multiple

branches of CN V.3.g allows for extensive neural connections within the head and neck, creating opportunities for distal pathologic abnormality to spread and invade neural structures. The inferior alveolar and auriculotemporal nerves are the most frequently involved branches in the setting of perineural spread of tumor,[51] as can be seen in the setting of malignant parotid tumors (Fig. 15). Similar to CN V.1.g, cutaneous lesions such as SCC, BCC, and melanoma may spread retrograde from distal CN V.3.g branches to involve the inferior alveolar nerve.[52] The auriculotemporal nerve travels and branches within the parotid gland, and has close communication with the facial nerve branches[52]; because of the neural network, salivary gland tumors can cause perineural spread along both extra-CNs.

CRANIAL NERVE VII.g: FACIAL NERVE, ANATOMY

The facial nerve is composed of a complex combination of motor, sensory, and parasympathetic fibers. The main extraforaminal trunk exits the temporal bone at the stylomastoid foramen along the posterior belly of the digastric muscle, and then immediately into the parotid gland.[53] Just

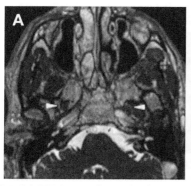
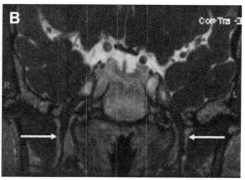

Fig. 12. (A) Axial CISS image shows the foraminal segment of V3 branch of the trigeminal nerve as it travels through the foramen ovale (arrowheads). (B) Coronal reconstructed CISS image shows the proximal extracranial course of V3 (arrows) before branching into the anterior and posterior divisions.

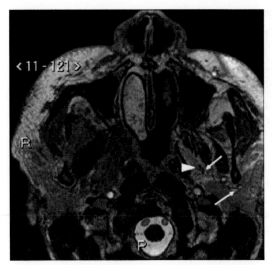

Fig. 13. Axial CISS image of the normal left auriculotemporal nerve (*white arrow*) as it travels in the retromandibular region of the parotid gland. The left lingual nerve (*arrowhead*) and inferior alveolar nerve (*yellow arrow*) are also clearly visible in the parapharyngeal space.

proximal to the parotid gland, the facial nerve gives off the posterior auricular nerve and branches to the posterior belly of the digastric and stylohyoid muscles.[3] Within the parotid gland, the facial nerve divides into the main temporofacial nerve and cervicofacial nerves that innervate the muscles of facial expression via multiple branches, including the temporal, zygomatic, buccal, marginal mandibular, and cervical branches[3,53,54] (**Fig. 16**). The ability of CISS to differentiate between multiple tissue types and characteristics, such as muscle and fat, and parenchymal tissue, such as the parotid gland, allows for striking anatomic detail.

Cranial Nerve VII.g: Selected Pathologic Abnormality

The central location of the extracranial facial nerve within the parotid gland with subsequent centripetal branching allows the parotid gland to be a main source for pathologic abnormality of CN VII.g. Perineural spread of malignancies, including salivary gland tumors, SCC, melanoma, and lymphoma, among others, can occur either via the parotid space into the facial canal, via the greater superficial petrosal nerve, or through distal superficial branches of the facial nerve. Enhancement within the buccal branch of the facial nerve may be an indicator of perineural spread in the setting of an adjacent SCC of the cheek (**Fig. 17**). Intrinsic tumors arising from the facial nerve, including schwannomas and rare entities, such as cellular

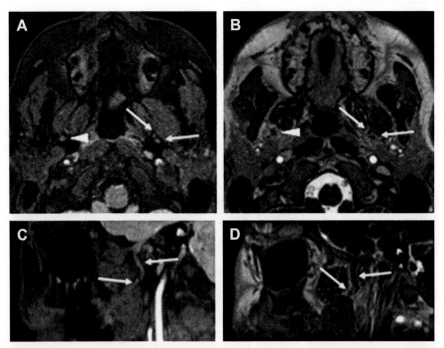

Fig. 14. Axial DESS sequence (*A*) and corresponding axial CE-CISS sequence (*B*) images at the level of the parapharyngeal space demonstrating corresponding representations of the lingual nerve (*white arrows*) and inferior alveolar nerve (*yellow arrows*). Note the contralateral posterior division of V3 (*arrowheads*) seen before branching. Sagittal reformatted DESS (*C*) and sagittal CE-CISS (*D*) show V3 giving off the inferior alveolar nerve (*yellow arrows*). A portion of the lingual nerve is seen just anteriorly (*white arrows*).

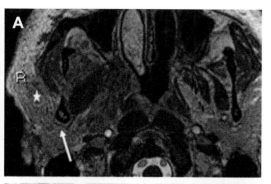

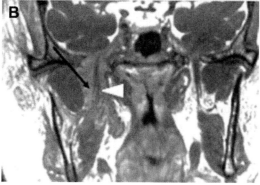

Fig. 15. (A) Axial CE-CISS images show an ill-defined enhancing mass arising from the parotid region (*star*) that extends along and engulfs the auriculotemporal branch of the right V3 nerve (*white arrow*). (B) On the coronal reformatted CE-CISS images, the infiltrating lesion is seen expanding the right parapharyngeal space. Perineural spread is also seen along the right lingual nerve (*black arrow*) and inferior alveolar nerve (*arrowhead*) branches of V3.

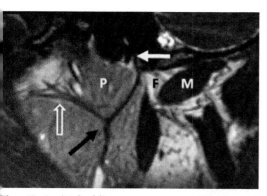

Fig. 16. Sagittal oblique postcontrast CISS through the region of the parotid gland. After exiting the stylomastoid foramen (*white solid arrow*), CN VII.g enters the parotid gland; the primary intraparotid branch point is then seen (*black arrow*), with division into the more anterior temporofacial branch (*open white arrow*) and the cervicofacial branch inferiorly. Differential tissue characteristics surrounding the CN, including fat (F), muscle (M), and parotid (P) tissue, allows for stark contrast anatomic detail.

myofibroblastic tumors (**Fig. 18**), may also involve the extracranial portion beyond the stylomastoid foramen. The isotropic high spatial resolution sequences obtained on CE-CISS can detect subtle features, including displacement of the facial nerve, which may suggest an extrinsic pathologic abnormality, such an intraparotid mass (**Fig. 19**); alternatively, CISS can also evaluate for internal enhancement or direct neural involvement by a lesion, suggesting that it originates from the facial nerve itself, such as a schwannoma (**Fig. 20**).

CRANIAL NERVE VIII

CN VIII alone does not extend beyond the skull and, for this reason, does not formally have an extraforaminal segment, rather it passes through foramina to innervate the inner ear within the temporal bone.

CRANIAL NERVES IX TO XI

Due to the close anatomic location of the extraforaminal segments of CNs IX to XI, they are discussed here together, with particular emphasis on the vagus nerve.

Cranial Nerve IX.g: Anatomy

The glossopharyngeal nerve exits the skull base via the jugular foramen in the pars nervosa,[3,55] subsequently giving off the carotid, pharyngeal, tonsillar, lingual, and muscular branches.

Cranial Nerve X.g: Vagus Nerve, Anatomy

The vagus nerve has the largest craniocaudal extent, spanning from the skull base through the neck and into the upper thorax carrying motor, sensory, and parasympathetic fibers. The extraforaminal segment begins at the outer limits of the jugular foramen and descends into the neck within the carotid sheath, where it is located posteriorly between the common carotid artery (CCA) and internal jugular vein (IJV) (**Fig. 21**).[56] Along its course, the CN X.g gives off multiple branches, including the recurrent laryngeal nerves.

Cranial Nerve XI.g: Spinal Accessory, Anatomy

The extraforaminal segment of the accessory nerve exits the jugular foramen. The motor spinal root innervates the sternocleidomastoid and trapezius, whereas the cranial root ascends toward the inferior vagal ganglion.[56]

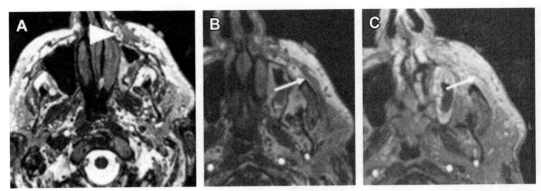

Fig. 17. (A) CE-CISS demonstrating SCC of the skin along the nasal fold (*arrowhead*). (B) Precontrast CISS shows thickening of the buccal branch (*arrow*) of the facial nerve. (C) Postcontrast CISS shows corresponding enhancement, compatible with perineural tumor spread (*arrow*).

Cranial Nerves IX.g, X.g, and XI.g: Selected Pathologic Abnormalities

The close anatomic location of CNs IX to XI often lead to symptoms affecting these nerves together from a single pathologic abnormality. Miscellaneous causes include vascular lesions, traumatic and iatrogenic injury, and infection.[57] Mass lesions of the jugular foramen may also simultaneously cause CNs IX to XI palsy, given their common foraminal course; these lesions include schwannomas, paragangliomas, and meningiomas.[58] Paragangliomas, or glomus tumors, arise from residual paraganglionic tissue; glomus jugulare and vagale are differentiated by the location of the paraganglionic rests.[3,58]

These lesions tend to be highly vascular, often exhibiting large internal flow voids, and may cause aggressive-appearing osseous changes. Their paraganglionic origin results in displacement rather than direct involvement of the nerve (Fig. 22). Schwannomas on the other hand are more homogeneous, although they may undergo degenerative fatty, cystic, and hemorrhagic changes,[59] and may cause expansion of the jugular foramen with surrounding sclerotic osseous changes.[57–60] Meningiomas may also cause expansion and remodeling of the jugular foramen with encasement of vessels and nerves. Determining the nerve of origin may be challenging; however, identifying the lesion's location and relationship to surrounding vascular and

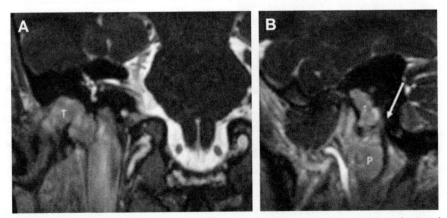

Fig. 18. (A) Coronal CE-CISS image shows a heterogeneous enhancing lesion (T) lateral to the jugular vein. (B) Sagittal reformatted image shows the extracranial portion of the facial nerve exiting the stylomastoid foramen before branching within the parotid (P) gland. The most superior portion of the nerve is in close relation to the lesion and demonstrates a faint degree of enhancement (*arrow*), suggesting invasion. The patient underwent successful surgical resection with preservation of the nerve that confirmed minor nerve involvement by tumor. Pathologic assessment revealed a rare entity: cellular myofibroblastic tumor.

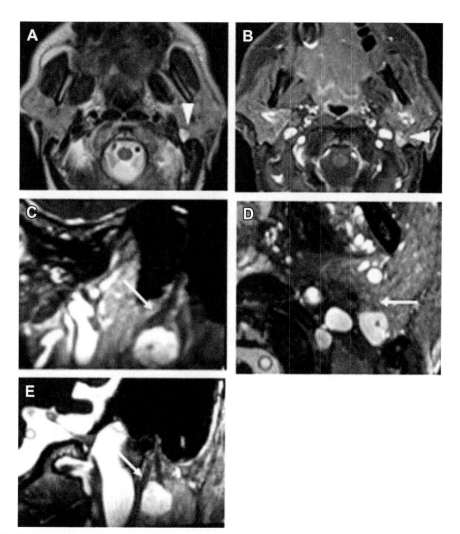

Fig. 19. (*A, B*) Conventional 2D MR imaging T2 and T1 postcontrast sequences demonstrate a T2 hyperintense and enhancing lesion (*arrowheads*). Sagittal (*C*), axial (*D*), and coronal (*E*) postcontrast CISS images demonstrate displacement of CN VII (*arrows*) superiorly, anteriorly, and medially along the margin of the lesion, suggesting that the tumor is originating from outside CN VII from the parotid gland. Biopsy confirmed the presence of a pleomorphic adenoma.

neural structures serves as diagnostic clues. For example, because CN X.g travels posteriorly in the carotid sheath between the carotid artery and IJV, CN X.g schwannomas may separate the CCA or internal carotid artery (ICA) and IJV[61,62]; cervical plexus schwannomas, because of their posterior and slightly medial location in the region of the carotid space, displace the vessels anteriorly and a little laterally.

CE-CISS can provide useful information in evaluating extracranial lesions of these CNs. This is especially true when a lesion is small without characteristic imaging features. The relationship of the lesion to the surrounding structures, in particular the adjacent vessels, and determining its origin, either intrinsically from or extrinsically compressing the nerve, can prove crucial to making the correct diagnosis.

Cranial Nerve XII.g: Hypoglossal Nerve, Anatomy

The extraforaminal hypoglossal nerve emerges from the hypoglossal canal surrounded by a venous plexus.[63] It then travels in the carotid space between the ICA and along with the vagus nerve.[3] CN XII.g exits the carotid space at the level of the mandible, supplying pure motor innervation to the intrinsic and extrinsic muscles of the tongue. Communication exists between CN XII.g and the

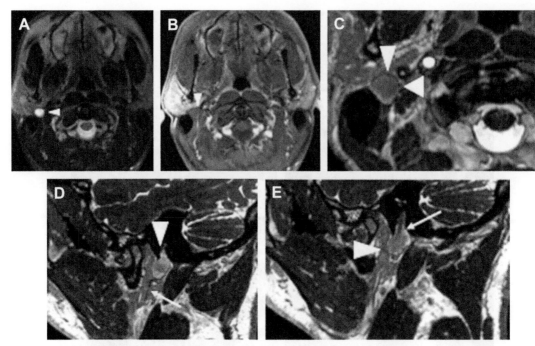

Fig. 20. (*A, B*) Conventional 2D T2-weighted and postcontrast images show a T2 hyperintense and mildly enhancing mass (*arrowhead*) in the region of the facial nerve and stylomastoid foramen. Differential considerations include a schwannoma and pleomorphic adenoma, given the location. Higher resolution 3D CISS imaging was performed to evaluate the relationship with CN VII. (*C*) CE-CISS shows the enhancing lesion (*arrowheads*) inferior to the stylomastoid foramen. (*D, E*) In sagittal reformatted images, the lesion (*arrowheads*) appears to arise directly from CN VII (*arrow*) without evidence of displacement. Findings are most consistent with a schwannoma.

inferior ganglion of the CN X.g, as well as the lingual nerve (a branch of CN V.3.g) at the level of the tongue[64]

CRANIAL NERVE XII:g: SELECTED PATHOLOGIC ABNORMALITY

CN XII.g can be affected anywhere along its course to produce classic symptoms of CN XII palsy, tongue weakness on protrusion, with particular pathologic abnormalities having a predilection for particular segments of the nerve. Given the location of CN XII.g, it has an extensive course in the head and neck, and it can be involved in

malignant processes originating from any of these spaces, including SCC; salivary gland tumors; such as adenoid cystic carcinoma[63,65]; and lymphoma, which may cause invasion of the nerve and/or perineural spread. Other causes of CN XII palsy include infection, demyelinating disorders, traumatic injury, and vascular abnormalities, including aneurysms within the carotid space[3,66]

Lesions involving the hypoglossal canal include paragangliomas, lymphoma, osseous lesions, chordomas, nerve sheath tumors, and metastases.[67] These should be accurately differentiated from each another. Of the head and neck schwannomas that make up to 25% to

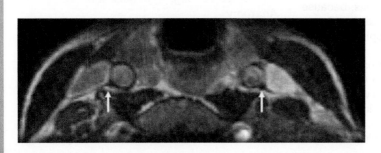

Fig. 21. Axial CISS images showing the location of the vagus nerves (*arrows*) within the carotid sheath, posterior to and in between the CCA and IJV.

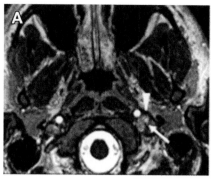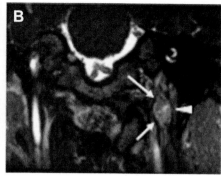

Fig. 22. (*A*) Axial CE-CISS image shows an enhancing lesion (*arrowhead*) displacing the carotid artery and IJV. The vagus nerve is also seen along the margin of the mass (*arrow*). Dots in (*A*) represent vasculature. (*B*) Coronal reformatted CE-CISS shows the enhancing mass (*arrowhead*) displacing the left vagus nerve medially (*arrows*). Findings suggest a glomus vagale tumor.

45% of all schwannomas,[68] most involve CN X.g or cervical plexus with very few originating from CN XII.g.[69,70]

SUMMARY

This article describes the normal high-resolution anatomy and appearance of several featured CNs, with specific emphasis on the extraforaminal portions. The superior visibility of many distal extraforaminal branches of these CNs on CISS sequences allows for assessment of involvement of these distal branches by pathologic assessment. The high signal-to-noise ratio, along with high spatial resolution with isotropic 3D images that can be reconstructed in multiple planes, makes this sequence superior to conventional 2D MR imaging sequences, as well as the high-resolution T1-weighted postcontrast sequences in current use. Contrast enhancement is an additional feature that can help diagnose and evaluate the extent of pathologic involvement. Crucial to accurate diagnosis is the relationship of a particular pathologic abnormality to the native CN, as highlighted in many previous examples. Abnormal enhancement of a CN or direct extension of a lesion from a particular CN are strong indicators of an intrinsic mass arising from or involving a particular CN. Displacement of the CN or a lesion clearly arising from a site adjacent or external to the CN is suggestive of an alternative extrinsic pathologic abnormality.

REFERENCES

1. Blitz AM, Choudhri AF, Chonka ZD, et al. Anatomic considerations, nomenclature, and advanced cross-sectional imaging techniques for visualization of the cranial nerve segments by MR imaging. Neuroimaging Clin N Am 2014;24(1):1–15.

2. Blitz AM, Macedo LL, Chonka ZD, et al. High-resolution CISS MR imaging with and without contrast for evaluation of the upper cranial nerves: segmental anatomy and selected pathologic conditions of the cisternal through extra-foraminal segments. Neuroimaging Clin N Am 2014;24(1):17–34.

3. Soldatos T, Batra K, Blitz AM, et al. Lower cranial nerves. Neuroimaging Clin N Am 2014;24(1):35–47.

4. Blitz AM, Aygun N, Herzka DA, et al. High resolution three-dimensional MR imaging of the skull base: compartments, boundaries, and critical structures. Radiol Clin North Am 2017;55(1):17–30.

5. Shigematsu Y, Korogi Y, Hirai T, et al. Contrast-enhanced CISS MRI of vestibular schwannomas: phantom and clinical studies. J Comput Assist Tomogr 1999;23(2):224–31.

6. Chavhan GB, Babyn PS, Jankharia BG, et al. Steady-state MR imaging sequences: physics, classification, and clinical applications. Radiographics 2008;28(4):1147–60.

7. Zhang Z, Meng Q, Chen Y, et al. 3-T imaging of the cranial nerves using three-dimensional reversed FISP with diffusion-weighted MR sequence. J Magn Reson Imaging 2008;27(3):454–8.

8. Qin Y, Zhang J, Li P, et al. 3D double-echo steady-state with water excitation MR imaging of the intraparotid facial nerve at 1.5T: a pilot study. AJNR Am J Neuroradiol 2011;32(7):1167–72.

9. Aiken AH, Mukherjee P, Green AJ, et al. MR imaging of optic neuropathy with extended echo-train acquisition fluid-attenuated inversion recovery. AJNR Am J Neuroradiol 2011;32(2):301–5.

10. Pollock JM, Greiner FG, Crowder JB, et al. Neurosarcoidosis mimicking a malignant optic glioma. J Neuroophthalmol 2008;28(3):214–6.

11. Millar WS, Tartaglino LM, Sergott RC, et al. MR of malignant optic glioma of adulthood. AJNR Am J Neuroradiol 1995;16(8):1673–6.

12. Ettl A, Zwrtek K, Daxer A, et al. Anatomy of the orbital apex and cavernous sinus on high-resolution magnetic resonance images. Surv Ophthalmol 2000;44(4):303–23.

13. Engel JM. Treatment and diagnosis of congenital fourth nerve palsies: an update. Curr Opin Ophthalmol 2015;26(5):353–6.

14. Kau H-C, Tsai C-C, Ortube MC, et al. High-resolution magnetic resonance imaging of the extraocular muscles and nerves demonstrates various etiologies of third nerve palsy. Am J Ophthalmol 2007;143(2):280–7.

15. Tamhankar MA, Volpe NJ. Management of acute cranial nerve 3, 4 and 6 palsies: role of neuroimaging. Curr Opin Ophthalmol 2015;26(6):464–8.

16. Kung NH, Van Stavern GP. Isolated ocular motor nerve palsies. Semin Neurol 2015;35(5):539–48.

17. Tantiwongkosi B, Hesselink JR. Imaging of ocular motor pathway. Neuroimaging Clin N Am 2015;25(3):425–38.

18. Wani NA, Jehangir M, Lone PA. Tolosa-hunt syndrome demonstrated by constructive interference steady state magnetic resonance imaging. J Ophthalmic Vis Res 2017;12(1):106–9.

19. García-Zamora M, Sánchez-Tocino H, Villanueva-Gómez A, et al. Isolated fourth nerve palsy in tuberculous meningitis. Neuroophthalmology 2016;40(1):40–3.

20. Ahlawat A, Jun-O'Connell A, Salameh J. Pearls & Oy-sters: an isolated cranial nerve 6 palsy as a presentation of polycythemia vera. Neurology 2015;85(11):e85–7.

21. Cantore WA. Neural orbital tumors. Curr Opin Ophthalmol 2000;11(5):367–71.

22. Cho Y-H, Sung K-S, Song Y-J, et al. Oculomotor nerve schwannoma: a case report. Brain Tumor Res Treat 2014;2(1):43–7.

23. Ohata K, Takami T, Goto T, et al. Schwannoma of the oculomotor nerve. Neurol India 2006;54(4):437–9.

24. Wang Q-J, Guo Y, Zhang Y, et al. 3D MRI of oculomotor nerve schwannoma in the prepontine cistern: a case report. Clin Imaging 2013;37(5):947–9.

25. Younes WM, Hermann EJ, Krauss JK. Cisternal trochlear nerve schwannoma: improvement of diplopia after subtotal tumour excision. Br J Neurosurg 2012;26(1):107–9.

26. Sanchez Dalmau BF. Young boy with progressive double vision. Surv Ophthalmol 1998;43(1):47–52.

27. Yang S-S, Li Z-J, Liu X, et al. Pediatric isolated oculomotor nerve schwannoma: a new case report and literature review. Pediatr Neurol 2013;48(4):321–4.

28. Kauser H, Rashid O, Anwar W, et al. Orbital oculomotor nerve schwannoma extending to the cavernous sinus: a rare cause of proptosis. J Ophthalmic Vis Res 2014;9(4):514–6.

29. Chaudhry NS, Ahmad FU, Morcos JJ. Pineal region schwannoma arising from the trochlear nerve. J Clin Neurosci 2016;32:159–61.

30. Elmalem VI, Younge BR, Biousse V, et al. Clinical course and prognosis of trochlear nerve schwannomas. Ophthalmology 2009;116(10):2011–6.

31. Irace C, Davì G, Corona C, et al. Isolated intraorbital schwannoma arising from the abducens nerve. Acta Neurochir 2008;150(11):1209–10.

32. Feichtinger M, Reinbacher KE, Pau M, et al. Intraorbital Schwannoma of the abducens nerve: case report. J Oral Maxillofac Surg 2013;71(2):443–5.

33. Bendszus M, Beck A, Koltzenburg M, et al. MRI in isolated sixth nerve palsies. Neuroradiology 2001;43(9):742–5.

34. Murchison AP, Gilbert ME, Savino PJ. Neuroimaging and acute ocular motor mononeuropathies: a prospective study. Arch Ophthalmol 2011;129(3):301–5.

35. Shah K, Esmaeli B, Ginsberg LE. Perineural tumor spread along the nasociliary branch of the ophthalmic nerve: imaging findings. J Comput Assist Tomogr 2013;37(2):282–5.

36. Badger D, Aygun N. Imaging of perineural spread in head and neck cancer. Radiol Clin North Am 2017;55(1):139–49.

37. Eneh A, Parsa K, Wright KW, et al. Pediatric adenoid cystic carcinoma of the lacrimal gland treated with intra-arterial cytoreductive chemotherapy. J AAPOS 2015;19(3):272–4.

38. Mardi K, Kaushal V, Uppal H. Cytodiagnosis of intracranial metastatic adenoid cystic carcinoma: Spread from a primary tumor in the lacrimal gland. J Cytol 2011;28(4):200–2.

39. Williams LS, Schmalfuss IM, Sistrom CL, et al. MR imaging of the trigeminal ganglion, nerve, and the perineural vascular plexus: normal appearance and variants with correlation to cadaver specimens. AJNR Am J Neuroradiol 2003;24(7):1317–23.

40. Yousry I, Moriggl B, Schmid UD, et al. Trigeminal ganglion and its divisions: detailed anatomic MR imaging with contrast-enhanced 3D constructive interference in the steady state sequences. AJNR Am J Neuroradiol 2005;26(5):1128–35.

41. Singh FM, Mak SY, Bonington SC. Patterns of spread of head and neck adenoid cystic carcinoma. Clin Radiol 2015;70(6):644–53.

42. Ferri A, Bergonzani M, Varazzani A, et al. Inflammatory Pseudotumor of the Infraorbital Nerve: A Rare Diagnosis to Be Aware of. J Craniofac Surg 2016;27(6):e554–7.

43. Francis M, Subramanian K, Sankari SL, et al. Herpes Zoster with Post Herpetic Neuralgia Involving the Right Maxillary Branch of Trigeminal Nerve: A Case Report and Review of Literature. J Clin Diagn Res 2017;11(1):ZD40–2.

44. Mazziotti S, Gaeta M, Blandino A, et al. Perineural spread in a case of sinonasal sarcoidosis: case report. AJNR Am J Neuroradiol 2001;22(6):1207–8.

45. Shah AT, Dagher WI, O'Leary MA, et al. Squamous cell carcinoma presenting with trigeminal anesthesia: an uncommon presentation of head & neck cancer with unknown primary. Am J Otolaryngol 2017;38(2):153–6.

46. Williams LS. Advanced concepts in the imaging of perineural spread of tumor to the trigeminal nerve. Top Magn Reson Imaging 1999;10(6):376–83.

47. Gandhi M, Sommerville J. The imaging of large nerve perineural spread. J Neurol Surg B Skull Base 2016;77(2):113–23.

48. Gadde J, Franck B, Liu X, et al. Inflammatory pseudotumor of the nasopharynx with spread along the trigeminal nerve. Am J Otolaryngol 2013;34(3):252–4.

49. Tejani N, Cooper A, Rezo A, et al. Numb chin syndrome: a case series of a clinical syndrome associated with malignancy. J Med Imaging Radiat Oncol 2014;58(6):700–5.

50. Motoori K, Hanazawa T, Yamakami I, et al. Intra- and extracranial solitary fibrous tumor of the trigeminal nerve: CT and MR imaging appearance. AJNR Am J Neuroradiol 2010;31(2):280–1.

51. Fernandes T, Lobo JC, Castro R, et al. Anatomy and pathology of the masticator space. Insights Imaging 2013;4(5):605–16.

52. Laine FJ, Braun IF, Jensen ME, et al. Perineural tumor extension through the foramen ovale: evaluation with MR imaging. Radiology 1990;174(1):65–71.

53. Cassetta M, Barchetti F, Pranno N, et al. High resolution 3-T MR imaging in the evaluation of the facial nerve course. G Chir 2014;35(1–2):15–9.

54. Raghavan P, Mukherjee S, Phillips CD. Imaging of the facial nerve. Neuroimaging Clin N Am 2009;19(3):407–25.

55. Rubinstein D, Burton BS, Walker AL. The anatomy of the inferior petrosal sinus, glossopharyngeal nerve, vagus nerve, and accessory nerve in the jugular foramen. AJNR Am J Neuroradiol 1995;16(1):185–94.

56. Lee JH, Cheng K-L, Choi YJ, et al. High-resolution Imaging of Neural Anatomy and Pathology of the Neck. Korean J Radiol 2017;18(1):180–93.

57. Gunbey HP, Kutlar G, Aslan K, et al. Magnetic resonance imaging evidence of varicella zoster virus polyneuropathy: involvement of the glossopharyngeal and vagus nerves associated with Ramsay Hunt syndrome. J Craniofac Surg 2016;27(3):721–3.

58. Makiese O, Chibbaro S, Marsella M, et al. Jugular foramen paragangliomas: management, outcome and avoidance of complications in a series of 75 cases. Neurosurg Rev 2012;35(2):185–94 [discussion: 194].

59. Sharma DK, Sohal BS, Parmar TL, et al. Schwannomas of head and neck and review of literature. Indian J Otolaryngol Head Neck Surg 2012;64(2):177–80.

60. Yasumatsu R, Nakashima T, Miyazaki R, et al. Diagnosis and management of extracranial head and neck schwannomas: a review of 27 cases. Int J Otolaryngol 2013;2013:973045.

61. Furukawa M, Furukawa MK, Katoh K, et al. Differentiation between schwannoma of the vagus nerve and schwannoma of the cervical sympathetic chain by imaging diagnosis. Laryngoscope 1996;106(12 Pt 1):1548–52.

62. Saito DM, Glastonbury CM, El-Sayed IH, et al. Parapharyngeal space schwannomas: preoperative imaging determination of the nerve of origin. Arch Otolaryngol Head Neck Surg 2007;133(7):662–7.

63. Alves P. Imaging the hypoglossal nerve. Eur J Radiol 2010;74(2):368–77.

64. Lin HC, Barkhaus PE. Cranial nerve XII: the hypoglossal nerve. Semin Neurol 2009;29(1):45–52.

65. Wee HE, Azhar R, Tang PY, et al. Diagnostic pitfall: adenoid cystic carcinoma of the tongue presenting as an isolated hypoglossal nerve palsy, case report and literature review. Int J Surg Case Rep 2016;25:102–5.

66. Learned KO, Thaler ER, O'Malley BW Jr, et al. Hypoglossal nerve palsy missed and misinterpreted: the hidden skull base. J Comput Assist Tomogr 2012;36(6):718–24.

67. Gursoy M, Orru E, Blitz AM, et al. Hypoglossal canal invasion by glomus jugulare tumors: clinicoradiological correlation. Clin Imaging 2014;38(5):655–8.

68. Ram H, Agrawal SP, Husain N, et al. Hypoglossal schwannoma of parapharyngeal space: an unusual case report. J Maxillofac Oral Surg 2015;14(Suppl 1):73–6.

69. Illuminati G, Pizzardi G, Pasqua R, et al. Schwannoma of the descending loop of the hypoglossal nerve: Case report. Int J Surg Case Rep 2017;34:20–2.

70. Oyama H, Kito A, Maki H, et al. Schwannoma originating from lower cranial nerves: report of 4 cases. Nagoya J Med Sci 2012;74(1–2):199–206.

Diffusion-Weighted Imaging in Head and Neck Cancer
Technique, Limitations, and Applications

Michael Connolly, MD[a], Ashok Srinivasan, MD[b],*

KEYWORDS

- Diffusion-weighted imaging • Intravoxel incoherent motion • Apparent diffusion coefficient
- Head and neck cancer • Head and neck squamous cell carcinoma (HNSCC)

KEY POINTS

- Diffusion-weighted imaging (DWI) of head and neck represents a distinct method of MR imaging with far ranging current and potential applications.
- New and better technology, scanners, and software have allowed DWI to become available across the globe.
- Research continues to hone the capabilities of DWI in characterization, prediction, monitoring, assessing response to treatment, and detecting posttreatment and recurrent changes.
- Pretreatment apparent diffusion coefficient values can suggest the likelihood of response to treatment, and delineate certain malignant masses from one another.

INTRODUCTION

The roots of diffusion-weighted imaging (DWI) of the head and neck owe their origin to the liver, where Turner and Le Bihan first hoped to use DWI to distinguish benign versus malignant lesions. DWI is an MR imaging sequence that measures the diffusion of water molecules in human tissues and attempts to assess the intrinsic cellularity of tissues by using the diffusion values as a surrogate marker for tissue cellularity. The amount of signal loss depends on the diffusion of water, and the intensity of that signal depends largely on the *b*-value of the diffusion encoding gradients. One of the factors contributing to this signal loss is the flow of water molecules through vascular structures such as capillaries. To this end, intravoxel incoherent motion (IVIM) is a technique used to account for the underlying perfusion, allowing the separation of perfusion and diffusion effects.

Although early studies and findings led DWI to the brain and detection of acute stroke, recent advancement in MR imaging technology has made routine use of DWI a widespread reality with use throughout the body. In the past 25 years, DWI has become more practical in its acquisition as higher performance field gradients have been introduced. The advent of echo planar imaging and IVIM allows for the rapid acquisition necessary to collect DWI data with significant reduction in motion artifact. Echo planar imaging has allowed DWI to branch out beyond the confines of brain imaging to head and neck, where limitations existed to good quality DWI owing to geometric variations in contour and patient motion (eg, swallowing). In addition, revisions to postprocessing software have also allowed for easier feasibility.

[a] Department of Radiology, University of Michigan, 1500 East Medical Center Drive, Ann Arbor, MI 48109, USA;
[b] Division of Neuroradiology, Department of Radiology, University of Michigan, 1500 East Medical Center Drive, Ann Arbor, MI 48109, USA
* Corresponding author.
E-mail address: ashoks@med.umich.edu

Magn Reson Imaging Clin N Am 26 (2018) 121–133
https://doi.org/10.1016/j.mric.2017.08.011
1064-9689/18/© 2017 Elsevier Inc. All rights reserved.

mri.theclinics.com

In simplistic terms, the data from a DWI sequence are used to quantify the average magnitude of diffusion for a specific voxel, and within each voxel this can be expressed as a metric called apparent diffusion coefficient (ADC). Although there are many factors that can influence the ADC of a voxel, it is generally accepted that the ADC of a voxel is inversely proportional to the cellularity of the tissue represented by that voxel. Therefore, highly cellular tissues typically restrict free diffusion of water, and would thus have a lower ADC owing to relatively decreased extracellular space and increased area of cell membranes that act as a boundary for water diffusion. Chen and colleagues[1] discussed the available research showing that higher ADC values for a specific voxel do in fact correlate with lower cellularity.

It is well-known that MR imaging can characterize tissues better than computed tomography owing to higher contrast resolution, and this is also applicable to head and neck mass characterization. DWI adds another dimension to conventional MR imaging sequences owing to its ability to act as a potential marker for tissue cellularity. We discuss how this underlying principle can potentially be used to characterize head and neck lesions as either benign or malignant, predict the response of head and neck cancer to various types of treatment, monitor tumor to determine the effectiveness of treatment, and determine whether a residual mass detected after treatment represents scar or recurrence.

TECHNIQUES

Routine DWI in the head and neck is performed as a single shot echo planar technique owing to its shorter acquisition time. There are advantages and disadvantages to performing both echo planar and non–echo planar diffusion techniques that are explained in detail.

Echo Planar Diffusion

Owing to its relative insensitivity to motion, echo planar diffusion is widely used for head and neck imaging. Single shot and multi shot echo planar sequences differ in the number of repetition times used for filling K-space, with the former using 1 repetition alone to fill K-space and the latter using many repetitions. The single shot technique, although shorter in acquisition time, suffers from greater susceptibility effects, geometric distortion, and reduced spatial resolution, which are all improved with the multishot technique.

Non–Echo Planar Diffusion

Non–echo planar diffusion can provide further improvement in image quality with lesser susceptibility artifacts and higher spatial resolution but take longer to acquire than echo planar diffusion (which can introduce more motions artifacts on the images owing to both gross patient motion and intrinsic visceral motion like vessel pulsatility) and have lower signal-to-noise ratio, which necessitates multiple averages and prolongs scanning time. Hence, non–echo planar diffusion is usually reserved for problem solving rather than routine clinical practice.

CLINICAL APPLICATIONS
Benign Versus Malignant

Biopsy with pathologic examination remains the gold standard for assessing the malignant potential of a head and neck lesion. However, tissue sampling in the head and neck is not without risk, and certain regions of head and neck are difficult or relatively impossible to access.

Multiple studies have tested the ability and reliability of DW in characterizing the malignant potential of a lesion based on ADC measurement. These were based on the hypothesis that malignant tumors would demonstrate lower ADC values compared with benign tumors owing to their relatively higher cellularity. Wang and colleagues[2] demonstrated that benign and malignant lesions at multiple sites in the head and neck (including parotids, thyroid, parathyroid, nasal cavity, lymph nodes) yielded significantly different ADC values, and when an ADC value of 1.22×10^{-3} mm^2/s was used to categorize lesions as benign (above the cutoff) or malignant (below the cutoff), the investigators were able to do so with an accuracy of 86%, sensitivity of 84%, and specificity of 91%.

In the orbit, Razek and colleagues[3] demonstrated an ADC cutoff value of 1.15×10^{-3} mm^2/s to distinguish benign from malignant tumors. This study yielded a sensitivity of 95%, a specificity of 91%, and an accuracy of 93%.

Similarly, Srinivasan and colleagues[4] compared 33 patients with head and neck masses on a 3T magnet and found that there was a significant difference between benign and malignant lesions, with the latter showing lower ADC values than the former. In their study, the threshold value of 1.3×10^{-3} mm^2/s provided the best differentiation.

Although these studies demonstrate the usefulness of ADC, it remains unclear whether there is a specific threshold that is applicable in different magnet strengths and with different 'b' values.

Hence, it may be better to use an internal reference standard, such as the adjacent brainstem or spinal cord to determine whether a lesion may be benign or malignant; those that seem to be darker on the ADC map than the brainstem and spinal cord can be expected to have higher cellularity and hence more likely malignant. Larger studies are, however, required before this method can be implemented in routine clinical practice. **Figs. 1–3** illustrate the differences in ADC maps between benign and malignant tumors and also emphasize why it is important to interpret ADC maps along with conventional MR images.

Furthermore, when initially imaging a patient for the workup of a head and neck lesion, a concomitant survey of surrounding lymph nodes would give radiologists, surgeons, and oncologists the data to locally stage, or at least definitively identify a metastatic lymph node for tissue sampling. In a study conducted by Abdel Razek and colleagues,[5] the usefulness of MR imaging evaluation of cervical lymphadenopathy to differentiate nodal metastases found that metastatic and lymphomatous lymph nodes had significantly lower mean ADC values than those of benign cervical lymph nodes. In this study, a threshold ADC value of 1.38×10^{-3} mm^2/s was chosen and when applied to the data, an accuracy of 96%, sensitivity of 98%, specificity of 88%, positive predictive value of 98.5%, and negative predictive value of 83.7% was achieved; the smallest lymph node able to be defined as metastatic measured 0.9 cm. **Fig. 4** illustrates the usefulness of DWI in lymph node imaging.

With regard to characterization of parotid tumors, Abdel Razek and colleagues[6] demonstrated that benign and malignant parotid masses showed significant difference in their mean ADC values, in keeping with prior studies of other head and neck lesions. When using a threshold ADC value of $(1.07 \times 10^{-3}$ mm^2/s) the authors achieved an accuracy of 77.1%, sensitivity of 88.9%, and specificity of 70%. It is important to note that an earlier study by Yerli and colleagues[7] found that, with respect to the MR imaging characterization of parotid tumors, the addition of DWI sequences added no value to diagnostic accuracy.

In terms of technique, Vidiri and colleagues[8] demonstrated that using a reduced field of view when imaging parotid and submandibular gland tumors, lymphoma, and metastatic lymph nodes of the head and neck allowed to significantly increase the accuracy of ADC measurements; such variations in technique will likely aid future studies and raises the potential for the widespread application of DWI for ADC characterization.

The potential of DWI is not just limited to differentiating benign versus malignant head and neck lesions; in some instances, DWI can help to distinguish different malignant tumors. **Fig. 5** demonstrates DWI and ADC maps in a patient with proven lymphoma. Driessen and colleagues[9] found that, in head and neck squamous cell cancer, positive human papillomavirus (HPV) status correlates with low mean ADC when compared with non-HPV squamous cell cancer. The favorable prognostic value of low pretreatment ADC might be partially attributed to patients with an

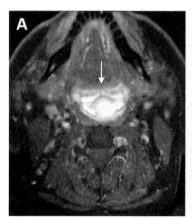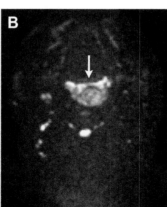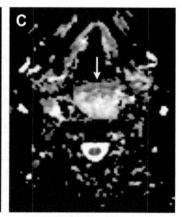

Fig. 1. Gadolinium-enhanced T1-weighted axial image (*A*) in a 63-year-old man with stridor and airway obstruction demonstrates a large enhancing mass (*arrow*) in the region of the tongue base. Although the corresponding trace diffusion image (*B*) shows increased signal (*arrow*), the apparent diffusion coefficient (ADC) map (*C*) shows high values, suggesting this is T2 shine-through (*arrow*). This was a biopsy-proven chronic inflammatory lesion. ADC values can help to distinguish benign and malignant neck lesions, with the latter typically demonstrating low ADC values owing to their hypercellularity.

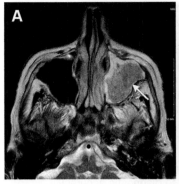 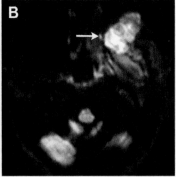 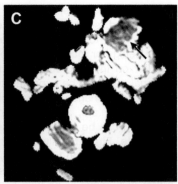

Fig. 2. Axial T2-weighted image (*A*) in a 48-year-old man demonstrates a large T2 hypointense mass (*arrow*) in the left maxillary sinus. There is high signal on the corresponding trace diffusion image (*B, arrow*) and low values on the apparent diffusion coefficient map (*C, arrow*), which are features suggestive of a hypercellular lesion such as a malignancy. Biopsy revealed a sinonasal squamous cell carcinoma.

HPV-positive status, which itself has a better prognosis than HPV-negative cancers. Given distinct differences in treatment response of HPV-positive and HPV-negative cancers, this distinction may lead to customization of treatment based on MR imaging findings.

As in other fields of medicine, there are exceptions to the general rule that ADC is low in malignant lesions and high in benign lesions. For instance, hypercellular benign tumors such as paragangliomas can demonstrate low ADC values (**Fig. 6**) and low-grade malignancies such as certain mucoepidermoid cancers in the parotid glands can demonstrate high ADC values. Therefore, it is important to always interpret the DWI images in conjunction with conventional MR imaging sequences. **Fig. 7** illustrates how DWI can be helpful in identifying skull base metastatic disease.

Prediction of Treatment Response

As stated, the findings from Driessen and colleagues[9] are part of another contribution DWI can make toward characterizing and defining head and neck masses; several past and current studies have explored the ability of DWI to predict a tumor's response to treatment before intervention.

Guo and colleagues[10] found that, when comparing treatment responders with nonresponders, a notably lower pretreatment ADC value, and D value (IVIM derived biexponential diffusion coefficient) were found in responders, as well as a higher posttreatment ADC; they concluded that lower pretreatment ADC value correlated with response to therapy.

Hatakenaka and colleagues[11] demonstrated a significant correlation between ADC, regional control, disease-free survival, and overall survival using certain b-values when ADC was examined as a sole prognostic factor. Furthermore, Kim and colleagues[12] found that complete responders to treatment had significantly lower ADC values than partial responders before treatment; when pretreatment ADC value was used to predict treatment response, the authors achieved a sensitivity of 65% and a specificity of 86%. Srinivasan and colleagues[13] further evaluated predictive value of ADC in head and neck squamous cell carcinoma (HNSCC), where they found that lesions with lower pretreatment ADC and more than 45% of their volume below a threshold of 1.15×10^{-3} mm^2/s had better response to chemoradiation 2 years after treatment.

Hauser and colleagues[14] used IVIM analyses of lymph node metastases to show that with regards to HNSCC, an elevated perfusion fraction (or *f*-value) at baseline examination may predict locoregional failure after treatment. Their results found that a high initial *f*-value in lymph nodes may predict poor treatment response in patients with HNSCC, namely locoregional failure.

Despite no apparent significant difference in ADC values between normal thyroid tissues and parathyroid cancers, Lu and colleagues[15] demonstrated that ADC values of parathyroid cancers without extrathyroidal extension were significantly higher than those that had extended beyond the thyroid. In addition, by using ADC values, 3 study patients were found to have extrathyroidal extension when ultrasound imaging had characterized their lesions as fit for observation. Ng and colleagues[16] found that ADC values are independent pretreatment prognostic factors for neck control in oropharyngeal and hypopharyngeal squamous cell carcinomas treated with chemoradiation.

It should be noted that some studies, for example, Huang and colleagues,[17] found no difference among pretreatment minimum ADC of the

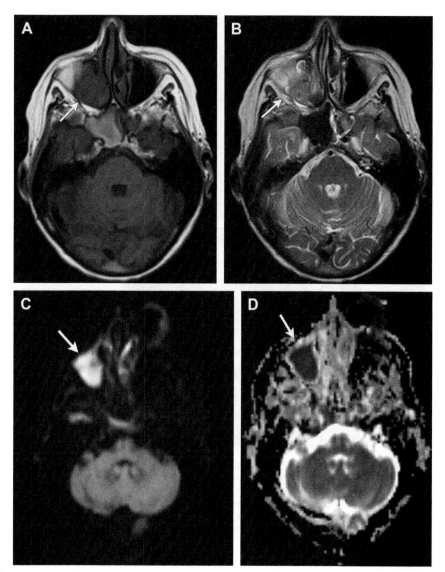

Fig. 3. Diffusion images should always be interpreted along with conventional images because there can be overlap of diffusion characteristics between benign and malignant neck pathologies. In this example, inspissated secretions (*arrow*) within the right maxillary sinus demonstrate low signal on both T1-weighted images (*A*) and T2-weighted images (*B*), and on corresponding high diffusion signal (*C, arrow*) and low apparent diffusion coefficient values (*D, arrow*) owing to dehydration resulting in reduced water mobility. Contrast-enhanced sequences can help distinguish tumors from inspissated secretions. Typically, tumors show homogenous or heterogenous enhancement, whereas inspissated secretions show peripheral enhancement reflecting the mucosal margin.

progressive disease group and that of the complete response and partial response groups. Other authors[15,16] also failed to demonstrate a significant correlation between pretreatment ADC and treatment response.

Despite such limitations, it is important for us to continue to explore the role played by ADC in prediction of treatment response, guide treatment strategies, and assess the overall prognosis.

Monitoring of Treatment Response

With so many different potential malignancies of the head and neck, and corresponding treatment, DWI may represent an avenue to quantify and serially assess the response of a tumor to treatment. Once treatment has commenced, be it radiation, chemotherapy, or a combination of both, it is desirable for radiation and medical oncologists to not only assess whether the treatment is effective, but also to quantify its efficacy and tailor further

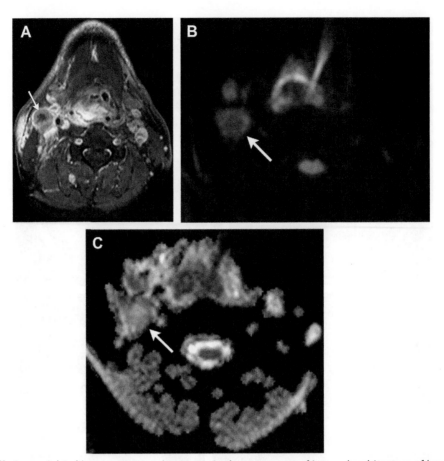

Fig. 4. Diffusion-weighted images are complementary in the assessment of internal architecture of lymph nodes. Axial gadolinium enhanced T1-weighted image (*A*) in a 55-year-old man with hypopharyngeal squamous cell carcinoma shows a centrally necrotic right level II lymph node (*arrow*), suspicious for metastatic disease. The trace diffusion image (*B, arrow*) and apparent diffusion coefficient (ADC) map (*C, arrow*) show a central area of low diffusion signal and high ADC, likely reflecting free water diffusion in the necrotic portion. Future research can help to determine if ADC values so generated from different components of the lymph node will allow for better prediction of treatment response.

treatment to the individual patient. Many studies have looked at ADC changes and their correlation to treatment response. Huang and colleagues[17] demonstrated that the minimum ADC after 1 cycle and minimum ADC after 5 cycles were significantly higher than the pretreatment minimum ADC, reflecting a decrease in cellularity (as tissue breakdown releases more free water in the tissues) and thus response to treatment. A significant positive correlation was observed between the percentages of minimum ADC change after 1 cycle of chemotherapy. The minimum ADC change and the percentage of minimum ADC change seemed to better differentiate final treatment response when comparing complete response and partial response from progressive disease.

Using IVIM, Paudyal and colleagues[18] found change in D (biexponential diffusion coefficient)

was significantly different between complete responders and incomplete responders. Their approach also identified subcategories in HPV-positive HNSCC patients, correlating with the known fact that tumors of this type have different radiotherapy sensitivities. The authors suggest that, with more research, MR imaging can not only assess response, but also characterize the magnitude of response to allow for individualized customization of treatment.

King and colleagues[19] investigated the role of DWI to predict and monitor chemoradiotherapy response in HNSCC. In their study, a significant correlation was found between locoregional failure and posttreatment ADC. Serial change in ADC was more significant, and when observing a decrease in ADC early (pretreatment to intratreatment) or late

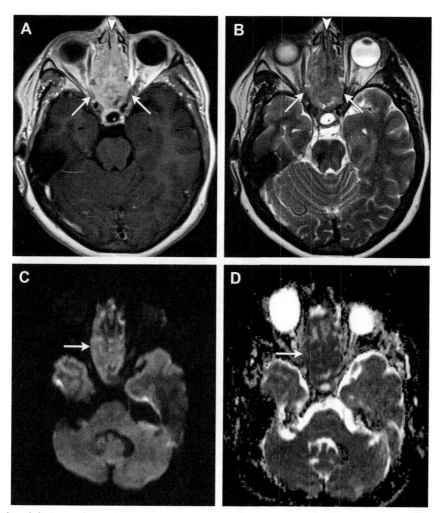

Fig. 5. Axial gadolinium-enhanced T1-weighted (*A*) and T2-weighted (*B*) images in a 43-year-old woman with nasal obstruction show a hyperenhancing (*arrowheads*), T2 hypointense mass (*arrows*) that was pathologically proven to be lymphoma. The trace diffusion image (*C*) shows increased diffusion signal (*arrow*) and the corresponding the apparent diffusion coefficient (ADC) map (*D*) shows significantly reduced ADC (compared with brain; *arrow*), which are features consistent with malignancy. In some studies, it has been shown that lymphoma tends to demonstrate lower ADC values compared with squamous cell carcinoma.

(intratreatment to posttreatment), the authors gained 100% specificity, 80% sensitivity, and 90% accuracy in predicting locoregional failure.

Kim and colleagues[12] found that complete responders had a significant increase in ADC after 1 week of treatment, which persisted until the end of treatment. Those who completely responded to treatment showed significantly higher increase in ADC than the partial responders by the first week of chemoradiation. They found that change in ADC within the first week of chemoradiation therapy predicted treatment response with 86% sensitivity and 83% specificity. **Fig. 8** shows how diffusion images can be used for the assessment of treatment response during early radiation in a patient with nasopharyngeal carcinoma.

Recurrence Versus Posttreatment Changes

DWI has also been investigated for its potential to distinguish posttreatment changes from recurrent neoplasm. Early laboratory research demonstrated that ADC correlated well with histologic changes, namely, increased extracellular space and decreased cellularity, occurring after treatment.[20] Conversely, when the remaining tumor cells multiplied and the tumor recurred, ADC returned to pretreatment levels.

Vaid and colleagues[21] examined 80 treated patients with head and neck cancer with a variety of malignancies to prospectively assess the viability of DWI as a tool to distinguish recurrence from posttreatment changes. Recurrent malignancy

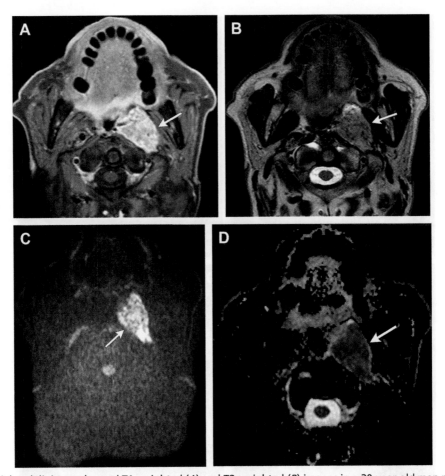

Fig. 6. Axial gadolinium-enhanced T1-weighted (*A*) and T2-weighted (*B*) images in a 30-year-old man presenting with a pulsatile neck mass demonstrate a large enhancing lesion with multiple flow voids (*arrow*) in the left carotid space suggestive of a paraganglioma. Although this is a benign entity, its higher cellularity probably explains the reason for restricted diffusion on the trace diffusion image (*C, arrow*) and low signal on the apparent diffusion coefficient (ADC) map (*D, arrow*). It should be noted that foci of hemorrhage within the paraganglioma often contribute to the low signal noted on the ADC map.

did show decreased ADC values when compared with posttreatment changes. Furthermore, they were able to achieve a sensitivity of 90.13% and a specificity of 82.5% using a threshold ADC value of 1.2×10^{-3} mm²/s. Desouky and colleagues[22] compared DWI and dynamic contrast enhanced imaging in 50 patients with laryngeal who underwent either surgery or chemoradiation and found that an ADC cutoff value of 0.9667×10^{-3} mm²/s effectively differentiated benign and malignant lesions with 100% sensitivity and 74.2% specificity.

Vandecaveye and colleagues[23] evaluated 26 patients with recurrent HNSCC, showing that DWI signal was significantly lower for recurrent HNSCC than for benign postradiotherapy tissue. Simply taking into account signal intensity on native *b*-1000 images, signal was significantly

higher for HNSCC than for nontumoral tissue, with a sensitivity of 71.6% and a specificity of 71.3%. ADC values were significantly lower for HNSCC than for benign tissue, providing a sensitivity of 94.6% and a specificity of 95.9%. When they compared these findings with computed tomography, turbo spin echo MR imaging, and PET with fludeoxyglucose F 18, DWI detected nodal metastases smaller than 1 cm, and gave fewer false-positive results in both the original tumor bed and in residual adenopathies. In a later study, Vandecaveye and colleagues[24] demonstrated that the observed change in ADC in primary tumors at 2 and 4 weeks after treatment initiation was significantly lower in lesions with recurrence than in lesions with complete remission. This same pattern was observed for primary tumors relative to nodal metastases. Beyond the

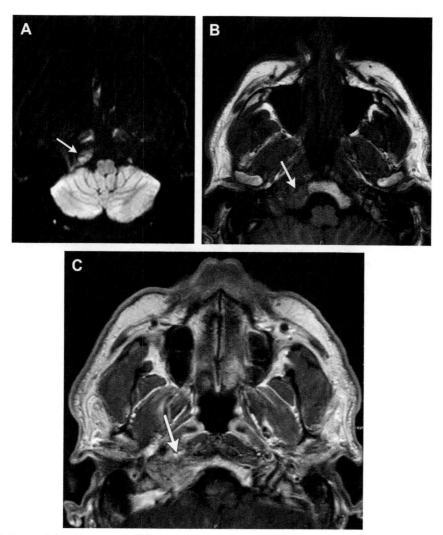

Fig. 7. Diffusion-weighted images can help to screen for potential sites of osseous metastasis in the skull base and calvarium in patients with primary carcinomas elsewhere. Increased diffusion signal is seen on the trace diffusion image (A) in the right clivus (arrow) in this patient with a primary renal cell carcinoma presenting with headaches. The precontrast and postcontrast (B, arrow; C, arrow) T1-weighted images at the same level confirm the presence of marrow signal replacement in the right clivus and patchy enhancement suggestive of osseous metastases.

immediate posttreatment period, the observed change in ADC correlated significantly with 2-year locoregional control. The current literature on DWI and the usefulness of ADC in differentiating recurrence from posttreatment changes is promising, although more research is needed to reach and validate a clear consensus on specific ADC values and thresholds. **Fig. 9** illustrates the usefulness of DWI in detection of tumor recurrence.

LIMITATIONS

Of course, the most obvious limitation in DWI is that, even though much of the available research

has sought ADC thresholds to evaluate head and neck cancers, there has been a reported non-negligible variability of ADC values with different MR imaging systems.[11] It will be cumbersome to try to validate ADC values for clinical use while different machines yield varying results. On the same vein, a standard DWI protocol must be validated and agreed on if the findings of DWI research are to be generalized and put into practice. As Vidiri and colleagues[8] had investigated smaller fields of view to increase the accuracy of ADC measurements, an agreed upon field of view when scanning for ADC measurements may need to be used to achieve sufficiently accurate ADC values. In a recent study focusing on

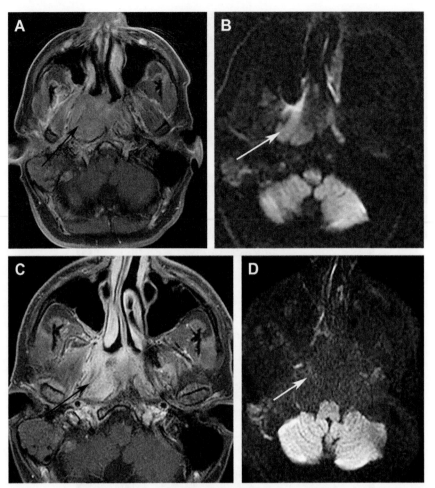

Fig. 8. Axial gadolinium enhanced T1-weighted image (*A*) with corresponding trace diffusion image (*B*) in a 33-year-old with biopsy-proven nasopharyngeal squamous cell carcinoma demonstrate restricted diffusion in a large enhancing mass involving the lateral and right posterior walls (*arrows*). After 2 cycles of radiation therapy, the mass demonstrates persistent enhancement on the axial gadolinium enhanced T1-weighted image (*C*), but complete resolution (*arrows*) of restricted diffusion on the trace diffusion image (*D*). This is indicative of good tumor response.

addressing this limitation, Koontz and Wiggins[25] compared ADC values of head and neck lesions with the medulla; by normalizing the observed ADC values attained by diffusion tensor imaging and DWI to an internal reference, similar ADC ratios on DWI and diffusion tensor imaging were achieved.

Schakel and colleagues,[26] as of 2013, had emphasized the limiting distortional effects of DWI. This was mainly with respect to using DWI for gross tumor volume imaging. This could be overcome by using other non-DWI sequences with better spatial resolution to define the borders of a lesion, with DWI being used for characterization.

In 1 study, data acquired from nodal sites was predictive of outcome, but not data acquired from the primary, for unknown reasons.[27] In addition, the *b*-value seems to have effects on how a mass is characterized in regards to ADC. Two studies have demonstrated that mean ADCs obtained with low *b* value ranges (0–100/300 s/mm^2) are not as predictive of treatment response when compared with ADCs obtained with high *b* value ranges (300/500–1000 s/mm^2).[28,29] However, within the higher range of *b* values, there is evidence that ADCs obtained at 0 to 750 and 0 to 2000 s/mm^2 are predictive of treatment response, whereas ADCs obtained at *b* values of 0 to 1000 s/mm^2 are not predictive, again for unknown reasons.[28,30] Therefore, further research includes identifying the best tumor sites in the head and neck to select for imaging, the optimum range

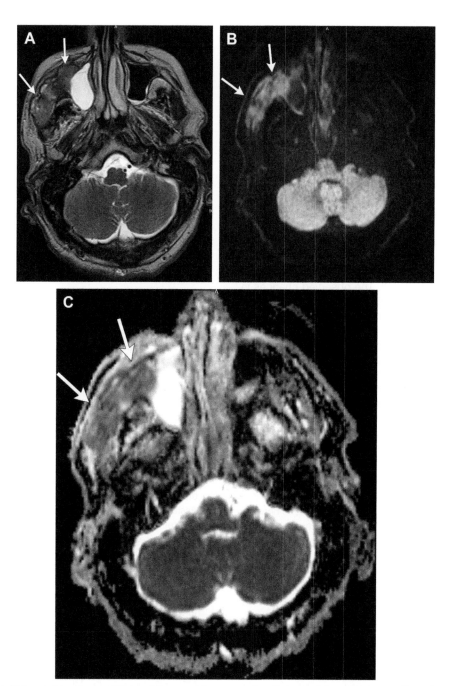

Fig. 9. Axial T2-weighted image (*A*) in a 60-year-old man previously treated for squamous cell carcinoma of the face demonstrates a heterogeneous, T2 hypointense area (*arrows*) overlying the right maxillary sinus. Owing to a significantly low glomerular filtration rate, no gadolinium was administered. The trace diffusion image (*B, arrows*) shows high diffusion signal with low apparent diffusion coefficient (ADC) values demonstrated on the corresponding ADC map (*C, arrows*). This was proven to be recurrent squamous cell carcinoma. In the post therapy setting, ADC values can help distinguish tumor recurrence from benign scar with the former demonstrating lower ADC and the latter higher ADC values.

of *b* values for DWI acquisition and analysis, and the optimum ADC parameters and thresholds.

Although echo planar DWI can suffer from image distortions and susceptibility artifacts in the head and neck, these can be reduced by switching to multishot echo planar or non–echo planar diffusion, and by using parallel imaging.

SUMMARY

DWI of head and neck represents a distinct method of MR imaging with far ranging current and potential applications. New and better technology, scanners, and software have allowed DWI to become available across the globe. Current research continues to hone the capabilities of DWI in characterizing masses as benign or malignant, predicting their response to treatment based on tissue characteristics, monitoring and assessing the response to treatment as therapy progresses, and surveilling areas of prior intervention to detect posttreatment and recurrent neoplastic changes. Pretreatment ADC values can suggest the likelihood of response to treatment, and delineate certain malignant masses from one another (namely HPV-positive from HPV-negative HNSCC). The observed changes in ADC and D (biexponential diffusion coefficient) occurring during treatment allow for assessment of response and degree of response, in addition to making further predictions of locoregional control or failure. Finally, DWI-obtained ADC values are able to look beyond the anatomy in posttreatment tumor beds and metastatic lymph nodes to evaluate for tumor recurrence. Further research should include large-scale, multiinstitutional studies to provide standardized ADC cutoff values for more widespread use.

REFERENCES

1. Chen L, Liu M, Bao J, et al. The correlation between apparent diffusion coefficient and tumor cellularity in patients: a meta-analysis. PLoS One 2013;8(11): e79008.

2. Wang J, Takashima S, Takayama F, et al. Head and neck lesions: characterization with diffusion-weighted echo-planar MR imaging. Radiology 2001;220(3):621–30.

3. Razek AA, Elkhamary S, Mousa A. Differentiation between benign and malignant orbital tumors at 3-T diffusion MR-imaging. Neuroradiology 2011;53(7):517–22.

4. Srinivasan A, Dvorak R, Perni K, et al. Differentiation of benign and malignant pathology in the head and neck using 3T apparent diffusion coefficient values: early experience. AJNR Am J Neuroradiol 2008; 29(1):40–4.

5. Abdel Razek AA, Soliman NY, Elkhamary S, et al. Role of diffusion-weighted MR imaging in cervical lymphadenopathy. Eur Radiol 2006;16(7):1468–77.

6. Abdel Razek AA, Samir S, Ashmalla GA. Characterization of parotid tumors with dynamic susceptibility contrast perfusion-weighted magnetic resonance imaging and diffusion-weighted MR imaging. J Comput Assist Tomogr 2017;41(1):131–6.

7. Yerli H, Aydin E, Haberal N, et al. Diagnosing common parotid tumours with magnetic resonance imaging including diffusion-weighted imaging vs fine-needle aspiration cytology: a comparative study. Dentomaxillofac Radiol 2010;39(6):349–55.

8. Vidiri A, Minosse S, Piludu F, et al. Feasibility study of reduced field of view diffusion-weighted magnetic resonance imaging in head and neck tumors. Acta Radiol 2017;58(3):292–300.

9. Driessen JP, van Bemmel AJ, van Kempen PM, et al. Correlation of human papillomavirus status with apparent diffusion coefficient of diffusion-weighted MRI in head and neck squamous cell carcinomas. Head Neck 2016;38(Suppl 1):E613–8.

10. Guo W, Luo D, Lin M, et al. Pretreatment intra-voxel incoherent motion diffusion-weighted imaging (IVIM-DWI) in Predicting induction chemotherapy response in locally advanced hypopharyngeal carcinoma. Medicine 2016;95(10):e3039.

11. Hatakenaka M, Nakamura K, Yabuuchi H, et al. Apparent diffusion coefficient is a prognostic factor of head and neck squamous cell carcinoma treated with radiotherapy. Jpn J Radiol 2014;32(2):80–9.

12. Kim S, Loevner L, Quon H, et al. Diffusion-weighted magnetic resonance imaging for predicting and detecting early response to chemoradiation therapy of squamous cell carcinomas of the head and neck. Clin Cancer Res 2009;15(3):986–94.

13. Srinivasan A, Chenevert TL, Dwamena BA, et al. Utility of pretreatment mean apparent diffusion coefficient and apparent diffusion coefficient histograms in prediction of outcome to chemoradiation in head and neck squamous cell carcinoma. J Comput Assist Tomogr 2012;36(1):131–7.

14. Hauser T, Essig M, Jensen A, et al. Prediction of treatment response in head and neck carcinomas using IVIM-DWI: evaluation of lymph node metastasis. Eur J Radiol 2014;83(5):783–7.

15. Lu Y, Moreira AL, Hatzoglou V, et al. Using diffusion-weighted MRI to predict aggressive histological features in papillary thyroid carcinoma: a novel tool for pre-operative risk stratification in thyroid cancer. Thyroid 2015;25(6):672–80.

16. Ng SH, Lin CY, Chan SC, et al. Clinical utility of multimodality imaging with dynamic contrast-enhanced MRI, diffusion-weighted MRI, and 18F-FDG PET/CT for the prediction of neck control in oropharyngeal or hypopharyngeal squamous cell carcinoma treated with chemoradiation. PLoS One 2014;9(12): e115933.

17. Huang WY, Wen JB, Wu G, et al. Diffusion-weighted imaging for predicting and monitoring primary central nervous system lymphoma treatment response. AJNR Am J Neuroradiol 2016. [Epub ahead of print].

18. Paudyal R, Oh JH, Riaz N, et al. Intravoxel incoherent motion diffusion-weighted MRI during chemoradiation therapy to characterize and monitor

treatment response in human papillomavirus head and neck squamous cell carcinoma. J Magn Reson Imaging 2017;45(4):1013–23.

19. King AD, Mo FK, Yu KH, et al. Squamous cell carcinoma of the head and neck: diffusion-weighted MR imaging for prediction and monitoring of treatment response. Eur Radiol 2010;20(9):2213–20.

20. Chenevert TL, McKeever PE, Ross BD. Monitoring early response of experimental brain tumors to therapy using diffusion magnetic resonance imaging. Clin Cancer Res 1997;3(9):1457–66.

21. Vaid S, Chandorkar A, Atre A, et al. Differentiating recurrent tumours from post-treatment changes in head and neck cancers: does diffusion-weighted MRI solve the eternal dilemma? Clin Radiol 2017; 72(1):74–83.

22. Desouky SE, Paudyal R, Oh JH. Role of dynamic contrast enhanced and diffusion weighted MRI in the differentiation between post treatment changes and recurrent laryngeal cancers. Egypt J Radiol Nucl Med 2015;46:379–89.

23. Vandecaveye V, De Keyzer F, Nuyts S, et al. Detection of head and neck squamous cell carcinoma with diffusion weighted MRI after (chemo)radiotherapy: correlation between radiologic and histopathologic findings. Int J Radiat Oncol Biol Phys 2007;67(4): 960–71.

24. Vandecaveye V, Dirix P, De Keyzer F, et al. Predictive value of diffusion-weighted magnetic resonance imaging during chemoradiotherapy for head and neck squamous cell carcinoma. Eur Radiol 2010;20(7): 1703–14.

25. Koontz NA, Wiggins RH 3rd. Differentiation of benign and malignant head and neck lesions with diffusion tensor imaging and DWI. AJR Am J Roentgenol 2017;208(5):1110–5.

26. Schakel T, Hoogduin JM, Terhaard CH, et al. Diffusion weighted MRI in head-and-neck cancer: geometrical accuracy. Radiother Oncol 2013; 109(3):394–7.

27. Noij DP, Pouwels PJ, Ljumanovic R, et al. Predictive value of diffusion-weighted imaging without and with including contrast-enhanced magnetic resonance imaging in image analysis of head and neck squamous cell carcinoma. Eur J Radiol 2015;84(1):108–16.

28. Hatakenaka M, Shioyama Y, Nakamura K, et al. Apparent diffusion coefficient calculated with relatively high b-values correlates with local failure of head and neck squamous cell carcinoma treated with radiotherapy. AJNR Am J Neuroradiol 2011; 32(10):1904–10.

29. Lambrecht M, Van Calster B, Vandecaveye V, et al. Integrating pretreatment diffusion weighted MRI into a multivariable prognostic model for head and neck squamous cell carcinoma. Radiother Oncol 2014;110(3):429–34.

30. Ryoo I, Kim JH, Choi SH, et al. Squamous cell carcinoma of the head and neck: comparison of diffusion-weighted MRI at b-values of 1,000 and 2,000 s/mm(2) to predict response to induction chemotherapy. Magn Reson Med Sci 2015;14(4): 337–45.

Dynamic Contrast-Enhanced MR Imaging in Head and Neck Cancer

Suraj J. Kabadi, MD[a],
Girish M. Fatterpekar, MBBS, DNB, MD[b],
Yoshimi Anzai, MD, MPH[c], Jonathan Mogen, MD[d],
Mari Hagiwara, MD[b], Sohil H. Patel, MD[e],*

KEYWORDS

- Head and neck cancer (HNC) • Squamous cell cancer (SCC)
- Dynamic contrast-enhanced MR imaging (DCE-MR imaging) • K(trans) • Time intensity curve (TIC)
- Permeability • Perfusion • Treatment response

KEY POINTS

- Dynamic contrast-enhanced (DCE) MR imaging serves as an adjunct to conventional imaging by delineating information on the microvascular biologic function of tissues through quantification of pharmacokinetic parameters.
- DCE-MR imaging allows for analysis of tissue kinetics using both quantitative analysis and semi-quantitative analysis, both of which provide information to discriminate between entities that otherwise appear similar by conventional imaging.
- When used to evaluate head and neck cancer (HNC), potential uses of DCE-MR imaging include predicting and evaluating treatment response, evaluating cervical adenopathy, distinguishing post-treatment changes from residual or recurrent tumor, and distinguishing between different types of HNC.
- The DCE-MR imaging parameter K(trans), which serves as a surrogate for permeability, appears to provide the most clinical utility in evaluating HNC, specifically with higher K(trans) in primary tumor sites and nodal metastases correlating with improved outcomes.
- DCE-MR imaging may also help to distinguish carotid spaces masses and parotid neoplasms.

INTRODUCTION

Head and neck cancer (HNC), which largely comprises malignant neoplasms of the pharynx and larynx, sinonasal and oral cavities, and glands and lymphatic system of the neck, is the sixth most common type of cancer worldwide and accounts for 2% of all cancer-related deaths in the United States.[1] Conventional imaging techniques used to evaluate HNC, including ultrasound computed tomography (CT), and MR imaging, can unfortunately be limited in terms of assessing underlying malignant potential due to overlapping conventional imaging features of malignant and

Disclosures: None.
[a] Diagnostic Radiology, University of Virginia Health System, PO Box 800170, 1215 Lee Street, Charlottesville, VA 22908, USA; [b] Department of Radiology, NYU Langone Medical Center, NYU Radiology Associates, 660 First Avenue, 2nd Floor, New York, NY 10016, USA; [c] University of Utah Health, 50 North Medical Drive, Salt Lake City, UT 84132, USA; [d] Neuroradiology, NYU Langone Medical Center, NYU Radiology Associates, 660 First Avenue, 2nd Floor, New York, NY 10016, USA; [e] Department of Radiology and Medical Imaging, University of Virginia Health System, PO Box 800170, 1215 Lee Street, Charlottesville, VA 22908, USA
* Corresponding author.
E-mail address: shp4k@virginia.edu

Magn Reson Imaging Clin N Am 26 (2018) 135–149
http://dx.doi.org/10.1016/j.mric.2017.08.008

benign diseases in the head and neck. Further-more, conventional imaging can also be limited in distinguishing tumor recurrence from posttreat-ment changes. Dynamic contrast-enhanced (DCE) MR imaging can supplement conventional imaging sequences by elucidating information on the microvascular biologic function of tissues through quantification of permeability parameters. These additional microvascular prop-erties revealed by DCE-MR imaging help discrim-inate between otherwise morphologically similar entities on conventional imaging.

TECHNIQUE
Dynamic Contrast-Enhanced MR Imaging

DCE-MR imaging is performed by obtaining rapid sequential T1-weighted MR images through an area of interest before, during, and after the intra-venous administration of a gadolinium-based contrast agent. This allows for temporal acquisi-tion of T1 intensity at each point in space within the area of interest. By incorporating baseline T1 mapping before contrast administration as well as the known relaxivity of the gadolinium contrast, DCE-MR imaging allows transformation of a time signal intensity curve into a time concentration curve. The time intensity or time concentration curve reflects the rate of uptake and clearance of contrast, which can be used to derive micro-vascular properties. These temporal kinetics can then be analyzed to obtain semiquantitative metrics, or quantified microvascular physiologic parameters through the use of a pharmacokinetic model and an arterial input function (AIF). Using the simple features of the time intensity or time concentration curve, time to peak or inte-grated area under the curve (AUC) is easily extracted without AIF or pharmacodynamic kinetic modeling. These semiquantitative metrics are used in diagnostic practice for some cancers.

The most universally accepted pharmacoki-netic model for quantitative analysis is the Tofts model, a simple 2-compartment model consisting of one tissue compartment (extravascular extra-cellular space [EES]) and one vascular compart-ment.[2] In this model, contrast agent travels through the microvasculature and leaks from the vascular space into the EES by passive diffusion (wash-in phase), altering T1 signal intensity of the tissue. The changes in signal depend on how the contrast agent distributes within the tis-sues, which depends on the local circulatory sys-tem. As the concentration of intravascular contrast agent decreases, contrast agent then starts moving back from the EES into the vascular space (wash-out phase). The concentration of

contrast agent in the EES in this model is assumed to be roughly proportional to T1 signal intensity.[3] Therefore, rapid T1-weighted acquisi-tion during this process allows for derivation of a time concentration curve, which reveals the dy-namics of contrast agent accumulation (wash-in) and dissipation (wash-out) over time, and subse-quent derivation of standard pharmacokinetic parameters. Among the kinetic parameters measured using the Tofts model are: K(trans), the volume transfer constant from the vascular space to the EES; K(ep), the rate constant from the EES to the vascular space; V(e), the volume of the EES per unit volume of tissue; PS, perme-ability surface area product per unit mass of tis-sue; F, flow of whole blood per unit mass of tissue; and V(p), total blood plasma volume.

In acquiring the dynamic dataset for the purpose of deriving pharmacokinetic parameters, a critical component of high-quality DCE-MR imaging is high temporal resolution.[4] High temporal resolu-tion, however, comes at the cost of decreased spatial resolution and SNR, both of which are addi-tional acquisition parameters that must be consid-ered for optimal evaluation of tumor vascular function. In this light, many different methods of fast 2D and 3D T1-weighted sequences have been described in the literature to achieve a reasonable balance of these parameters in clinical practice.[5–8]

Beyond dynamic acquisition, there are 2 other datasets that must be acquired and fed into the Tofts model in order to obtain accurate pharmaco-kinetic parameters: (1) baseline T1 mapping, and (2) AIF. Baseline T1 mapping is done before the administration of contrast agent in order to correct for the nonlinear relationship between the T1 signal intensity and tissue contrast concentration. There are various techniques for T1 mapping, including variable flip angle techniques, inversion recovery technique, and the Look-Locker technique.[9–11] The second additional dataset necessary for quantitative analysis is the AIF. The AIF provides data on the enhancement kinetics of the afferent artery supplying the area of interest, typically achieved by placing a region of interest (ROI) over any visible large artery (eg, carotid artery) in the dynamic dataset.[12]

In summary, quantitative DCE-MR image acqui-sition consists of 3 steps: (1) baseline T1 mapping before administration of contrast agent; (2) dy-namic data acquisition; and (3) AIF assessment. These data are then fit to a model, most commonly the extended Tofts model, to calculate standard pharmacokinetic parameters based upon the ki-netics of contrast agent concentration within the vascular space and EES.

Of note, in addition to quantitative analysis, semiquantitative analysis can also be performed on the obtained dynamic data. In semiquantitative analysis, rather than fitting derived time concentration curves to a model, the observed time intensity curves (TICs) of the tissue of interest are used to derive clinically salient parameters, including wash-in slope, maximum peak enhancement, time to peak enhancement (TTP), wash-out slope, maximum signal enhancement ratio, and AUC.[3] Semiquantitative analysis offers the advantage of easier implementation, because it does not require the acquisition of baseline T1 mapping or AIF, nor does it rely on the assumptions of a pharmacokinetic model. However, unlike in quantitative analysis, semiquantitative parameters do not correlate to a specific biologic property, and thus, their true physiologic meaning may be confounded by the effects of multiple tissue properties.[13] Nonetheless, semiquantitative analysis still has important clinical applications for tumor characterization, as discussed later.

Dynamic Susceptibility Contrast MR Imaging

For head and neck applications, a less commonly used method of MR perfusion imaging is DSC-MR imaging. In contrast to DCE-MR imaging, which uses T1-weighted imaging, DSC-MR imaging uses either T2*- or T2-weighted imaging for performing dynamic image acquisition.[14] A series of precontrast images are first acquired to enable an estimate of baseline signal intensity. Rapid loss of MR signal on T2- or T2*-weighted images is then measured during first pass contrast tissue transit through a series of rapid image acquisitions, usually using either echo-planar imaging (EPI) or fast low angle shot (FLASH) techniques.[15,16] The TICs are then transformed into a measure of contrast agent concentration by calculating the change in the effective transverse relaxation rate (R2*). Unlike in DCE-MR imaging, quantitative tissue kinetic analysis using DSC-MR imaging is relatively unreliable due to underlying problems of T1 shine-through, as well as image distortion due to susceptibility effects from airways or paranasal sinuses.[14] However, tissue perfusion can still be assessed, yielding standard parameters of blood volume (BV) and blood flow (BF) that are typically normalized to standard soft tissue structures.[17]

Arterial Spin Labeling

Arterial spin labeling (ASL) perfusion imaging has also been investigated in head and neck applications. ASL offers a unique method of measuring tissue perfusion without administration of an intravenous contrast agent. Water in the blood is labeled magnetically using a radiofrequency inversion pulse, which can be done as either continuous labeling or pulsed labeling.[18] The concentration of the magnetically labeled arterial water tracked over time as it passes through the tissue of interest is measured using serial MR acquisition.[19] The image acquisition technique involves collection of a pair of images, a labeled image, and a control image, with the labeled image including additional signal from labeled blood. On subtraction of the 2 images, a purely perfusion-weighted image is then obtained. Acquisition is performed with an echo-planar imaging sequence.[20] The temporal kinetics of perfusion can then be analyzed, usually performed using a single tissue compartment model. Semiquantitative parameters, analogous to those discussed earlier with DSC-MR imaging and DCE-MR imaging, can also be derived. Like DSC-MR imaging, however, ASL is limited to assessment of tissue perfusion (BF) only, and not tissue permeability as can be assessed with DCE-MR imaging.

CLINICAL APPLICATIONS
Tumor Hypoxia, Prediction, and Evaluation of Treatment Response

An important potential application of DCE-MR imaging for HNC is in characterizing tumor hypoxia, and using this characterization to predict treatment response of chemoradiation. It is well known that impaired tumor perfusion, which leads to tumor hypoxia, increases the likelihood of treatment failure. Specifically, tumor hypoxia is often the result of disordered angiogenesis through the release of VEGF. Rather than producing normal vessels, VEGF causes the formation of tortuous, leaky vessels supplying the tumor, resulting in variable and heterogeneous perfusion. This ultimately leads to poor supply of nutrients and oxygen to parts of the tumor and to the development of areas of hypoxia as well as decreased delivery of chemotherapeutic agents resulting in treatment failure.[21]

Unfortunately, conventional imaging provides no rigorous information on tumor perfusion, hypoxia, or angiogenesis, a shortcoming that DCE-MR imaging can potentially overcome. Newbold and colleagues[22] were able to show several statistically significant negative correlations between tumor hypoxia (identified through the bioreductive agent pimonidazole, which binds to hypoxic cells) and DCE-MR imaging parameters such as K(trans) and V(e). Specifically, they were able to show that tumors showing high K(trans) values and high V(e) values had low fractions of hypoxic cells, and vice versa. This correlates with existing literature in regards to other cancers,[23] and also the expected pathophysiology of well-perfused tumors with high permeability. Donaldson and colleagues[24] were able to show similar correlations of DCE-MR imaging parameters with pimonidazole-labeled hypoxic tissue, specifically that more hypoxic tumors had lower values of perfusion ($P = .033$) and capillary permeability ($P = .049$), providing an inverse correlation between typical DCE-MR imaging parameters and tumor hypoxia as would be expected based on pathophysiology.

Jansen and colleagues[25] examined DCE-MR imaging parameters of neck nodal metastases of HNC and how they correlated with immunohistochemistry assays of the corresponding surgical specimens and were able to show 2 significant correlations in regards to hypoxia. First, a strong positive correlation was observed between VEGF and standard deviation of K(ep), which is in keeping with the notion that promotion of angiogenic growth factor pathways, that is, VEGF production, promotes tumor heterogeneity. Second, a strong negative correlation was observed between Ki-67 (a marker of cellular proliferation) and tumor heterogeneity markers standard deviation of K(trans) and V(e), reflecting that heterogeneous tumors contain areas of low proliferation and often highly necrotic regions. As a summative argument, DCE-MR imaging parameters may reflect the expected pathophysiology of VEGF in promoting the formation of tortuous vessels, which are ineffective in appropriately perfusing a tumor and result in heterogeneous distribution of tumor necrosis and areas of low cellular proliferation.

More than just establishing evidence for the use of DCE-MR imaging as a noninvasive method for depicting tumor hypoxia, the more apt clinical question stems around whether this tumor characterization can ultimately be used to predict treatment response, as would be expected on a pathophysiologic basis. This has been shown in other malignancies, most convincingly by Jensen and colleagues[26] in gliomas, where they were able to show that higher pretreatment V(e) in areas of peritumoral edema correlated with patient overall survival ($P = .007$) and that capillary heterogeneity within active tumor ($P = .014$) also correlated with patient overall survival. This follows intuition as both of these DCE-MR imaging parameters are markers for accessibility of contrast material to the tissue, reflecting breakdown in the blood-brain barrier, which would similarly allow accessibility of chemotherapeutic drugs and increase treatment effectiveness and overall survival.

Similar results have been found in HNC. Bernstein and colleagues[27] studied whether baseline tumor plasma flow F(p) determined by DCE-MR imaging would predict induction chemotherapy response for HNC. Indeed, they found that median baseline F(p) was greater in responders than nonresponders in both the primary tumor (53.2 vs 23.9 mL/100 mL/min, $P = .027$) and also nodal metastases (25.8 vs 17.1 mL/100 mL/min, $P = .066$). Ng and colleagues[28] looked at the relationship of K(trans) in responders and nonresponders after treatment for HNC. They found that patients with a high pretreatment K(trans) value (≥ 0.62 min^{-1}) had a significantly higher 2-year local control rate than those with a low K(trans) value ($P = .03$), indicating that pretreatment K(trans) of the primary tumor may help predict local control in HNC patients treated with chemoradiation. Agrawal and colleagues[7] demonstrated that pretreatment BF (mL/100 g/min) and BV (mL/100 g) were both higher at the primary site in patients who showed complete response versus partial response (22.01 vs 12.10, $P = .06$, and 21.13 vs 12.08, $P = .05$, respectively). Similar results have also been demonstrated with other perfusion MR imaging techniques, particularly ASL, where Fujima and colleagues[29] found that pretreatment tumor BF (mL/100 g/min) in patients in the failure group was significantly lower than that in patients in the local control group (109.6 vs 142.3, $P<.01$). These results all point to the same conclusion that increased pretreatment tumor perfusion as reflected by various DCE-MR imaging parameters are associated with better outcomes (**Fig. 1**), likely through improved delivery of chemotherapeutic agents and oxygen to the tumor.

More than just predicting response of HNC based on pretreatment DCE-MR imaging, DCE-MR imaging can also be used posttreatment as a potential method of noninvasively reflecting treatment response immediately after radiotherapy or chemotherapy. Agrawal and colleagues[7] showed a significantly higher BV and BF of the complete response patients compared with partial response patients after treatment ($P = .002$ and $P = .03$, respectively). Wang and colleagues[30] examined regions and subvolumes within primary tumors of HNC and reached a similar conclusion when examining BF and BV. By performing both pretreatment and posttreatment DCE-MR imaging, they were able to show that increase in the size of subvolume of tumor with low BV 2 weeks after initiation of treatment was predictive of local failure ($P<.05$). Cao and colleagues[31] reached a corroborative conclusion when examining pre-chemoradiation and

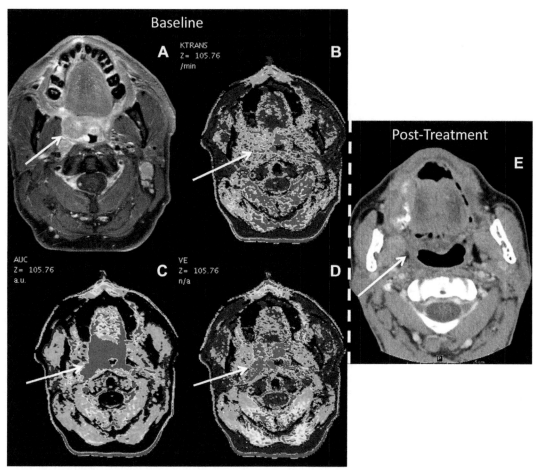

Fig. 1. Axial postcontrast T1 fat-saturated image (*A*) demonstrates a right tonsillar SCC (*arrow*). Corresponding parametric maps demonstrate elevated K(trans) (*B*), elevated AUC (*C*), and elevated V(e) (*D*), which are favorable pretreatment imaging features. (*E*) Axial contrast-enhanced CT image 8 months after completion of chemoradiation demonstrates significant interval decrease in size of the right tonsillar mass.

post-chemoradiation BV, namely that there was a statistically significant interval increase in BV in the primary tumor after 2 weeks of chemoradiation in the local control patients compared with the local failure patients (*P*<.03). In summary, these 3 studies show that those tumors that are well perfused on DCE-MR imaging after initial treatment (as evidence by high posttreatment BV or interval increase in BV from pretreatment values) were reflective of local control. Conversely, those which are poorly perfused on DCE-MR imaging during the early course of chemoradiation were indicative of local failure and thus could be candidates for local dose intensification.

A few other studies have also examined different DCE-MR imaging parameters and their relationship to treatment response. Chikui and colleagues[32] were able to show a statistically significant increase in V(e) and K(trans) in responders versus nonresponders status post-

chemoradiation (*P* = .001), strongly suggesting that an increase in V(e) and K(trans) is reflective of good tumor response to chemoradiation and corroborating the previously discussed studies demonstrating that well-perfused tumors (as demonstrated by DCE-MR imaging parameters V(e) and K(trans) in this case) are reflective of treatment response. Tomura and colleagues[33] performed DCE-MR imaging in tumors histologically classified as having either viable tumor cells, nonviable tumor cells, or no tumor cells. They were able to find a significant difference in maximum slope of increase (MSI) on TIC of patients with no tumor cells after radiotherapy, concluding that MSI quantitatively reflects response to radiotherapy for HNC. Finally, Baba and colleagues[34] examined the efficacy of using DCE-MR imaging for evaluation of HNCs treated with radiation therapy, which were subsequently histologically examined. They found that

DCE correctly diagnosed 17 of the 18 complete remission cases, 33 of the 36 partial response cases, and all of the 7 no-response cases, with accuracy of 94.4%, proving that DCE-MR imaging may be useful in the evaluation of radiation therapy in HNC.

In summary, although the relationship between tumor perfusion, permeability, and response to chemoradiation is complex on a biologic basis, current evidence supports a general conclusion that tumors with good baseline perfusion and permeability as demonstrated by higher DCE-MR imaging K(trans) values have less tumor hypoxia, and thus better sensitivity to chemoradiation treatment and better survival. As a result, DCE-MR imaging can be an effective method of characterizing these dynamics to better predict treatment response in HNC. Future work may be targeted at how DCE-MR imaging can prospectively be applied at an individual patient level, and what cut-off values of K(trans), BF, BV, and V(e) to apply.

Lymph Node Imaging

Metastatic lymph node involvement is one of the most important prognostic factors for HNC, and the nodal status is critical for treatment planning. Routine anatomic imaging relies predominantly on the assessment of lymph node size, morphology, and the presence of necrosis in determining possible lymph node involvement. Unfortunately, each of these imaging features has a limited sensitivity or specificity in predicting metastatic lymph node involvement, making staging with routine imaging imprecise. DCE-MR imaging offers an additional noninvasive method that might improve upon the diagnostic accuracy of morphology imaging in nodal staging of HNC.

DCE-MR imaging has shown promise in characterizing lymph node status on the initial staging scans in patients with HNC. One of the most convincing of such studies was performed by Fischbein and colleagues.[35] In their study, DCE-MR imaging was performed in patients who had HNC and subsequently underwent a clinically indicated neck dissection. In comparison to normal lymph nodes, metastatic lymph nodes demonstrated significantly longer TTP ($P<.001$), lower peak enhancement ($P<.05$), lower maximum slope ($P<.01$), and slower wash-out slope ($P<.05$). These DCE-MR imaging results indicated decreased transfer of contrast agent to tissue and reduced volume of the EES in tumor-involved nodes as compared with normal or reactive lymph nodes. They concluded that DCE-MR imaging can be performed as a fairly simple add-on to routine MR imaging and may provide additional useful physiologic information regarding nodal staging in patients with squamous cell carcinoma (SCC) of the head and neck. Other perfusion MR imaging methods, particularly DSC-MR imaging, have also been studied to differentiate benign from malignant lymph nodes. Abdel Razek and colleagues[36] looked at the parameter DSC%, calculated as $(S0 - SI)/S0 \times 100\%$, where S0 represents the signal intensity of the lesion just before descent of signal intensity, and SI represents the signal intensity at peak descent. This is analogous to maximum signal enhancement ratio of DCE-MR imaging. They found that the mean DSC% of malignant HNC nodes was significantly higher than that of benign nodes ($P = .001$) and lymphoma ($P = .001$), showing the ability of DSC-MR imaging to characterize untreated lymph nodes.

In addition to helping to determine the N stage of patients initially presenting with HNC, DCE-MR imaging may also have a role in evaluating and predicting lymph node response to treatment in metastatic HNC. In patients who received chemoradiation for HNC, Kim and colleagues[37] were able to show that the average pretreatment K(trans) in metastatic lymph nodes of the complete response group (ie, no evidence of disease after chemoradiation) was significantly higher than that of the residual disease group (0.64 vs 0.21 min^{-1}, $P = .001$), suggesting that pretreatment K(trans) can be potentially used for prediction of nodal response to chemoradiation treatment of HNC. Using an ROI of the largest metastatic cervical lymph node, Chawla and colleagues[38] achieved a similar result, showing that patients with higher pretreatment K(trans) values (≥ 0.41 min^{-1}) had prolonged disease-free survival compared with patients with lower K(trans) values ($P = .029$), concluding that pretreatment K(trans) may be a useful prognostic marker in HNC. Shukla-Dave and colleagues[39] further showed that in a stepwise Cox regression, skewness of K(trans) of nodal metastases was the strongest predictor of progression-free survival and overall survival for stage IV HNC patients ($P<.001$). These results are in keeping with similar results found using DCE-MR imaging regarding nodal response to treatment and predicting long-term survival for multiple other malignancies, including cervical, colorectal, breast, and lung cancer.[40–44] Through a different approach using both DCE-MR imaging and PET and comparing DCE-MR imaging and 18F-fluoromisonidazole uptake in nodal metastases of HNC, Jansen and colleagues[45] were additionally able to show that hypoxic nodes had significantly lower median K(trans) ($P = .049$) values than did nonhypoxic nodes.

In keeping with previously described DCE-MR imaging findings regarding tumor hypoxia and treatment response, nodal metastases with good baseline perfusion and permeability as demonstrated by higher DCE-MR imaging K(trans) values have better sensitivity to chemoradiation treatment (**Fig. 2**), and ultimately, better survival. Conversely, those tumors with nodal metastases demonstrating low K(trans) values generally have poorer prognoses (**Fig. 3**). In addition, DCE-MR imaging may also have a role in differentiating metastatic nodes from benign nodes on the basis of decreased EES volume and slower contrast transfer, potentially improving the diagnostic accuracy of nodal staging.[35]

Differentiating Residual or Recurrent Head and Neck Cancer from Benign Posttreatment Change

Distinguishing posttreatment changes (from either radiation or chemotherapy) from residual or recurrent tumor in HNC is challenging using conventional imaging techniques, with often overlapping appearance between these entities. Recent studies have evaluated the potential of DCE-MR imaging for making this distinction.

Ishiyama and colleagues[46] found that posttreatment benign changes in the head and neck region had significantly higher permeability surface area than newly diagnosed or previously treated recurrent tumor (P = .031). In semiquantitative analysis, Furukawa and colleagues[47] showed that benign postradiation changes of the head and neck had a significantly longer time to peak (P = .024) and lower relative wash-out ratio (P = .007) than did recurrent tumors. Semiz Oysu and colleagues[48]

found significantly greater contrast uptake and enhancement ratio in posttreatment tumor-positive tissue compared with posttreatment fibrotic tissue (P<.05). Apart from DCE-MR imaging, Abdel Razek and colleagues[49] investigated the use of DSC-MR imaging to differentiate benign from malignant posttreatment tissue in the head and neck. In keeping with DCE-MR imaging results, they found significantly higher DSC% in recurrent cancer compared with postradiation changes (P = .001), and further, that using a combination of ADC and DSC% had an accuracy of 97.6% in differentiating the 2.

These results all point to residual tumor tissue having early and more intense enhancement when compared with posttreatment benign tissue. These results align with the commonly observed subjective finding of fibrotic tissue demonstrating delayed and less avid contrast enhancement on routine imaging. DCE-MR imaging, and possibly DSC-MR imaging, may provide more specificity than conventional imaging in this regard by quantitatively delineating these temporal enhancement characteristics, and thus, potentially improving differentiation of benign posttreatment changes from residual or recurrent HNC.

Differentiating Squamous Cell Carcinoma from Other Head and Neck Malignancy

Differentiating SCC of the head and neck from other head and neck malignancies is another potential application of DCE-MR imaging that has been investigated.

Lee and colleagues[50] examined differences in DCE-MR imaging parameters in SCC, undifferentiated carcinoma (UD), and lymphoma. They

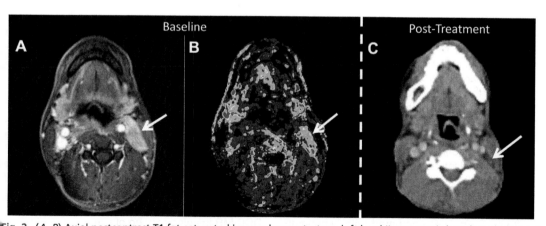

Fig. 2. (A, B) Axial postcontrast T1 fat-saturated image demonstrates a left level II metastatic lymph node (*arrow*) in a patient with nasopharyngeal carcinoma pretreatment, with corresponding parametric map showing elevated K(trans) = 0.48 min^{-1} (*arrow*). (C) Axial contrast-enhanced CT image 8 months post-chemoradiation demonstrates markedly decreased size of the left level II lymph node (*arrow*). Lymph nodes with higher pretreatment K(trans) have been found to be more responsive to treatment.

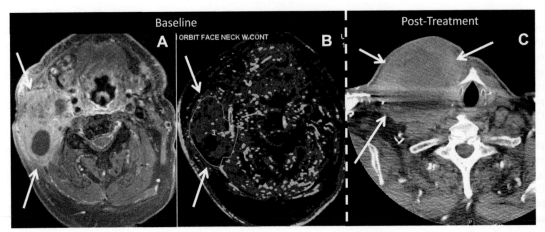

Fig. 3. (A) Axial postcontrast T1 fat-saturated image demonstrates extensive right cervical necrotic adenopathy with extracapsular spread (*arrows*) in a patient with T4N3M0 SCC of the base of the tongue. (B) Corresponding parametric map shows low K(trans) = 0.04 min^{-1} of the necrotic adenopathy (*arrows*). (C) Axial contrast-enhanced CT image 2 months following right neck dissection, flap reconstruction, and chemoradiation demonstrates bulky tumor recurrence inferior to the flap (*arrows*). Lymph nodes with lower pretreatment K(trans) have been found to be poor responders to treatment.

found statistically significant differences in K(trans), AUC in the initial 60 seconds, and AUC in the initial 90 seconds (*P*<.01) between UD and SCC (K(trans) 1.26 vs 0.78 min^{-1}) and UD and lymphoma (K(trans) 1.26 vs 0.59 min^{-1}), but no statistically significant differences between SCC and lymphoma, concluding that DCE has the potential for distinguishing UD from SCC or lymphoma, but not necessarily between SCC and lymphoma. Park and colleagues,[51] however, found that DCE can be useful for differentiating SCC from malignant lymphoma of the oropharynx. Specifically, they found that the median K(trans) was significantly higher in SCC than in lymphoma (0.20 vs 0.13 min^{-1}, *P* = .039), and the skewness and kurtosis of V(e) were significantly different in SCC than in lymphoma (*P* = .039 and .032, respectively). Similar results were also found by Kitamoto and colleagues[52] regarding V(e), specifically that lymphoma had lower V(e) than SCC (0.143 vs 0.199, *P* = .028), concluding that V(e) could be used for establishing a diagnosis of lymphoma. Semiquantitative methods as examined by Asaumi and colleagues[53] focused on contrast index (CI), calculated as CI = (SI[t] − SI[0])/SI[0], where SI[t] is the mean signal intensity at the time t after the injection of contrast medium, and SI[0] is the mean signal intensity before the injection of contrast medium. They showed significantly higher maximum CI in SCC compared with lymphoma (*P*<.001) as well as faster time to reach the maximum CI in SCC (*P* = .0177). However, in their study, there was overlap between SCC and lymphoma DCE-MR imaging features, with

several lymphoma masses demonstrating a TIC indistinguishable from SCC.

In summary, prior DCE-MR imaging studies attempting to differentiate SCC from lymphoma have used variable DCE-MR imaging techniques and demonstrated somewhat mixed results. The overall findings in the literature appear to indicate that SCC has increased tumor perfusion and capillary permeability when compared with lymphoma, as evidenced by higher K(trans) and V(e), as well as higher peak contrast uptake and earlier time to peak based on TIC analysis (**Fig. 4**). The lower K(trans) and V(e) found in lymphoma may be the result of the comparatively higher cellular content of lymphoma, as often demonstrated by conventional imaging. In fact, diffusion imaging with assessment of ADC plays a potentially larger role in differentiation of SCC from lymphoma. More work will be required to confidently establish differences in perfusion parameters between SCC and lymphoma before routine clinical application.

Evaluation of Carotid Space Masses

The 2 most common masses of the carotid space are schwannomas and paragangliomas.[54] Although paragangliomas and schwannomas are often successfully discriminated by conventional CT and MR imaging, they may occasionally share conventional imaging features. In this setting, DCE-MR imaging may be of use.

Two studies to date have examined the role that DCE-MR imaging could play in differentiating paraganglioma versus schwannoma. In an analysis of 6 patients with carotid space tumors

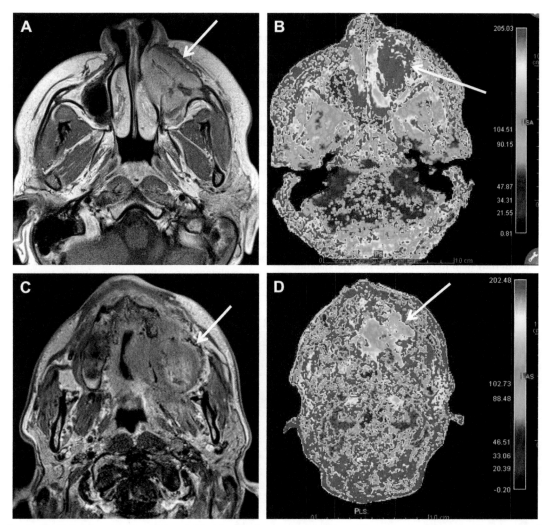

Fig. 4. (*A, B*) Axial postcontrast T1-weighted image demonstrates left maxillary sinus lymphoma with corresponding parametric map of time to peak (*arrows*). (*C, D*) Axial postcontrast T1-weighted image demonstrates left maxillary sinus SCC with corresponding parametric map of time to peak (*arrows*). Note that SCC (*D, green,* 114 s) has lower time to peak when compared with lymphoma (*B, red,* 201 s).

(4 schwannomas and 2 paraganglioma), Gaddikeri and colleagues[55] found that although conventional MR imaging was not sufficient to differentiate the 2 (all hypointense on T1, hyperintense on T2, and avidly enhancing), there were DCE-MR imaging parameters that demonstrated significant differences. First, paragangliomas had lower K(trans) (0.001 vs 0.35 min^{-1}), K(ep) (0.10 vs 0.63 min^{-1}), and V(e) (0.01 vs 0.44) than schwannomas. Second, in semiquantitative analysis, paragangliomas had visibly higher peak enhancement, shorter time for maximum enhancement, and higher signal-enhancement ratio compared with schwannomas. This agrees with semiquantitative data obtained by Yuan and colleagues[56] when examining DCE-MR imaging characteristics of paragangliomas, whereby they also found

higher peak enhancement, shorter time to peak, and higher maximum enhancement ratio than is commonly found with other benign tumors.

The pathophysiologic basis for these results is that the internal vascular architecture of paragangliomas is starkly different than other benign tumors. Although other benign tumors, such as schwannomas, have microvascular proliferation with effective perfusion and diffusion into the tumor tissue, paragangliomas are instead composed of much denser, extensive pathologic vessels with arteriovenous shunting that behave similarly to arteriovenous malformations, with significant arterial supply, but ineffective perfusion. DCE-MR imaging results for paragangliomas described above, including low K(trans), K(ep), and V(e), appear to reflect the ineffective tumor perfusion. The unique microvasculature architecture of paragangliomas compared with other benign tumors has also been demonstrated with DSC-MR imaging analysis. Razek and colleagues[57] showed that paragangliomas had a significantly increased DSC% among benign tumors ($P = .001$) owing to its prominent density of blood vessels, so much so that paragangliomas were mistaken for malignant tumors in their analysis.

Overall, these early results suggest that DCE-MR imaging may provide added diagnostic information in differentiating carotid space tumors, both through semiquantitative analysis (**Fig. 5**) and quantitative analysis. Specifically, paragangliomas have a microvascular makeup that is not commonly seen in other benign tumors, and actually more comparable to that seen in malignant tumors. This internal vascular architecture is reflected in DCE-MR imaging parameters that may help to differentiate paragangliomas from other benign carotid space tumors.

Other Clinical Applications

Multiple other applications of DCE-MR imaging of the head and neck have been examined, although with more limited results at the present. Among the more promising of these applications has been in differentiating benign from malignant salivary gland tumors. Alibek and colleagues[58] used semiquantitative analysis to show a statistically significantly longer TTP of pleomorphic adenomas compared with other parotid tumors ($P = .0011$). Malignant tumors had significantly higher maximum peak enhancement compared with all benign tumors ($P = .0049$) and compared specifically with pleomorphic adenomas ($P = .0033$). They also showed qualitative differences in TIC between pleomorphic adenomas (slow wash-in, plateau at low intensity) versus Warthin tumors and malignant parotid tumors (rapid wash-in,

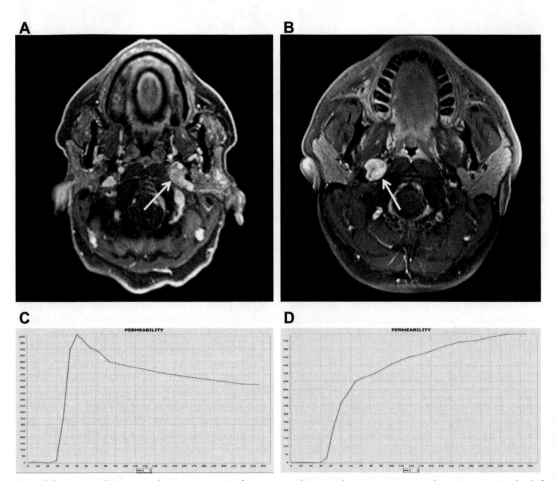

Fig. 5. (A) Paraganglioma. Axial postcontrast T1 fat-saturated image demonstrates an enhancing mass in the left carotid space (arrow). (B) Schwannoma. Axial postcontrast T1 fat-saturated image demonstrates a heterogeneously enhancing mass in the right carotid space (arrow). (C) TIC of the left carotid space paraganglioma demonstrates higher peak enhancement, shorter time to peak, and rapid wash-in and wash-out in comparison to the right carotid space schwannoma (D), which demonstrates progressive, gradual wash-in.

plateau at high intensity). Lam and colleagues[59] found that using a TTP less than 150 seconds and wash-out ratio (defined as (SI[max] − SI[5 min])/(SI [max] − SI[pre])) < 30% provided 79% sensitivity and 95% specificity in predicting salivary gland malignancy. They also found identical qualitative differences in TIC between pleomorphic adenomas and malignant tumors as above. Similarly, Matsuzaki and colleagues[60] found significantly lower TTP in malignant tumors versus benign tumors (*P* = .004). In contrast, however, a review by Assili and colleagues[61] concluded that DCE-MR imaging alone could not be reliably used to differentiate benign from malignant salivary gland tumors, although in combination with DWI could be used to increase the accuracy of discrimination between different tumor types. Thus, further investigation is needed to validate the use of DCE-MR imaging for the evaluation of salivary gland tumors, although early results indicate malignant salivary gland tumors of having faster wash-in, shorter TTP, and higher maximum peak enhancement when compared with benign tumors. However, the TIC of Warthin tumors may mimic that of malignant salivary tumors (**Fig. 6**).

Thyroid nodules have also been examined with DCE-MR imaging. Ben-David and colleagues[62] found no significant difference in both quantitative and semiquantitative parameters between benign and malignant lesions of the thyroid. However, Yuan and colleagues[63] found that thyroid carcinoma showed significantly lower wash-in slope and longer TTP (*P*<.05) than benign nodules. Qualitatively, carcinomas demonstrated a slow wash-in pattern, whereas benign nodules demonstrated rapid wash-in and rapid wash-out. These disparate study results suggest no clearly defined role for DCE-MR imaging in differentiating malignant from benign thyroid nodules at the present time (**Fig. 7**).

The role of DCE-MR imaging in evaluating orbital tumors has been studied as well. Sun and colleagues[64] found numerous statistically significant differences in DCE-MR imaging parameters when comparing lymphoma to inflammation of the orbit: shorter TTP, lower CI (defined as CI = (SI[end] − SI[pre])/SI[pre]), lower Enhancement Ratio (defined as ER = (SI[max] − SI[pre])/ SI[pre]), and higher Wash-out Ratio (defined as WR = (SI[max] − SI[end])/(SI[max] − SI[pre])).

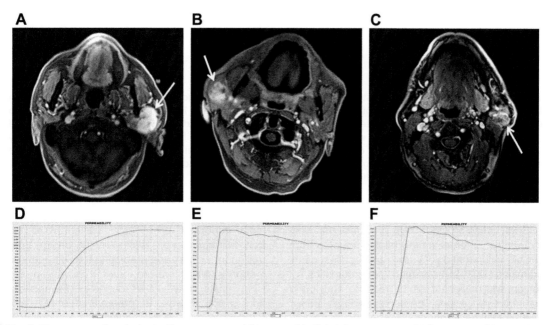

Fig. 6. Three cases of pathologically proven parotid tumors. (*A–C*) Axial postcontrast T1 fat-saturated images in 3 patients show enhancing parotid masses (*arrows*). Image A is a pleomorphic adenoma; B is an adenoid cystic carcinoma, and C is a Warthin tumor. Note the overlapping and nonspecific imaging appearances. (*D–F*) TICs of each lesion. Note the characteristic gradual progressive wash-in of contrast material associated with the pleomorphic adenoma (image D). The adenoid cystic carcinoma has a steep wash-in slope, early time to peak, and washout of contrast material (image E), characteristic of a malignant neoplasm. However, note that the Warthin tumor is associated with a TIC that appears very similar to that of the adenoid cystic carcinoma (image F). In general, DCE-MR imaging performs well in differentiating pleomorphic adenomas from all other parotid neoplasms. The performance of DCE-MR imaging in differentiating all benign parotid neoplasms from malignant parotid neoplasms is hindered by the permeability features of Warthin tumors (a benign neoplasm) that can overlap with malignancies.

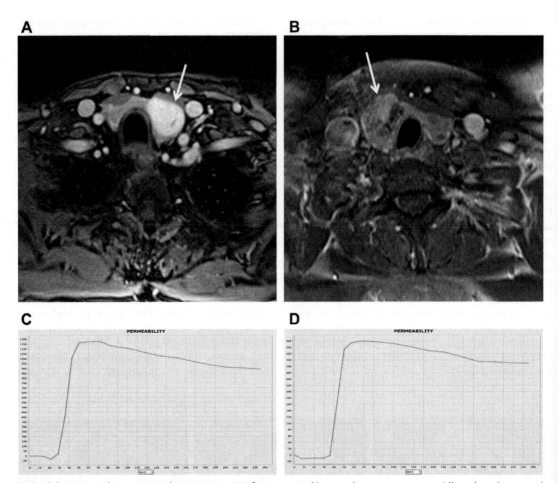

Fig. 7. (*A*) Benign adenoma. Axial postcontrast T1 fat-saturated image demonstrates an avidly enhancing mass in the left thyroid gland (*arrow*). (*B*) Papillary carcinoma. Axial postcontrast T1 fat-saturated image demonstrates a heterogeneous, predominantly isointense mass in the right thyroid gland (*arrow*). (*C*) TIC of the left thyroid benign adenoma demonstrates rapid wash-in with short time to peak, similar to that of the malignant papillary carcinoma (*D*), although with higher degree of peak contrast enhancement than the papillary carcinoma. The authors have not found DCE-MR imaging to be sufficiently accurate in discriminating between benign and malignant thyroid nodules for routine clinical use as of yet.

They further concluded that the combination of DCE-MR imaging and DWI provided the best accuracy in differentiating orbital lymphoma from orbital inflammation. Yuan and colleagues[65] examined DCE-MR imaging characteristics of benign and malignant orbital masses and found that benign lesions demonstrated a slower wash-in slope and longer TTP of contrast material compared with malignant lesions.

SUMMARY

DCE-MR imaging serves as an adjunct to conventional head and neck imaging and demonstrates the potential to discriminate between entities that are otherwise indistinguishable by conventional imaging through the quantification of microvascular permeability parameters. The most important prospective clinical roles for DCE-MR imaging are distinguishing benign from malignant entities and predicting future treatment response, with literature thus far showing promising results. However, its routine clinical application is still a work in progress due to many factors, most of all the varied image acquisition protocols and postprocessing methods used currently in the literature. Efforts to standardize the data acquisition processes of DCE-MR imaging may lead to increased clinical use. DCE-MR imaging results also need to be validated on much larger sample sizes to demonstrate consistently significant results. In addition, DCE-MR imaging results must be interpreted in a specific clinical context, because permeability parameters have different, sometimes nonintuitive meanings depending on the tissue being studied. For example, DCE-MR imaging parameters indicating increased tissue perfusion are considered favorable in the pretreatment setting, because they are an indicator of better response to chemoradiation. However, in the posttreatment setting, the interpretation of increased tissue perfusion can be challenging, with some studies favoring a treatment response and some favoring residual disease. Therefore, these nuances must be delineated clearly to clinicians, who may use DCE-MR imaging data to make important treatment decisions. Nonetheless, DCE-MR imaging constitutes an emerging application of MR imaging, which has shown the potential to add diagnostic value where conventional imaging alone may have limitations.

REFERENCES

1. Jemal A, Bray F, Center MM, et al. Global cancer statistics. CA Cancer J Clin 2011;61:69–90.
2. Tofts PS, Brix G, Buckley DL, et al. Estimating kinetic parameters from dynamic contrast enhanced T(1)-weighted MRI of a diffusable tracer: standardized quantities and symbols. J Magn Reson Imaging 1999;10:223–32.
3. Cheng HL. Investigation and optimization of parameter accuracy in dynamic contrast-enhanced MRI. J Magn Reson Imaging 2008;28:736–43.
4. Gaddikeri S, Gaddikeri RS, Tailor T, et al. Dynamic contrast-enhanced MR imaging in head and neck cancer: techniques and clinical applications. AJNR Am J Neuroradiol 2016;37(4):588–95.
5. Yabuuchi H, Fukuya T, Tajima T, et al. Salivary gland tumors: diagnostic value of gadolinium-enhanced dynamic MR imaging with histopathologic correlation. Radiology 2003;226:345–54.
6. Asaumi J, Hisatomi M, Yanagi Y, et al. Assessment of ameloblastomas using MRI and dynamic contrast-enhanced MRI. Eur J Radiol 2005;56:25–30.
7. Agrawal S, Awasthi R, Singh A, et al. An exploratory study into the role of dynamic contrast-enhanced (DCE) MRI metrics as predictors of response in head and neck cancers. Clin Radiol 2012;67:e1–5.
8. Van Cann EM, Rijpkema M, Heerschap A, et al. Quantitative dynamic contrast-enhanced MRI for the assessment of mandibular invasion by squamous cell carcinoma. Oral Oncol 2008;44:1147–54.
9. Wang HZ, Riederer SJ, Lee JN. Optimizing the precision in T1 relaxation estimation using limited flip angles. Magn Reson Med 1987;5:399–416.
10. Ogg RJ, Kingsley PB. Optimized precision of inversion-recovery T1 measurements for constrained scan time. Magn Reson Med 2004;51:625–30.
11. Freeman AJ, Gowland PA, Mansfield P. Optimization of the ultrafast Look-Locker echo-planar imaging T1 mapping sequence. Magn Reson Imaging 1998;16:765–72.
12. Cuenod CA, Balvay D. Perfusion and vascular permeability: basic concepts and measurement in DCE-CT and DCE-MRI. Diagn Interv Imaging 2013;94(12):1187–204.
13. Yankeelov TE, Gore JC. Dynamic contrast enhanced magnetic resonance imaging in oncology: theory, data acquisition, analysis, and examples. Curr Med Imaging Rev 2009;3:91–107.
14. O'Connor JP, Tofts PS, Miles KA, et al. Dynamic contrast-enhanced imaging techniques: CT and MRI. Br J Radiol 2011;84:S112–20.
15. Calamante F, Thomas DL, Pell GS, et al. Measuring cerebral blood flow using magnetic resonance imaging techniques. J Cereb Blood Flow Metab 1999;19:701–35.
16. Li KL, Zhu XP, Jackson A. Parametric mapping of scaled fitting error in dynamic susceptibility contrast enhanced MR perfusion imaging. Br J Radiol 2000;73:470–81.
17. Chavhan GB, Babyn PS, Thomas B, et al. Principles, techniques, and applications of T2*-based MR imaging and its special applications. Radiographics 2009;29:1433–49.
18. Detre JA, Leigh JS, Williams DS, et al. Perfusion imaging. Magn Reson Med 1992;23:37–45.
19. Detre JA, Zhang W, Roberts DA, et al. Tissue specific perfusion imaging using arterial spin labeling. NMR Biomed 1994;7:75–82.
20. Fujima N, Kudo K, Tsukahara A, et al. Measurement of tumor blood flow in head and neck squamous cell carcinoma by pseudo-continuous arterial spin labeling: comparison with dynamic contrast-enhanced MRI. J Magn Reson Imaging 2015;41:983–91.
21. Vaupel P, Kallinowski F, Okunieff P. Blood flow, oxygen and nutrient supply, and metabolic microenvironment of human tumors: a review. Cancer Res 1989;49:6449–65.
22. Newbold K, Castellano I, Charles-Edwards E, et al. An exploratory study into the role of dynamic contrast-enhanced magnetic resonance imaging or perfusion computed tomography for detection of intratumoral hypoxia in head-and-neck cancer. Int J Radiat Oncol Biol Phys 2009;74:29–37.
23. Egeland TA, Gulliksrud K, Gaustad JV, et al. Dynamic contrast-enhanced-MRI of tumor hypoxia. Magn Reson Med 2012;67(2):519–30.
24. Donaldson SB, Betts G, Bonington SC, et al. Perfusion estimated with rapid dynamic contrast-enhanced magnetic resonance imaging correlates inversely with vascular endothelial growth factor expression and pimonidazole staining in head-and-neck cancer: a pilot study. Int J Radiat Oncol Biol Phys 2011;81:1176–83.

25. Jansen JF, Carlson DL, Lu Y, et al. Correlation of a priori DCE-MRI and 1H MRS data with molecular markers in neck nodal metastases: initial analysis. Oral Oncol 2012;48:717–22.

26. Jensen RL, Mumert ML, Gillespie DL, et al. Preoperative dynamic contrast-enhanced MRI correlates with molecular markers of hypoxia and vascularity in specific areas of intratumoral microenvironment and is predictive of patient outcome. Neuro Oncol 2014;16(2):280–91.

27. Bernstein JM, Kershaw LE, Withey SB, et al. Tumor plasma flow determined by dynamic contrast-enhanced MRI predicts response to induction chemotherapy in head and neck cancer. Oral Oncol 2015;51(5):508–13.

28. Ng SH, Lin CY, Chan SC, et al. Dynamic contrast-enhanced MR imaging predicts local control in oropharyngeal or hypopharyngeal squamous cell carcinoma treated with chemoradiotherapy. PLoS One 2013;8:e72230.

29. Fujima N, Yoshida D, Sakashita T, et al. Usefulness of pseudocontinuous arterial spin-labeling for the assessment of patients with head and neck squamous cell carcinoma by measuring tumor blood flow in the pretreatment and early treatment period. AJNR Am J Neuroradiol 2016;37(2):342–8.

30. Wang P, Popovtzer A, Eisbruch A, et al. An approach to identify, from DCE MRI, significant subvolumes of tumors related to outcomes in advanced head-and-neck cancer. Med Phys 2012;39:5277–85.

31. Cao Y, Popovtzer A, Li D, et al. Early prediction of outcome in advanced head and neck cancer based on tumor blood volume alterations during therapy: a prospective study. Int J Radiat Oncol Biol Phys 2008;72:1287–90.

32. Chikui T, Kitamoto E, Kawano S, et al. Pharmacokinetic analysis based on dynamic contrast-enhanced MRI for evaluating tumor response to preoperative therapy for oral cancer. J Magn Reson Imaging 2012;36:589–97.

33. Tomura N, Omachi K, Sakuma I, et al. Dynamic contrast-enhanced magnetic resonance imaging in radiotherapeutic efficacy in the head and neck tumors. Am J Otolaryngol 2005;26:163–7.

34. Baba Y, Furusawa M, Murakami R, et al. Role of dynamic MRI in the evaluation of head and neck cancers treated with radiation therapy. Int J Radiat Oncol Biol Phys 1997;37:783–7.

35. Fischbein NJ, Noworolski SM, Henry RG, et al. Assessment of metastatic cervical adenopathy using dynamic contrast-enhanced MR imaging. AJNR Am J Neuroradiol 2003;24(3):301–11.

36. Abdel Razek AA, Gaballa G. Role of perfusion magnetic resonance imaging in cervical lymphadenopathy. J Comput Assist Tomogr 2011;35:21–5.

37. Kim S, Loevner LA, Quon H, et al. Prediction of response to chemoradiation therapy in squamous cell carcinomas of the head and neck using dynamic contrast-enhanced MR imaging. AJNR Am J Neuroradiol 2010;31:262–8.

38. Chawla S, Kim S, Loevner LA, et al. Prediction of disease-free survival in patients with squamous cell carcinomas of the head and neck using dynamic contrast-enhanced MR imaging. AJNR Am J Neuroradiol 2011;32:778–84.

39. Shukla-Dave A, Lee NY, Jansen JF, et al. Dynamic contrast-enhanced magnetic resonance imaging as a predictor of outcome in head-and-neck squamous cell carcinoma patients with nodal metastases. Int J Radiat Oncol Biol Phys 2012;82:1837–44.

40. Yamashita Y, Baba T, Baba Y, et al. Dynamic contrast-enhanced MR imaging of uterine cervical cancer: pharmacokinetic analysis with histopathologic correlation and its importance in predicting the outcome of radiation therapy. Radiology 2000;216:803–9.

41. George ML, Dzik-Jurasz AS, Padhani AR, et al. Non-invasive methods of assessing angiogenesis and their value in predicting response to treatment in colorectal cancer. Br J Surg 2001;88:1628–36.

42. Loncaster JA, Carrington BM, Sykes JR, et al. Prediction of radiotherapy outcome using dynamic contrast enhanced MRI of carcinoma of the cervix. Int J Radiat Oncol Biol Phys 2002;54:759–67.

43. Bone B, Szabo BK, Perbeck LG, et al. Can contrast-enhanced MR imaging predict survival in breast cancer? Acta Radiol 2003;44:373–8.

44. Ohno Y, Nogami M, Higashino T, et al. Prognostic value of dynamic MR imaging for non-small-cell lung cancer patients after chemoradiotherapy. J Magn Reson Imaging 2005;21:775–83.

45. Jansen JF, Schöder H, Lee NY, et al. Noninvasive assessment of tumor microenvironment using dynamic contrast-enhanced magnetic resonance imaging and 18F-fluoromisonidazole positron emission tomography imaging in neck nodal metastases. Int J Radiat Oncol Biol Phys 2010;77(5):1403–10.

46. Ishiyama M, Richards T, Parvathaneni U, et al. Dynamic contrast-enhanced magnetic resonance imaging in head and neck cancer: differentiation of new H&N cancer, recurrent disease, and benign post-treatment changes. Clin Imaging 2015;39(4):566–70.

47. Furukawa M, Parvathaneni U, Maravilla K, et al. Dynamic contrast-enhanced MR perfusion imaging of head and neck tumors at 3 Tesla. Head Neck 2013;35(7):923–9.

48. Semiz Oysu A, Ayanoglu E, Kodalli N, et al. Dynamic contrast-enhanced MRI in the differentiation of post-treatment fibrosis from recurrent carcinoma of the head and neck. Clin Imaging 2005;29(5):307–12.

49. Abdel Razek AA, Gaballa G, Ashamalla G, et al. Dynamic susceptibility contrast perfusion-weighted magnetic resonance imaging and diffusion-weighted

magnetic resonance imaging in differentiating recurrent head and neck cancer from postradiation changes. J Comput Assist Tomogr 2015;39(6): 849–54.

50. Lee FK, King AD, Ma BB, et al. Dynamic contrast enhancement magnetic resonance imaging (DCE-MRI) for differential diagnosis in head and neck cancers. Eur J Radiol 2012;81:784–8.

51. Park M, Kim J, Choi YS, et al. Application of dynamic contrast-enhanced MRI parameters for differentiating squamous cell carcinoma and malignant lymphoma of the oropharynx. AJR Am J Roentgenol 2016;206(2):401–7.

52. Kitamoto E, Chikui T, Kawano S, et al. The application of dynamic contrast-enhanced MRI and diffusion-weighted MRI in patients with maxillofacial tumors. Acad Radiol 2015;22(2):210–6.

53. Asaumi J, Yanagi Y, Konouchi H, et al. Application of dynamic contrast-enhanced MRI to differentiate malignant lymphoma from squamous cell carcinoma in the head and neck. Oral Oncol 2004;40: 579–84.

54. Dimitrijevic MV, Jesic SD, Mikic AA, et al. Parapharyngeal space tumors: 61 case reviews. Int J Oral Maxillofac Surg 2010;39(10):983–9.

55. Gaddikeri S, Hippe DS, Anzai Y, et al. Dynamic contrast-enhanced MRI in the evaluation of carotid space paraganglioma versus schwannoma. J Neuroimaging 2016;26(6):618–25.

56. Yuan Y, Shi H, Tao X, et al. Head and neck paragangliomas: diffusion weighted and dynamic contrast enhanced magnetic resonance imaging characteristics. BMC Med Imaging 2016;16:12.

57. Razek AA, Elsorogy LG, Soliman NY, et al. Dynamic susceptibility contrast perfusion MR imaging in distinguishing malignant from benign head and neck tumors: a pilot study. Eur J Radiol 2011;77:73–9.

58. Alibek S, Zenk J, Bozzato A, et al. The value of dynamic MRI studies in parotid tumors. Acad Radiol 2007;14(6):701–10.

59. Lam PD, Kuribayashi A, Imaizumi A, et al. Differentiating benign and malignant salivary gland tumours: diagnostic criteria and the accuracy of dynamic contrast-enhanced MRI with high temporal resolution. Br J Radiol 2015;88(1049):20140685.

60. Matsuzaki H, Yanagi Y, Hara M, et al. Minor salivary gland tumors in the oral cavity: diagnostic value of dynamic contrast-enhanced MRI. Eur J Radiol 2012;81(10):2684–91.

61. Assili S, Fathi Kazerooni A, Aghaghazvini L, et al. Dynamic contrast magnetic resonance imaging (DCE-MRI) and diffusion weighted MR imaging (DWI) for differentiation between benign and malignant salivary gland tumors. J Biomed Phys Eng 2015;5(4):157–68.

62. Ben-David E, Sadeghi N, Rezaei MK, et al. Semiquantitative and quantitative analyses of dynamic contrast-enhanced magnetic resonance imaging of thyroid nodules. J Comput Assist Tomogr 2015; 39(6):855–9.

63. Yuan Y, Yue XH, Tao XF. The diagnostic value of dynamic contrast-enhanced MRI for thyroid tumors. Eur J Radiol 2012;81(11):3313–8.

64. Sun B, Song L, Wang X, et al. Lymphoma and inflammation in the orbit: diagnostic performance with diffusion-weighted imaging and dynamic contrast-enhanced MRI. J Magn Reson Imaging 2017;45(5):1438–45.

65. Yuan Y, Kuai XP, Chen XS, et al. Assessment of dynamic contrast-enhanced magnetic resonance imaging in the differentiation of malignant from benign orbital masses. Eur J Radiol 2013;82(9): 1506–11.

Update in Parathyroid Imaging

Samuel J. Kuzminski, MD[a], Julie A. Sosa, MD[b], Jenny K. Hoang, MD[c],*

KEYWORDS

- Parathyroid • Primary hyperparathyroidism • 4D-CT • Sestamibi • Parathyroid ultrasound
- Parathyroid MR imaging

KEY POINTS

- Primary hyperparathyroidism is a clinical diagnosis based on biochemical evaluation; imaging is reserved for patients who have the established diagnosis for parathyroid localization to facilitate focused exploration or exclude ectopic disease.
- Ultrasound imaging has multiple advantages as a first-line modality; however, it performs poorly at visualizing parathyroid pathology within the mediastinum or in retroesophageal or retropharyngeal locations.
- Nuclear scintigraphy is a first-line imaging modality sensitive for both ectopic and eutopic glands, and is often used with ultrasound imaging for preoperative localization.
- Multiphase computed tomography is becoming a viable first-line imaging option, as it has analogous to superior sensitivity for parathyroid localization when compared with scintigraphy and ultrasound imaging.
- Currently, the choice of imaging algorithm is largely based on local expertise and institutional norms.

INTRODUCTION

Primary hyperparathyroidism (PHPT) is characterized by excessive, dysregulated production of parathyroid hormone (PTH) that results in the disruption of normal calcium homeostasis. Overproduction of PTH can be due to an adenomatous, hyperplastic, or carcinomatous parathyroid gland(s) and can be surgically cured. In the last decade, the development of focused surgical techniques using a small incision and limited dissection for removal of a single pathologic parathyroid gland has created the need for more precise localization of the parathyroid lesion(s) by imaging. A variety of imaging protocols and techniques have been used for this purpose. Nuclear medicine scintigraphy and ultrasound are established modalities. Recently, multiphase or 4-dimensional computed tomography (4D-CT) has emerged as modality with several advantages and has become the first-line study in several institutions. MR imaging is used less commonly, although it can be used as a second- or third-line option.

This review provides a background of PHPT and key anatomy, and discusses the parathyroid imaging modalities with updates.

Disclosure Statement: Dr J.A. Sosa is a member of the Data Monitoring Committee of the Medullary Thyroid Cancer Consortium Registry supported by Novo Nordisk, GlaxoSmithKline, AstraZeneca, and Eli Lilly. Drs S.J. Kuzminski and J.K. Hoang have nothing to disclose.
^a Department of Radiological Sciences, University of Oklahoma Health Sciences Center, College of Medicine, PO Box 2690, Garrison Tower, Suite 4G4250, Oklahoma City, OK 73126, USA; ^b Department of Surgery, Duke University, Duke University Medical Center, Box 2945, Durham, NC 27710, USA; ^c Department of Radiology, Duke University, Duke University Medical Center, Box 3808, Erwin Road, Durham, NC 27710, USA
* Corresponding author.
E-mail address: jennykh@gmail.com

Magn Reson Imaging Clin N Am 26 (2018) 151–166
https://doi.org/10.1016/j.mric.2017.08.009
1064-9689/18/© 2017 Elsevier Inc. All rights reserved.

CLINICAL CONCEPTS FOR PRIMARY HYPERPARATHYROIDISM

PHPT is 2 to 4 times more common in women than men, more common in Caucasians, and usually presents in the fifth through seventh decades of life. A solitary parathyroid adenoma is the most common cause of primary hyperparathyroidism (89%), followed by 4-gland hyperplasia (6%), double adenoma (4%), and parathyroid carcinoma (1%).[1] Most cases are sporadic, although hereditary causes exist, including multiple endocrine neoplasia types 1 and 2A, and familial isolated hyperparathyroidism.[2] A history of prior neck radiation as a child or adolescent is also a risk factor for PHPT.

According to 1 study, 85% of PHPT patients are asymptomatic at presentation,[3] with some estimates being even higher. Although asymptomatic, these patients are at risk for osteoporosis and pathologic fractures, nephrolithiasis, pancreatitis, peptic ulcer disease, renal dysfunction, and cardiovascular disease. For those with clinical manifestations, the classic mnemonic *bones, stones, groans, moans, and psychic overtones*[4] illustrates some of the more common potential symptoms. These include arthralgias, myalgias, constipation, gastrointestinal upset, weakness, and psychiatric and neurocognitive disability, including problems with memory, mood, and concentration.

The diagnosis of primary hyperparathyroidism is established based on biochemical evaluation and criteria rather than imaging; typically, increased serum calcium levels are encountered in the setting of elevated or inappropriately high normal intact PTH levels and normal renal function (**Box 1**). Normocalcemic primary hyperparathyroidism is a subtype of PHPT where PTH levels are increased despite normal serum albumin-adjusted and ionized calcium concentrations, which is confirmed on at least 2 additional occasions over a course of 3 to 6 months.[5,6] Secondary and hereditary causes of hyperparathyroidism should be excluded, including chronic renal failure or insufficiency, vitamin D deficiency, various medications such as lithium and thiazide diuretics, and benign familial hypocalciuric hypercalcemia.

Tertiary hyperparathyroidism is a unique circumstance for which imaging localization may be required. Like secondary hyperparathyroidism, tertiary hyperparathyroidism is associated with chronic renal disease. In these patients, however, persistent parathyroid stimulation related to renal disease is accompanied by autonomously functioning parathyroid tissue that is unresponsive to medical therapy. In this subset of patients, preoperative localization may be necessary to assess for a single adenoma, or in the setting of recurrent or residual disease.

Definitive treatment for primary hyperparathyroidism is surgery, although medical management and surveillance strategies can be used for many asymptomatic patients. The Fourth International Workshop released guidelines for the management of asymptomatic primary hyperparathyroidism to aid in decision making with regard to surgery versus medical management and surveillance (**Box 2**).[7] Recommendations are for all symptomatic patients with PHPT to proceed to surgery, as well as selected asymptomatic patients who meet the criteria outlined in **Box 2**. Note that some opt for surgery over medical surveillance regardless, because parathyroidectomy has a high cure rate.[1]

Broadly speaking, the 2 surgical options to consider are the traditional 4-gland exploration or

---

Box 1
What the referring clinician needs to know

- The diagnosis of primary hyperparathyroidism is based on clinical and laboratory analysis.
- Imaging is reserved for those for whom surgery is considered.
- Approximately 85% of patients with primary hyperparathyroidism have a single parathyroid adenoma that is amenable to minimally invasive parathyroidectomy. The remainder might require more extensive neck dissection.
- The choice of imaging modality is largely site specific and should be based on the experience and comfort level of the surgeons and radiologists. There is no universally accepted imaging algorithm.
- Patients undergoing reoperation run a higher risk of having an adverse outcome, generally recurrent laryngeal nerve injury. Often surgeons will require 2 concordant imaging studies before performing a repeat parathyroidectomy.
- The sensitivity for detecting smaller glands, multigland disease, and localizing patients who have had previous parathyroid surgery is lower for all available modalities, although multiphase computed tomography seems to be superior in these situations.

Box 2
Guidelines for surgery in asymptomatic hyperparathyroidism

- Serum calcium >1 mg/dL (0.25 mmol/L) above upper limit of normal.
- Decreased bone mineral density by dual-energy x-ray absorptiometry.
  ○ T-score of less than −2.5 at lumbar spine, total hip, femoral neck, or distal one-third of the radius.
- Vertebral fracture.
- Renal dysfunction, creatinine clearance of less than 60 mL/min.
- Twenty-four-hour urine calcium greater than 400 mg/d.
- Nephrolithiasis or nephrocalcinosis, increased stone risk by biochemical stone risk analysis.
- Age less than 50 years.

Data from Bilezikian JP, Brandi ML, Eastell R, et al. Guidelines for the management of asymptomatic primary hyperparathyroidism: summary statement from the Fourth International Workshop. J Clin Endocrinol Metab 2014;99(10):3562.

a focused parathyroidectomy; the latter is often facilitated by adjunctive intraoperative technologies such as rapid PTH assay testing. Focused parathyroidectomy is generally most appropriate for patients with a suspected single parathyroid adenoma, although it can be extended to bilateral exploration if an appropriate decrease in PTH is not achieved after resection of the suspected culprit gland. Minimally invasive parathyroidectomy is a commonly performed subtype of focused parathyroidectomy in which a limited incision and targeted resection is achieved with locoregional anesthesia and intravenous sedation.[8] Focused parathyroidectomy has a comparable cure rate with 4-gland exploration, and has added benefits of shorter duration of stay, shorter operative time, less postoperative pain, and lower rates of postoperative hypocalcemia.[8,9] The emergence of focused parathyroidectomy techniques has placed new importance on successful preoperative localization of culprit parathyroid pathology, and imaging becomes of vital importance for informing the surgical strategy.

Preoperative imaging is also essential for those with persistent or recurrent PHPT. There are increased risks of recurrent laryngeal nerve (RLN) injury, permanent hypoparathyroidism, and failure to cure when reoperation is required.[10] Multigland disease, ectopic, and supernumerary glands are also more commonly seen in the setting of persistent or recurrent disease and likely explain, in part, the failed primary exploration. For these reasons, most surgeons require 2 concordant confirmatory imaging studies before a repeat operation to improve localization. With adequate preoperative imaging, the success of remedial parathyroidectomy is reported to be greater than 95% in the hands of experienced, high-volume endocrine surgeons.[11]

KEY ANATOMY AND EMBRYOLOGY

Understanding parathyroid gland embryology and anatomy helps the radiologist to identify parathyroid lesions, especially when there is variant anatomy. A normal parathyroid gland is approximately $5 \times 4 \times 2$ mm, weighs 35 to 50 mg, and is generally not visible on imaging.[12] The overwhelming majority of individuals have 4 parathyroid glands, 2 superior and 2 inferior, whereas between 2.5% and 13.0% have supernumerary glands, and 3% have fewer than 4 glands.[12,13] An important surgical landmark in locating and differentiating superior from inferior glands is the RLN within the tracheoesophageal groove.

Superior parathyroid glands
- Arise from the fourth branchial pouch.
- A majority are posterior to thyroid gland at or above the level of the cricothyroid junction.
- Ectopic glands will be found in a retropharyngeal or retroesophageal location, even extending inferiorly into the mediastinum.
- Located posterior to the RLN, typically 1 cm or so above the point where the RLN crosses the inferior thyroidal artery.
- When enlarged, they may fall inferiorly and posteriorly. If a parathyroid adenoma is encountered at or below the level of the inferior pole of the thyroid gland, but is in a location posterior to the RLN, it is likely to be a descended superior parathyroid gland.

Inferior parathyroid glands
- Arise from the third branchial pouch with the thymus and have a long descent during development.

- Greater variability in location compared with superior glands.
- The majority are associated with the inferior pole of the thyroid gland, either posterior, anterior, lateral, or inferior to it, and they can be intrathyroidal.
- Ectopic locations include the thyrothymic ligament and thymus, with some descending into the anterior mediastinum as far as the pericardium. A minority have arrested descent, and can occur in close approximation to the carotid space as far cranially as the angle of the mandible.
- Tend to be anterior to the RLN.

Blood supply to the parathyroid glands is usually via the inferior thyroid artery, and often an enlarged inferior thyroid artery will be observed with an adenomatous gland. In a minority of cases, the superior thyroid artery will supply the superior parathyroid glands. Venous drainage is via the superior, middle, and inferior parathyroid veins.

COMPARING IMAGING TECHNIQUES: WHICH ONE TO PERFORM FIRST?

There is no universally accepted algorithm for imaging of the parathyroid glands, and the choice of imaging approach is largely based on surgeon preference and expertise at the radiology practice. Reported sensitivities of the imaging modalities vary depending on the study cohort and bias. In practice, nuclear medicine scintigraphy and ultrasound imaging are the most commonly used first-line modalities. However, a recent survey found that 4D-CT scanning is gaining acceptance as a first-line study, because its usefulness is more widely recognized.[14]

Comparing the relative effectiveness of the different imaging modalities is challenging, and no one technique or imaging algorithm has proven to be clearly superior in localizing parathyroid lesions; however, 4D-CT scanning has some advantageous qualities, most notably in predicting multigland disease and in the setting of remedial parathyroidectomy.[15–18] According to one metaanalysis, the pooled sensitivities and positive predictive values of ultrasound, sestamibi-single photon emission computed tomography (SPECT) scans, and 4D-CT scanning were as follows:

- Ultrasound had a sensitivity of 76.1% and a positive predictive value of 93.2%.
- Sestamibi-SPECT scanning had a sensitivity of 78.9% and a positive predictive value of 90.7%.
- Four-dimensional-CT had a sensitivity of 89.4% and a positive predictive value of

93.5%.[19] There were only two 4D-CT studies included in this analysis. A more recent meta-analysis of 4D-CT concluded that the pooled sensitivity of localizing the parathyroid adenoma to the correct quadrant was 73%, and the sensitivity of 4D-CT for correctly lateralizing the parathyroid adenoma was 81%.[20]

There are 2 clinical scenarios for which parathyroid imaging is particularly challenging. Multigland disease occurs in approximately 10% to 15% of patients, and preoperative recognition of multigland disease is important, because it necessitates more extensive surgery.[1,21,22] Unfortunately, none of the available modalities perform particularly well at identifying multigland disease, although 4D-CT scanning is likely superior in this regard.[16,18] Reported sensitivities for multigland disease are 4D-CT scanning (32%–55%), ultrasound imaging (15%–35%), and 99mTc-sestamibi imaging (30%–44%).[18,20] Parathyroid lesions in multigland disease tend to be smaller, often less than 1 cm in greatest diameter. In 1 study, 36% of abnormal parathyroid glands in multigland disease remained imperceptible by 4D-CT scanning, despite knowledge of surgical localization. These same investigators developed a tool for predicting multigland disease based on lesion size, number of candidate lesions on 4D-CT, and biochemical markers, which improved their ability to classify patients as single versus multigland disease.[18]

The second challenging subgroup are those with persistent or recurrent disease, and 4D-CT scanning seems to be advantageous compared with the other modalities.[17,23] This subset of patients presents challenges owing to altered anatomy related to prior neck dissection, as well as the increased prevalence of multigland disease and ectopic glands. A direct comparison of 4D-CT scanning, sestamibi parathyroid imaging, and ultrasound imaging revealed 4D-CT scanning to be much more sensitive and accurate than the other modalities for lateralizing and localizing hyperfunctioning parathyroid tissue in patients undergoing reoperation.[17]

A comparison of the 3 main imaging modalities also should include costs. Ultrasound imaging is the least costly, followed by 4D-CT scans, and then sestamibi studies. The most cost-effective strategy, according to one model, seems to be ultrasound examination, with 4D-CT scanning in selected patients if the ultrasound examination is negative or indeterminate.[24] In this model, strategies using nuclear scintigraphy were more expensive, and bilateral neck exploration was the most expensive. This model accounted for the widely variable sensitivities of the modalities that have been reported in the literature as well as the potential risks involved with radiation exposure.

IMAGING MODALITIES: TECHNIQUE, IMAGING FINDINGS, AND UPDATES
Ultrasound Imaging

Technique
The patient is imaged with a high-frequency linear transducer, and B-mode scanning is performed from the carotid bifurcation to the thoracic inlet in the craniocaudal direction and from the carotid to carotid in the mediolateral direction (**Table 1**). Color and power Doppler imaging are used as adjuncts in the imaging evaluation once a candidate lesion is identified.

Imaging findings
On ultrasound examination, normal parathyroid glands are typically invisible. However, when a parathyroid gland becomes adenomatous or hyperplastic, it enlarges and usually decreases in echogenicity (**Fig. 1**). A hyperplastic or adenomatous parathyroid gland usually appears as a hypoechoic oval, rounded, or lobulated solid lesion with a well-defined echogenic capsule. Some parathyroid lesions, and especially larger ones, can undergo cystic degeneration, fat deposition, fibrosis, calcification, or hemorrhage, thereby altering the classic appearance. Cystic degeneration results in some portion of the parathyroid gland becoming anechoic with posterior acoustic enhancement. Internal fat, hemorrhage, calcifications, and fibrosis, in contrast, result in a heterogeneous-appearing gland with regions of increased echogenicity.

When color or power Doppler imaging is used, adenomas often have a ring or arc of vascularity.[25] Sometimes, an enlarged vessel can be observed entering the end of the elongated abnormal parathyroid gland, a finding termed the "polar vessel sign." This finding discriminates parathyroid glands from lymph nodes, because lymph nodes lack a ring of vascularity and have vessels entering at the hilum rather than the pole. Increased vascularity in the thyroid gland ipsilateral to a parathyroid adenoma is also a common finding, and can be useful for confirming the identity of a suspected lesion.[26]

Advantages

- No ionizing radiation or contrast administration.
- Noninvasive, fast, and inexpensive.
- The ability to evaluate the thyroid gland for lesions that may require further evaluation or removal.
- Can be performed by the surgeon, and can be used immediately before, or during surgery to aid in successful lesion localization and removal.
- Ultrasound imaging also can be used to guide fine needle aspiration biopsy of a suspected lesion before surgery in selected cases.[27]

Limitations

- Thyroid nodules and lymph nodes may mimic adenomas, and the presence of thyroid nodules decreases the sensitivity of the imaging study.[28,29]
- Visualizing parathyroid adenomas within the mediastinum or in retroesophageal or retropharyngeal locations where bone and air, respectively, prevent visualization of deeper structures.
- The sensitivity for small parathyroid glands is generally poor, and it has limited sensitivity in multigland disease and reoperative cases.[1,17,28,29]
- Body habitus also influences the performance of parathyroid ultrasound imaging, with decreased sensitivity in obese patients.

Updates
Ultrasound elastography is a method to quantify the stiffness of tissues, and initial data suggest that it may have some usefulness in parathyroid imaging with regard to discriminating a parathyroid adenoma from a thyroid nodule or hyperplastic parathyroid gland. When comparing parathyroid adenomas to parathyroid hyperplasia or benign thyroid nodules, adenomas display significantly greater stiffness. Conversely, malignant thyroid nodules tend to have greater stiffness than parathyroid adenomas.[30] Preoperative differentiation of these entities would be of great benefit to the surgeon and potentially increase the value of preoperative ultrasound, although the application of this technique to parathyroid imaging is recent, and it remains to be seen if this affects clinical or surgical outcomes.

Nuclear Scintigraphy

Technique
Nuclear scintigraphy uses the preferential uptake of a radionuclide by 1 or more hyperfunctioning parathyroid glands for preoperative localization. Over time, the techniques for scintigraphic imaging of the parathyroid gland have been refined, and the protocol varies by site (see **Table 1**). Planar imaging is still in use, although at many centers it has been augmented by SPECT scans, often times with coregistration to computed tomography images (SPECT-CT).

Table 1
Sample parathyroid imaging protocols

Modality	Protocol
Ultrasound imaging[57]	• Patient is supine, neck hyperextended. • Image with a high frequency, >10 MHz, linear transducer. • B-mode scanning from carotid bifurcation to thoracic inlet in the longitudinal plane, from carotid to carotid in the transverse plane. • Color or power Doppler technique to evaluate vascularity.

Nuclear scintigraphy[32]	Imaging parameters
	• Planar images with a high-resolution collimator, include both the neck and mediastinum
	  ○ Additional imaging can be performed with a pinhole or converging collimator.
	• Planar images obtained first, followed by SPECT or SPECT/CT for each time point.
	Dual phase, single isotope
	• 20–30 mCi ^{99m}Tc-sestamibi administered intravenously.
	• Two phases of imaging
	  ○ Early: 10–30 min after injection.
	  ○ Delayed: 1.5–2.5 h after injection.
	Single phase, dual isotope
	• Agents without parathyroid uptake
	  ○ 2–10 mCi ^{99m}Tc-pertechnitate or
	  ○ 200–600 μCi ^{123}I.
	• Agents with parathyroid uptake
	  ○ 20–30 mCi ^{99m}Tc-sestamibi (typically) or ^{99m}Tc-tetrofosmin are administered intravenously.
	• The 2 acquisitions are subtracted, yielding a parathyroid-only image.
	• If ^{99m}Tc-pertechnitate is used, it may be administered before or after ^{99m}Tc-sestamibi. ^{123}I must be given before ^{99m}Tc-sestamibi.
	  ○ ^{99m}Tc-pertechnitate then ^{99m}Tc-sestamibi
	    ■ High count, 10 min, images are obtained 30 min after ^{99m}Tc-pertechnitate injection.
	    ■ After imaging is completed, ^{99m}Tc-sestamibi is injected and high-count images are obtained 10 min later.
	  ○ ^{99m}Tc-sestamibi then ^{99m}Tc-pertechnitate
	    ■ ^{99m}Tc-sestamibi is injected and high-count images are obtained 10 min later.
	    ■ After ^{99m}Tc-pertechnitate injection, the patient is immobilized for 15–30 min, then imaging is performed.
	  ○ ^{123}I then ^{99m}Tc-sestamibi
	    High count images are obtained 4 h after ^{123}I injection, then ^{99m}Tc-sestamibi is injected and images are performed 10 min later.

4D-CT[45]	• 0.625 mm section thickness, 0.4 s tube rotation time, 0.516:1 pitch factor, 20 cm field of view.
	• 120 kVp with automatic tube current modulation, noise index 8, minimum of 100 mÅ and maximum 400 mÅ (nonenhanced and delayed phases) or 600 mÅ (arterial phase).
	• Contrast injection of 75 mL of iopamidol at 4 mL/s, right antecubital fossa vein
	• Scanning
	  ○ Nonenhanced phase from the hyoid bone to clavicular head
	  ○ Arterial and delayed phases from the angle of the mandible to the carina at 25 and 80 s after the start of the contrast injection, respectively
	    ■ Bolus tracking if significantly decreased cardiac output
	• 1 mm thick contiguous axial images in all 3 phases
	• 2.5 mm thick contiguous axial, coronal, and sagittal reformations in all 3 phases

(continued on next page)

Table 1
(continued)

Modality	Protocol

MR imaging	• Protocols and scan parameters vary by site, magnet, and vendor.
	• Field of view to include the area from the carotid bifurcation to the level of the carina
	• Three-plane localizer
	• Fat saturated T2-weighted FSE
	  ○ Chemical fat saturation or inversion recovery.
	  ○ Many advocate Dixon fat suppression technique, more homogeneous fat suppression.
	  ○ Can be acquired in >1 scan plane
	• Axial T1-weighted
	• Postcontrast (optional)
	  ○ Fat saturated T1-weighted FSE.
	  ○ Dynamic contrast-enhanced images.

Abbreviations: CT, computed tomography; 4D-CT, 4-dimensional computed tomography; FSE, fast spin echo.

The most common radiotracer used for parathyroid imaging is ^{99m}Tc-sestamibi. ^{99m}Tc-sestamibi is concentrated in mitochondria in various metabolically active tissues including thyroid gland, heart, liver, salivary glands, and abnormal parathyroid glands (**Fig. 2**).[31] Parathyroid scintigraphy is performed as a dual phase, single isotope study or dual isotope, single phase study (see **Table 1**). There is no clear consensus as to the superiority of the 2 techniques,[32] although dual

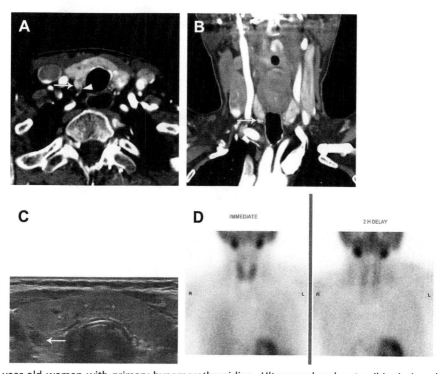

Fig. 1. 79-year-old woman with primary hyperparathyroidism. Ultrasound and sestamibi scintigraphy were reported as negative. (*A*) Axial and (*B*) coronal arterial phase images show a candidate lesion in the right lower location (*arrow*). The confidence score for the lesion is "consistent with" based on Type A relative enhancement pattern, and a polar vessel (*arrowhead*). (*C*) In retrospect, the lesion was present on ultrasound (*arrows*) and hypoechogenic relative to the thyroid gland. Note an incidental thyroid nodule (*cursors*). (*D*) The lesion was not seen on the scintigraphy study.

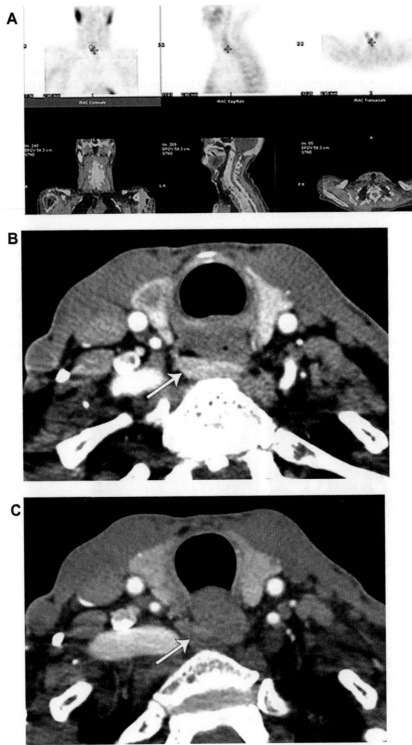

Fig. 2. 70-year-old man with primary hyperparathyroidism. (*A*) Sestamibi scintigraphy shows a focal area of tracer uptake on the right posterior to the esophagus (*red cursors*). (*B*) Axial arterial phase image shows a corresponding vividly enhancing mass (*arrow*). (*C*) Axial delayed phase image shows wash out of contrast from the mass (*arrow*) greater than the thyroid. The confidence score for the lesion is "consistent with" based on Type B relative enhancement pattern, and size of 25 mm.

isotope technique results in a higher radiation dose to the patient and requires that the patient remain in the same position for both phases.

The use of SPECT scanning improves parathyroid lesion localization.[33] Furthermore, registering the SPECT imaging to grayscale CT images (SPECT-CT) provides additional anatomic information, although with the cost of increased radiation dose. SPECT and SPECT-CT scans are particularly useful for ectopic gland localization, such as those extending into the mediastinum.[32] Some contradictory data exist with regard to whether SPECT and SPECT-CT scans improve the sensitivity for the detection of abnormal parathyroid glands over planar imaging alone, although a number of studies indicate that they do.[33–35]

Imaging findings

The detection of abnormal parathyroid glands depends on both increased focal uptake and prolonged retention of ^{99m}Tc-sestamibi. Initially, the abnormal parathyroid gland is visible as a focus of increased activity superimposed on the background of normal, physiologic uptake (see **Fig. 2**). If delayed imaging is performed, more of the activity washes out of the surrounding tissues than the hyperfunctioning parathyroid gland(s), improving identification of the parathyroid lesion(s).

Advantages

- Relatively operator independent in comparison with ultrasound examination.
- Detects ectopic and posterior glands that ultrasound examination may miss.
- SPECT-CT provides the surgeon with valuable anatomic landmarks.
- Lower radiation dose than with 4D-CT.[36]
- Can be used as a tool in the operating room for parathyroid localization, a technique termed radioguided parathyroidectomy. ^{99m}Tc-sestamibi is injected 1 to 2 hours before surgery, and a handheld gamma probe is used intraoperatively to localize the abnormal gland. Radionuclide counts of greater than 20% higher than background within the resected tissue is verification that the parathyroid lesion has been removed.[22,37] Some investigators find this technique to be a useful adjunct to preoperative imaging localization and intraoperative PTH monitoring.

Limitations

- Duration of time for study acquisition. Patients must remain relatively motionless for extended periods of time, especially if a dual isotope protocol is used.
- It is more expensive than ultrasound or 4D-CT scans.[24]
- Radiation dose, with a small estimated lifetime attributable risk of cancer increase of 0.19%.[36]
- Scintigraphy performs poorly at detecting small glands, multigland disease, and in the remedial setting.[18,38]
- Parathyroid adenoma subtypes with fewer oxyphil cells take up less radiotracer and, thus, decrease the sensitivity of the study.[31]
- On single isotope, dual phase imaging, some lesions do not follow the classic pattern with delayed washout compared with the thyroid. This pattern is particularly true in the setting of parathyroid hyperplasia, making accurate identification more difficult.[32]
- There are a number of parathyroid mimics on nuclear scintigraphy. Parathyroid carcinoma, thyroid nodules, thyroid malignancies, asymmetric thyroid tissue, asymmetrically enlarged submandibular gland tissue, lymphadenopathy, sarcoidosis, and Graves' disease are all potential causes of false positive studies (**Box 3**).[39–42] Correlation with anatomic imaging such as SPECT-CT, 4D-CT, ultrasound, or MR imaging can often aid in correctly identifying the cause of the spurious uptake.

Updates

Recently, PET scanning has been described in parathyroid imaging, although data are limited and PET scanning has yet to find widespread clinical use for parathyroid lesion localization. A number of radiopharmaceuticals have been used, including ^{18}F-fluorochlorine, ^{18}F-fluorodeoxyglucose, and most commonly ^{11}C-methionine. There are major limitations to parathyroid PET imaging, including concomitant thyroid uptake of ^{11}C-methionine, resulting in decreased sensitivity for lesions adjacent to the thyroid, and the widely discrepant sensitivities of ^{18}F-fluorodeoxyglucose, ranging from 0% to 94%.[43,44] Expense, radiation

---

Box 3
Differential considerations for a parathyroid lesion

- Lymph node
- Thyroid nodule
- Lobule of normal thyroid gland, asymmetric, or ectopic thyroid tissue
- Ectopic thymic tissue

dose, and limitations of radiotracer production (^{11}C-methionine requires a cyclotron) all limit the usefulness of this modality. A restricted role for PET-CT may exist as a problem solving tool in evaluating discrepant or false-negative results after an imaging evaluation with more conventional modalities is exhausted.[44]

Four-Dimensional Computed Tomography

Multiphase parathyroid CT scanning, also referred to as 4D-CT scanning, is a relatively newer technique for preoperative parathyroid imaging compared with ultrasound imaging and scintigraphy. Because there are some inherent advantages to this technique, the use of 4D-CT scans is increasing. At a majority of institutions, it remains a second- or third-line study, although a recent survey suggested that approximately 10% have adopted it as the first-line study. It is anticipated that use will likely only increase.[14]

Technique

The name 4D-CT scan originates from the number of phases of imaging, typically 3, and the change over time, the fourth dimension. As with scintigraphy, 4D-CT protocols vary by site. In reality, only approximately one-half of institutions with parathyroid CT scanners use a 3-phase protocol, whereas others image with 2 or 4 phases.[14]

The initial phase of a 3-phase protocol is nonenhanced, extending from the hyoid bone to the clavicular heads. The purpose of the nonenhanced phase is to differentiate parathyroid tissue, which is low in attenuation, from the high attenuation of the thyroid gland. Intravenous contrast is administered at a rate of 4 mL/s, and imaging is performed at 25 and 80 seconds after the initiation of the contrast injection. These arterial and venous contrast-enhanced phases are imaged from the angle of the mandible to the carina to include the potential locations for ectopic parathyroid lesions in the neck and thorax within the imaging field.[45]

Imaging findings

The characteristic appearance of an adenomatous or hyperplastic parathyroid gland on 4D-CT scans is a soft tissue nodule with enhancement peaking in the arterial phase and diminishing, or washing out, in the venous phase. This enhancement pattern differentiates parathyroid lesions from lymph nodes, which progressively enhance. Findings that are often but not uniformly present are a polar vessel and internal cystic degeneration. The polar vessel on CT scans is the analog to the finding described on ultrasound imaging, an enlarged vessel entering one end of the elongated parathyroid gland. When present, these signs are useful to confirm the identity of a candidate lesion and increase the radiologist's confidence in interpretation of the imaging findings.

Advantages

- Rapid acquisition times, which means that 4D-CT scanning is much less motion sensitive compared with MR imaging (in particular).
- Provides superior anatomic information compared with the other modalities, a factor that may be useful in operative planning.
- There are data to suggest that the sensitivity of 4D-CT scanning for preoperative localization of abnormal parathyroid glands is superior to ultrasound imaging and scintigraphy.
- Four-dimensional CT seems to be more sensitive than ultrasound imaging and scintigraphy for small glands (see **Fig. 1**), multigland disease (**Fig. 3**), and in the remedial setting.[19,46]

Limitations

- The radiation dose from a 4D-CT scan using a standard, 3-phase protocol results in an effective dose of 28 mSv, more than double that of scintigraphy, with an increase in lifetime incidence of cancer of 0.52%.[36] Dose reduction techniques, such as dual-energy CT scans, have the potential to mitigate some of the concern. A recent study found similar sensitivity for parathyroid adenomas using dual-energy CT scans compared with conventional 4D-CT scans, with a dose reduction of greater than 50%.[47]
- Intravenous contrast administration carried related risks of contrast-induced nephropathy and contrast allergy.
- Artifact related to metal or concentrated contrast material within the neck veins can obscure adjacent structures and result in missed lesions.

Updates

Recently, the necessity of the 3-phase protocol has been brought into question; the primary concern is the radiation dose incurred by the patient during the additional phase.[20,48] Eliminating one of the phases, typically the nonenhanced phase, may come at the cost of decreased sensitivity and accuracy in lesion localization. The reason for this is that a substantial number of lesions (approximately 20%) do not exhibit the typical enhancement characteristics and could be missed on a 2-phase study.[49] This concern is particularly true for smaller lesions, the detection of which is one of the advantageous qualities

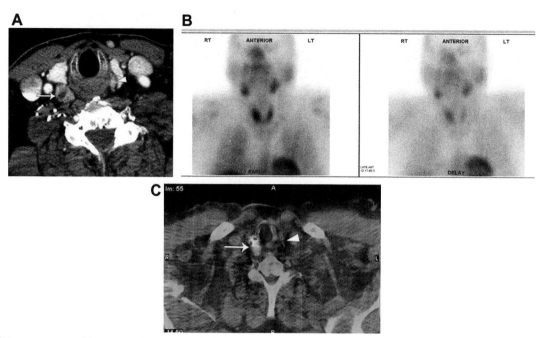

Fig. 3. 77-year-old man with primary hyperparathyroidism. (*A*) Axial arterial phase image shows a vividly enhancing mass posterior to the right thyroid lobe (*arrow*) with cystic change. There is an additional lesion on the left (*arrowhead*). (*B*) Sestamibi scintigraphy planar images with immediate and delayed images was interpreted as normal. Persistent uptake was thought to represent thyroid tissue. (*C*) In retrospect, the double adenomas (*arrow and arrowhead*) were better seen on the SPECT-CT images, but mistaken for thyroid tissue.

of 4D-CT scans. A recent publication described 3 patterns of contrast enhancement (termed types A, B, and C) for parathyroid lesions based on a visual assessment using the thyroid gland as an internal control (**Table 2**). Types A and B enhancement conform to the characteristic enhancement pattern of parathyroid adenomas, whereas type C lesions neither hyperenhance nor washout. Differentiating these atypical lesions from the adjacent thyroid gland would be difficult if not impossible for some of these lesions without the nonenhanced series of images (**Fig. 4**).[49]

Additional findings, like the presence of an enlarged polar vessel or cystic degeneration, are morphologic factors that can aid in accurate interpretation. A confidence scoring system was recently developed to combine the enhancement pattern and morphologic features to provide a standardized method for reporting the radiologist's confidence in lesion localization by 4D-CT scan (see **Table 2**; see **Figs. 1–4**; **Fig. 5**). Although limited to a single institution's experience at this time, this scoring system has been well-received by referring surgeons. Using this scoring system, a patient with only 1 high confidence lesion could presumably proceed to surgery using a focused approach, whereas those with multiple or no high

Table 2 Duke 4-dimensional computed tomography scoring system	
Score	**Imaging Features**
Consistent with	Type A or B enhancement plus at least one additional finding
Suspicious for	Type A or B enhancement without an additional finding *Or* Type C enhancement plus at least one additional finding
Possible	Type C enhancement without an additional finding

Enhancement types: All use the thyroid as a reference
A. Greater in attenuation than thyroid on arterial phase (hyperenhance), can have any appearance on delayed phase
B. Similar or lower in attenuation than thyroid on arterial phase, lower in attenuation (washout) on delayed phase.
C. Neither hyperenhance on arterial phase nor washout on delayed phase.
Additional findings: Size ≥1 cm, cystic change, polar vessel

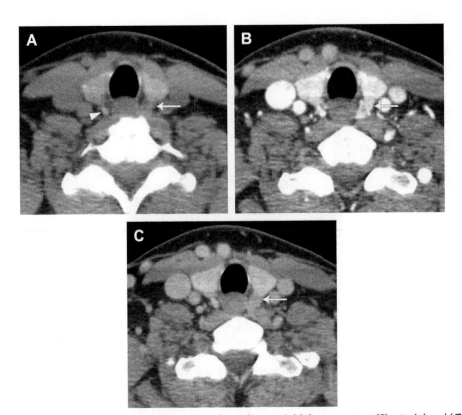

Fig. 4. A 64-year-old woman with primary hyperparathyroidism. Axial (*A*) noncontrast (*B*) arterial and (*C*) delayed phase images show a candidate lesion in the left para-esophageal location (*arrows*). The confidence score for the lesion is "consistent with" based on Type B relative enhancement pattern, and size 15 mm. Another right sided lesion (*arrowhead*) has high attenuation on the noncontrast phase. This represents thyroid tissue.

confidence lesions might require additional imaging or an anticipated 4-gland exploration. This scoring system could change the threshold for surgical intervention, placement of the incision, or anesthetic approach (local anesthesia with sedation vs general anesthesia).

MR Imaging

The use of MR imaging for parathyroid imaging has been limited in scope. New sequences, technology, and techniques show promise in improving MR imaging of the parathyroid glands, although some challenges remain. Currently, it remains a second- or third-line modality reserved for problem solving, reoperative cases, or as an adjunct to more established modalities.[50] Like the other modalities listed, the sensitivities of MR imaging for parathyroid detection cited in the literature are highly variable and range from 43% to 94%.[22,51–53]

Technique

The basic imaging protocol for parathyroid MR imaging includes both T1- and T2-weighted images, typically fast spin echo sequences, with a field of view extending from the carotid bifurcation to the carina.[53] Fat saturation is generally performed on T2-weighted images, and both inversion recovery and chemical fat suppression techniques have been described.[53–55] A common technique used in the literature is a chemical shift-based Dixon water–fat separation method, which reportedly provides more homogenous fat suppression than alternative techniques.[53,55] The usefulness of gadolinium-based contrast administration is debatable.[51]

Imaging findings

Adenomatous and hyperplastic parathyroid glands typically have high signal on T2-weighted images, which may manifest as a relatively homogenous appearance or one that has been described as "marbled."[53] On T1-weighted images, parathyroid lesions are usually intermediate to low in intensity. The presence of remote hemorrhage or fibrosis can decrease signal intensity on both T1 and T2 weighting, whereas more recent hemorrhage can result in increased signal intensity on both sequences.

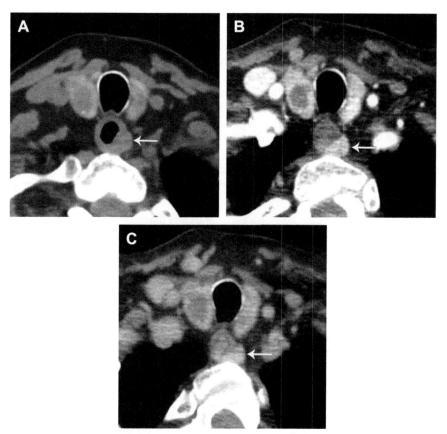

Fig. 5. 68-year-old woman with primary hyperparathyroidism. Axial (*A*) noncontrast (*B*) arterial and (*C*) delayed phase images show a candidate lesion in the left para-esophageal location (*arrows*). The low attenuation on non-contrast phase helps to differentiate this lesion from thyroid tissue. The confidence score for the lesion is "highly suspicious" based on Type C relative enhancement pattern, and size of 26 mm.

Advantages

- Lacks ionizing radiation.
- Superior anatomic information inherent to cross-sectional imaging.
- Intravenous contrast material is not necessary for parathyroid detection; therefore, this technique can be used in pregnant patients, those with renal dysfunction, contrast allergy, or any other predisposing factor making iodinated or gadolinium based contrast material administration contraindicated.

Limitations

- MR imaging is expensive and time consuming.
- MR imaging is contraindicated in a number of patients with metallic foreign bodies or implant incompatible with MR imaging.
- Lack of specificity of the imaging characteristics of parathyroid lesions. Lymph nodes and thyroid nodules, the primary differential considerations in parathyroid imaging, often

have similar signal characteristics. Contrast is of limited usefulness to further discriminate between these differential considerations, because most MR imaging sequences lack the temporal resolution over the large field of view.[50] There are newer techniques, discussed elsewhere in this article, that aim to solve that problem.

Updates

Recent advances in MR imaging might have the ability to improve the usefulness of MR imaging for para-thyroid imaging. Improvements in fat suppression sequences result in more homogeneous fat suppression, with the most commonly described technique being a Dixon fat suppression method.[55] Advances in dynamic contrast-enhanced imaging and parallel imaging present solutions to some of the limitations of traditional contrast-enhanced imaging.[54,55] Using these techniques, the rapidly peaking enhancement and subsequent washout characteristic of many parathyroid lesions can

---

Box 4
Pearls, pitfalls, and variants

- For all imaging modalities, it is important to extend the field of imaging to cover potential ectopic parathyroid sites.
- Differentiation of intrathyroidal parathyroid glands from thyroid nodules can be difficult, because the imaging appearances can overlap.
- Parathyroid adenomas may undergo cystic degeneration, hemorrhage, calcification, fibrosis, or have fat deposition. All of these changes may alter the imaging appearance.
- Hyperplastic glands, which are often smaller than adenomatous glands, may have atypical imaging appearances and are often more difficult to detect.

---

be observed. As imaging after contrast administration is continuous, contrast–time curves can be generated that allow for quantitative analysis of the perfusion parameters, including time-to-peak enhancement, washin, and washout. In 1 study, the application of dynamic contrast-enhanced MR imaging allowed for a diagnostic accuracy of 96% in differentiating parathyroid lesions from lymph nodes and thyroid nodules.[55] Although these newer techniques show promise, further study is necessary before MR imaging can regularly supplant ultrasound, scintigraphy, or 4D-CT examination in the imaging evaluation of primary hyperparathyroidism.

Fine Needle Aspiration

Fine needle aspiration of potential parathyroid lesions is sometimes necessary in challenging cases to confirm the parathyroid origin of a potential lesion before surgery. Thyroid nodules and abnormal parathyroid glands have overlapping imaging appearances, and even cytology cannot reliably differentiate follicular thyroid from parathyroid tissue.[22] Imaging guidance, typically ultrasound imaging, is used to direct the needle, and an intact PTH level is measured from the aspirate.[56] An elevated PTH is specific for parathyroid tissue, although further characterization (ie, parathyroid adenoma vs carcinoma) is often impossible.[22]

Selective Arteriography and Selective Venous Sampling

The preoperative evaluation of PHPT patients is dominated by noninvasive imaging; however, selective arteriography and selective venous sampling are invasive techniques that may be useful in remedial cases. Selective arteriography relies on visualizing the increased vascularity of an abnormal parathyroid gland, whereas selective venous sampling attempts to localize the hyperfunctioning gland by measuring PTH levels in multiple cervical veins, and comparing these values with PTH levels in peripheral veins. These techniques are expensive

and carry the risks inherent to invasive vascular procedures, including vascular injury, stroke (for arteriography), bleeding, and radiation exposure. Both techniques require great technical skill to perform, and are typically reserved for remedial cases.

SUMMARY

Parathyroid imaging continues to evolve with the emergence of new techniques, although, at this time, no modality has demonstrated clear superiority. The choice of imaging algorithm is largely based on local experience and institutional norms; however, there are some commonalities that can be applied to any of the available imaging modalities (**Box 4**). Ultrasound imaging and nuclear scintigraphy are well-established studies and are most commonly used. A newer modality, 4D-CT is gaining acceptance as either a first- or second-line examination. It has high sensitivity, and some studies suggest it has a sensitivity that is the highest of all of the available modalities, potentially allowing it to outperform the alternative modalities at imaging reoperative patients, small glands, and multigland disease. As technology continues to evolve and experience with MR imaging and 4D-CT scanning grows, it is possible that one or a combination of modalities becomes predominant.

REFERENCES

1. Ruda JM, Hollenbeak CS, Stack BC Jr. A systematic review of the diagnosis and treatment of primary hyperparathyroidism from 1995 to 2003. Otolaryngol Head Neck Surg 2005;132(3):359–72.
2. Kraimps JL, Duh QY, Demeure M, et al. Hyperparathyroidism in multiple endocrine neoplasia syndrome. Surgery 1992;112(6):1080–6 [discussion: 1086–8].
3. Rubin MR, Bilezikian JP, McMahon DJ, et al. The natural history of primary hyperparathyroidism with or

without parathyroid surgery after 15 years. J Clin Endocrinol Metab 2008;93(9):3462–70.

4. Mysliwiec J. Mnemonics for endocrinologists - hyperparathyroidism. Endokrynol Pol 2012;63(6):504–5.

5. Pawlowska M, Cusano NE. An overview of normocalcemic primary hyperparathyroidism. Curr Opin Endocrinol Diabetes Obes 2015;22(6):413–21.

6. Eastell R, Brandi ML, Costa AG, et al. Diagnosis of asymptomatic primary hyperparathyroidism: proceedings of the Fourth International Workshop. J Clin Endocrinol Metab 2014;99(10):3570–9.

7. Bilezikian JP, Brandi ML, Eastell R, et al. Guidelines for the management of asymptomatic primary hyperparathyroidism: summary statement from the Fourth International Workshop. J Clin Endocrinol Metab 2014;99(10):3561–9.

8. Udelsman R, Lin Z, Donovan P. The superiority of minimally invasive parathyroidectomy based on 1650 consecutive patients with primary hyperparathyroidism. Ann Surg 2011;253(3):585–91.

9. Jinih M, O'Connell E, O'Leary DP, et al. Focused versus bilateral parathyroid exploration for primary hyperparathyroidism: a systematic review and meta-analysis. Ann Surg Oncol 2017;24(7): 1924–34.

10. Wells SA Jr, Debenedetti MK, Doherty GM. Recurrent or persistent hyperparathyroidism. J Bone Miner Res 2002;17(Suppl 2):N158–62.

11. Udelsman R, Donovan PI. Remedial parathyroid surgery: changing trends in 130 consecutive cases. Ann Surg 2006;244(3):471–9.

12. Akerstrom G, Malmaeus J, Bergstrom R. Surgical anatomy of human parathyroid glands. Surgery 1984;95(1):14–21.

13. Nakatsuka K, Nishizawa Y, Ishimura E, et al. The fifth hyperfunctioning parathyroid gland in end-stage renal disease. Nephron 1989;51(1):140–2.

14. Hoang JK, Williams K, Gaillard F, et al. Parathyroid 4D-CT: multi-institutional international survey of use and trends. Otolaryngol Head Neck Surg 2016; 155(6):956–60.

15. Kukar M, Platz TA, Schaffner TJ, et al. The use of modified four-dimensional computed tomography in patients with primary hyperparathyroidism: an argument for the abandonment of routine sestamibi single-positron emission computed tomography (SPECT). Ann Surg Oncol 2015;22(1): 139–45.

16. Galvin L, Oldan JD, Bahl M, et al. Parathyroid 4D CT and scintigraphy: what factors contribute to missed parathyroid lesions? Otolaryngol Head Neck Surg 2016;154(5):847–53.

17. Mortenson MM, Evans DB, Lee JE, et al. Parathyroid exploration in the reoperative neck: improved preoperative localization with 4D-computed tomography. J Am Coll Surg 2008;206(5):888–95 [discussion: 895–6].

18. Sepahdari AR, Bahl M, Harari A, et al. Predictors of multigland disease in primary hyperparathyroidism: a scoring system with 4D-CT imaging and biochemical markers. AJNR Am J Neuroradiol 2015;36(5): 987–92.

19. Cheung K, Wang TS, Farrokhyar F, et al. A meta-analysis of preoperative localization techniques for patients with primary hyperparathyroidism. Ann Surg Oncol 2012;19(2):577–83.

20. Kluijfhout WP, Pasternak JD, Beninato T, et al. Diagnostic performance of computed tomography for parathyroid adenoma localization; a systematic review and meta-analysis. Eur J Radiol 2017;88:117–28.

21. Fraker DL, Harsono H, Lewis R. Minimally invasive parathyroidectomy: benefits and requirements of localization, diagnosis, and intraoperative PTH monitoring. Long-term results. World J Surg 2009; 33(11):2256–65.

22. Wilhelm SM, Wang TS, Ruan DT, et al. The American Association of Endocrine Surgeons Guidelines for definitive management of primary hyperparathyroidism. JAMA Surg 2016;151(10):959–68.

23. Kelly HR, Hamberg LM, Hunter GJ. 4D-CT for preoperative localization of abnormal parathyroid glands in patients with hyperparathyroidism: accuracy and ability to stratify patients by unilateral versus bilateral disease in surgery-naive and reexploration patients. AJNR Am J Neuroradiol 2014;35(1):176–81.

24. Lubitz CC, Stephen AE, Hodin RA, et al. Preoperative localization strategies for primary hyperparathyroidism: an economic analysis. Ann Surg Oncol 2012;19(13):4202–9.

25. Lane MJ, Desser TS, Weigel RJ, et al. Use of color and power Doppler sonography to identify feeding arteries associated with parathyroid adenomas. AJR Am J Roentgenol 1998;171(3):819–23.

26. Reeder SB, Desser TS, Weigel RJ, et al. Sonography in primary hyperparathyroidism: review with emphasis on scanning technique. J Ultrasound Med 2002;21(5):539–52 [quiz: 553–4].

27. Bancos I, Grant CS, Nadeem S, et al. Risks and benefits of parathyroid fine-needle aspiration with parathyroid hormone washout. Endocr Pract 2012;18(4): 441–9.

28. Ghaheri BA, Koslin DB, Wood AH, et al. Preoperative ultrasound is worthwhile for reoperative parathyroid surgery. Laryngoscope 2004;114(12):2168–71.

29. Kamaya A, Quon A, Jeffrey RB. Sonography of the abnormal parathyroid gland. Ultrasound Q 2006; 22(4):253–62.

30. Batur A, Atmaca M, Yavuz A, et al. Ultrasound elastography for distinction between parathyroid adenomas and thyroid nodules. J Ultrasound Med 2016;35(6):1277–82.

31. Bleier BS, LiVolsi VA, Chalian AA, et al. 99m sestamibi sensitivity in oxyphil cell-dominant parathyroid

adenomas. Arch Otolaryngol Head Neck Surg 2006; 132(7):779–82.

32. Greenspan BS, Dillehay G, Intenzo C, et al. SNM practice guideline for parathyroid scintigraphy 4.0. J Nucl Med Technol 2012;40(2):111–8.

33. Thomas DL, Bartel T, Menda Y, et al. Single photon emission computed tomography (SPECT) should be routinely performed for the detection of parathyroid abnormalities utilizing technetium-99m sestamibi parathyroid scintigraphy. Clin Nucl Med 2009; 34(10):651–5.

34. Slater A, Gleeson FV. Increased sensitivity and confidence of SPECT over planar imaging in dual-phase sestamibi for parathyroid adenoma detection. Clin Nucl Med 2005;30(1):1–3.

35. Nichols KJ, Tomas MB, Tronco GG, et al. Preoperative parathyroid scintigraphic lesion localization: accuracy of various types of readings. Radiology 2008;248(1):221–32.

36. Hoang JK, Reiman RE, Nguyen GB, et al. Lifetime attributable risk of cancer from radiation exposure during parathyroid imaging: comparison of 4D CT and parathyroid scintigraphy. AJR Am J Roentgenol 2015;204(5):W579–85.

37. Chen H, Mack E, Starling JR. Radioguided parathyroidectomy is equally effective for both adenomatous and hyperplastic glands. Ann Surg 2003; 238(3):332–8.

38. Jones JM, Russell CF, Ferguson WR, et al. Pre-operative sestamibi-technetium subtraction scintigraphy in primary hyperparathyroidism: experience with 156 consecutive patients. Clin Radiol 2001;56(7):556–9.

39. Palazzo FF, Delbridge LW. Minimal-access/minimally invasive parathyroidectomy for primary hyperparathyroidism. Surg Clin North Am 2004;84(3):717–34.

40. Vattimo A, Bertelli P, Cintorino M, et al. Hurthle cell tumor dwelling in hot thyroid nodules: preoperative detection with technetium-99m-MIBI dual-phase scintigraphy. J Nucl Med 1998;39(5):822.

41. Erbil Y, Barbaros U, Yanik BT, et al. Impact of gland morphology and concomitant thyroid nodules on preoperative localization of parathyroid adenomas. Laryngoscope 2006;116(4):580–5.

42. Smith JR, Oates ME. Radionuclide imaging of the parathyroid glands: patterns, pearls, and pitfalls. Radiographics 2004;24(4):1101–15.

43. Herrmann K, Takei T, Kanegae K, et al. Clinical value and limitations of [11C]-methionine PET for detection and localization of suspected parathyroid adenomas. Mol Imaging Biol 2009;11(5):356–63.

44. Kluijfhout WP, Pasternak JD, Drake FT, et al. Use of PET tracers for parathyroid localization: a systematic review and meta-analysis. Langenbecks Arch Surg 2016;401(7):925–35.

45. Hoang JK, Sung WK, Bahl M, et al. How to perform parathyroid 4D CT: tips and traps for technique and interpretation. Radiology 2014;270(1):15–24.

46. Eichhorn-Wharry LI, Carlin AM, Talpos GB. Mild hypercalcemia: an indication to select 4-dimensional computed tomography scan for preoperative localization of parathyroid adenomas. Am J Surg 2011; 201(3):334–8 [discussion: 338].

47. Leiva-Salinas C, Flors L, Durst CR, et al. Detection of parathyroid adenomas using a monophasic dual-energy computed tomography acquisition: diagnostic performance and potential radiation dose reduction. Neuroradiology 2016;58(11): 1135–41.

48. Noureldine SI, Aygun N, Walden MJ, et al. Multiphase computed tomography for localization of parathyroid disease in patients with primary hyperparathyroidism: how many phases do we really need? Surgery 2014;156(6):1300–6 [discussion: 13006–7].

49. Bahl M, Sepahdari AR, Sosa JA, et al. Parathyroid adenomas and hyperplasia on four-dimensional CT scans: three patterns of enhancement relative to the thyroid gland justify a three-phase protocol. Radiology 2015;277(2):454–62.

50. Grayev AM, Gentry LR, Hartman MJ, et al. Presurgical localization of parathyroid adenomas with magnetic resonance imaging at 3.0 T: an adjunct method to supplement traditional imaging. Ann Surg Oncol 2012;19(3):981–9.

51. Lopez Hanninen E, Vogl TJ, Steinmuller T, et al. Preoperative contrast-enhanced MRI of the parathyroid glands in hyperparathyroidism. Invest Radiol 2000; 35(7):426–30.

52. Michel L, Dupont M, Rosiere A, et al. The rationale for performing MR imaging before surgery for primary hyperparathyroidism. Acta Chir Belg 2013; 113(2):112–22.

53. Sacconi B, Argiro R, Diacinti D, et al. MR appearance of parathyroid adenomas at 3 T in patients with primary hyperparathyroidism: what radiologists need to know for pre-operative localization. Eur Radiol 2016;26(3):664–73.

54. Aschenbach R, Tuda S, Lamster E, et al. Dynamic magnetic resonance angiography for localization of hyperfunctioning parathyroid glands in the reoperative neck. Eur J Radiol 2012;81(11):3371–7.

55. Nael K, Hur J, Bauer A, et al. Dynamic 4D MRI characterization of parathyroid adenomas: multiparametric analysis. AJNR Am J Neuroradiol 2015; 36(11):2147–52.

56. Triggiani V, Resta F, Giagulli VA, et al. Parathyroid hormone determination in ultrasound-guided fine needle aspirates allows the differentiation between thyroid and parathyroid lesions: our experience and review of the literature. Endocr Metab immune Disord Drug Targets 2013;13(4):351–8.

57. AIUM practice guideline for the performance of a thyroid and parathyroid ultrasound examination. J Ultrasound Med 2013;32(7):1319–29.

PET/MR Imaging in Head and Neck Cancer
Current Applications and Future Directions

Samuel J. Galgano, MD[a],*, Ryan V. Marshall, MD[b],
Erik H. Middlebrooks, MD[c],
Jonathan E. McConathy, MD, PhD[d],
Pradeep Bhambhvani, MD[e]

KEYWORDS

- PET/MR Imaging • FDG-PET • Oncologic imaging • Melanoma • Squamous cell carcinoma
- Thyroid cancer • Head and neck oncology

KEY POINTS

- PET/MR imaging is part of routine clinical use at multiple institutions in the United States, Asia, and Europe.
- Clinical PET/MR imaging protocols include whole-body PET/MR imaging, regional PET/MR imaging, and a combination of both.
- Essential to the performance of PET/MR imaging is the execution of a high-quality diagnostic MR imaging in the region of interest.
- Although published research is sparse, it appears that for primary head and neck tumors PET/MR imaging is not inferior to PET/CT and may prove advantageous in certain scenarios.
- PET/MR imaging allows for comprehensive staging of advanced stage melanoma in a single setting, allowing the patient to undergo a single imaging examination.

INTRODUCTION

Primary malignancies of the head and neck are initially evaluated by physical examination and direct visualization, such as endoscopy.[1–4] Physical examination is often accompanied by computed tomography (CT) in the initial workup of most head and neck cancers. PET/CT is a well-established modality in certain head and neck cancers, particularly for posttreatment assessment, as well as pretreatment staging. Certain malignancies of the head and neck can benefit from pretreatment MR imaging. For instance, MR imaging may better delineate soft tissue extent of tumors and is superior to CT in sinonasal or nasopharyngeal tumors.[5,6] MR imaging also has a higher sensitivity and negative predictive value for bone and cartilage invasion.[7,8] MR imaging is also more sensitive for detecting perineural tumor spread. In contrast to sequential

Dr J. McConathy is a consultant for Siemens Healthcare, GE Healthcare, Blue Earth Diagnostics, and Eli Lilly/Avid. The remaining authors have nothing to disclose.

[a] Department of Radiology, The University of Alabama at Birmingham, 619 19th Street South, JTN 338, Birmingham, AL 35249, USA; [b] Department of Otolaryngology, The University of Alabama at Birmingham, 619 19th Street South, JT 136, Birmingham, AL 35249, USA; [c] Department of Radiology, The University of Alabama at Birmingham, 619 19th Street South, JT N409, Birmingham, AL 35249, USA; [d] Department of Radiology, The University of Alabama at Birmingham, 619 19th Street South, JT 773, Birmingham, AL 35249, USA; [e] Department of Radiology, The University of Alabama at Birmingham, 619 19th Street South, JT 777, Birmingham, AL 35249, USA
* Corresponding author.
E-mail address: samuelgalgano@uabmc.edu

imaging with PET/CT, the PET and MR imaging sequences in integrated PET/MR imaging systems are acquired simultaneously, which may reduce registration error between images.

Given the complementary nature of these imaging modalities, the emergence of simultaneous PET/MR imaging may play a beneficial role in evaluation of some head and neck cancers. As PET/MR imaging scanners are acquired and used by an increasing number of institutions worldwide along with development of novel radiotracers, the role of PET/MR imaging in head and neck malignancies in both the pretreatment and posttreatment settings will likely expand. The primary aim of this article was to review the current literature pertaining to PET/MR imaging for head and neck cancers and to evaluate potential future directions for research in the field.

PROTOCOLS, TECHNICAL CHALLENGES, AND REIMBURSEMENT

Given the relative paucity of research regarding PET/MR imaging for the evaluation of head and neck cancer, few established dedicated PET/MR imaging protocols have been published.[9–12] The readers are, however, urged to look up a comprehensive and well-written review article that provides a selection of partial-body (skull base to mid-thighs) and whole-body (skull vertex to toes) PET/MR imaging protocols, including one for head and neck cancer.[13] Essential to the value of PET/MR imaging in head and neck cancer is the performance of a high-quality diagnostic MR imaging of the neck. Important MR imaging sequences to include in a protocol include precontrast T1 (preferably without fat suppression), short tau inversion recovery (STIR), diffusion-weighted imaging (DWI), and T2 images, along with multiplanar fat-suppressed T1 postcontrast sequences. Similar to oncologic applications for other regions of the body, the PET and MR imaging portions of the examination provide complementary information. The metabolic evaluation by fluorodeoxyglucose (FDG)-PET plays an important role in staging of nodal and distant metastases for patients with head and neck cancer, whereas MR imaging plays an important role in the precise T staging of the primary tumor and evaluating posttreatment changes from recurrent or residual disease. Thus, a cornerstone of PET/MR imaging evaluation of the head and neck involves execution of a high-quality MR imaging, including both diffusion-weighted and contrast-enhanced images. A significant technical challenge in the performance of both PET/MR imaging and MR imaging alone of the neck is respiratory motion, which is difficult to correct given the long acquisition times. In the posttreatment setting, PET/MR imaging may be difficult to correctly interpret due to susceptibility artifact from surgical clips following neck dissection. Ultimately, the PET/MR imaging examination should be tailored to answer the specific clinical question and if inappropriate, should not be performed in light of other available options (such as PET/CT).

Billing and reimbursement for PET/MR imaging examinations remains a challenge in current practice, largely due to the relative newness of the hybrid modality. Patients who are being considered for PET/MR imaging are often selected on the basis of needing a dedicated diagnostic MR imaging of the region of interest and comprehensive whole-body staging with PET. Unlike PET/CT, no current procedural terminology (CPT) codes exist to bill for PET/MR imaging examinations. Instead, billing is performed using the appropriate PET-only (78811, 78812, 78813) and MR imaging CPT code(s). Therefore, to be completely reimbursed for a PET/MR imaging examination, it is essential that patients meet criteria for need for both diagnostic MR imaging and PET scans. As PET/MR imaging usage continues to increase in the United States, it is likely that specific CPT codes will be developed for this hybrid modality. These codes could facilitate more widespread patient eligibility and increase utilization of PET/MR imaging for both oncologic and nononcologic indications.

CUTANEOUS MELANOMA OF THE HEAD AND NECK

In clinical practice, PET/CT is often used for the initial staging and follow-up of advanced stages of cutaneous melanoma. For patients at higher risk of metastatic disease (T3 and T4 tumors), sentinel lymph node biopsy and locoregional lymphadenectomy if positive node biopsy is the standard-of-care treatment. Additionally, both pretreatment and posttreatment serum lactate dehydrogenase values play a role in prognosticating successful response to treatment and monitoring for disease recurrence.[14] In patients with positive lymph nodes at the time of surgery, subsequent imaging is needed to evaluate for additional nodal and distant metastases. Several studies have investigated the performance of whole-body MR imaging with PET/CT for melanoma staging.[15–17] When DWI sequences are included in the whole-body MR imaging, sensitivity and specificity are comparable to PET/CT (approximately 82%–84% and 87%–97% for MR imaging, respectively, compared with 73%–80% and 92%–93% for PET/CT, respectively).[15,16] However, there are no prospective studies examining the diagnostic performance of simultaneous PET/MR imaging for the staging or restaging of melanoma. A significant limitation of PET/MR imaging is the detection of subcentimeter pulmonary nodules, an important site of potential metastatic disease in head and neck cutaneous melanoma (**Fig. 1**). To overcome this problem, ultrashort echo time sequences are being developed as part of PET/MR imaging protocols to specifically increase detection of pulmonary nodules measuring less than 1 cm.[18] Additionally, the potential benefit of whole-body PET/MR imaging staging for melanoma lies in its theoretic superiority of detecting subcutaneous, osseous, hepatic, and intracranial metastases and in its ability to provide comprehensive whole-body staging in a single examination. Finally, in the era of immunotherapy for metastatic melanoma, there is potential benefit in assessing tumor characteristics with PET/MR imaging to evaluate response to therapy beyond the traditional RECIST (Response Evaluation Criteria in Solid Tumors) imaging criteria and serum S100 level.[19,20] Although the role of PET/MR imaging in the staging of melanoma is not well-established, its potential benefits and applications are apparent and further research is needed.

SQUAMOUS CELL CARCINOMA OF THE HEAD AND NECK

Squamous cell carcinoma (SCCa) is the most common malignancy of the head and neck. The primary site of SCCa varies widely, primarily arising from the skin or mucosal surfaces of the aerodigestive tract. The most common primary site is the oral cavity, which accounts for approximately 30% of all head and neck cancers. As a result of its heterogeneity, these cancers are often studied as a conglomerate group. The use of PET/CT and MR imaging for the staging and restaging of head and neck SCCa provides complementary information. PET/CT has excellent accuracy for staging nodal and distant metastases, whereas MR imaging is useful for more accurate T staging of the primary lesion, evaluation of perineural tumor spread, bone and cartilage invasion, and intracranial spread of tumor[5–8,21,22] (**Fig. 2**). Traditionally, MR imaging was considered inferior to CT in detecting nodal disease and extracapsular spread; however, more recent studies have suggested MR imaging and CT may be comparable.[23–25] In the posttreatment setting, PET/CT is useful in the whole-body restaging of metastatic disease, whereas MR imaging is useful in differentiating postradiation changes of the neck from recurrent/residual tumor.[26–28] Therefore, it is logical that PET/MR imaging can potentially be

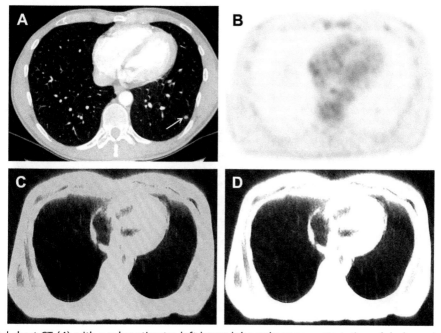

Fig. 1. Axial chest CT (*A*) with a subcentimeter left lower lobe pulmonary metastatic nodule (*arrow*) that is not visualized on attenuation-corrected axial FDG-PET (*B*), axial fused PET/MR imaging (*C*), or axial single-hot fast spin echo (SS-FSE) MR imaging (*D*).

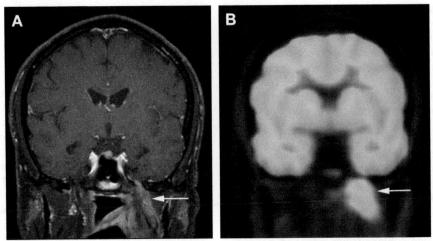

Fig. 2. Perineural tumor spread (*arrows*) into the foramen ovale in a patient with nasopharyngeal carcinoma (not shown). (*A*) Post-gadolinium coronal T1 fat-suppressed MR imaging. (*B*) Fused coronal FDG-PET/MR imaging. (*Courtesy of* Dr Michelle M. Miller-Thomas, Washington University in St. Louis, Mallinckrodt Institute of Radiology, St Louis, MO.)

used to evaluate locally recurrent disease in the posttreatment setting. We show a case of sinonasal melanoma that was resected and treated with definitive radiotherapy, PET/MR imaging demonstrated focal FDG activity in the left maxillary sinus at the resection site, suspicious for recurrent tumor and prompting nasal endoscopy (**Fig. 3**). **Figs. 4** and **5** depict additional cases with posttreatment changes on PET/MR imaging.

Several studies have examined the potential role of PET/MR imaging in the staging and restaging of SCCa of the head and neck. A single study

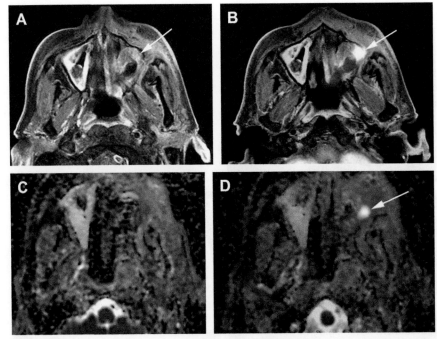

Fig. 3. Previously treated left maxillary sinus melanoma with contrast enhancement (*A*), focal hypermetabolism (*B* and *D*), and low apparent diffusion coefficient (ADC) values (*C*) suspicious for locally recurrent tumor (*arrows*). PET/MR images can be used to guide biopsy. (*A*) Post-gadolinium T1 axial fat-suppressed MR imaging, (*B*) axial fused FDG-PET/MR imaging, (*C*) ADC map, (*D*) axial fused FDG-PET/ADC map.

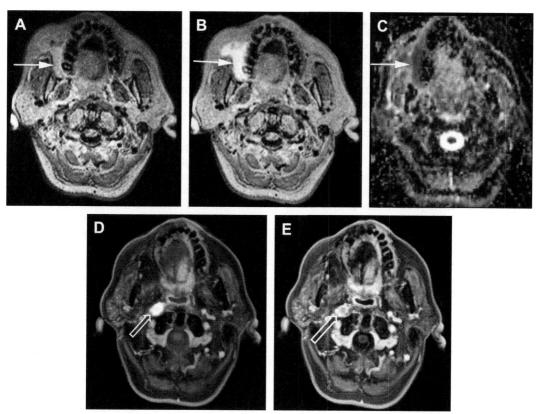

Fig. 4. Hypermetabolic right buccal mucosa SSCa with corresponding low ADC values (*arrows, A, B, C*). One-year posttreatment PET/MR imaging shows an FDG avid necrotic right lateral retropharyngeal lymph node (*open arrow*), consistent with recurrent tumor (*D, E*). (*A*) Post-gadolinium axial T1 non–fat-suppressed MR imaging, (*B*) axial fused FDG-PET/MR imaging, (*C*) ADC map, (*D*) axial fused FDG-PET/MR imaging, (*E*) post-gadolinium axial T1 fat-suppressed MR imaging. (*Courtesy of* Dr Michelle M. Miller-Thomas, Washington University in St. Louis, Mallinckrodt Institute of Radiology, St Louis, MO.)

examining initial staging of SCCa of the head and neck with PET/MR imaging demonstrated a significant increase in the number of cervical lymph nodes detected when compared with stand-alone PET; a

finding that may partly be due to PET/MR imaging being performed during a more delayed phase compared with stand-alone PET, following FDG administration.[10] An additional benefit of PET/MR

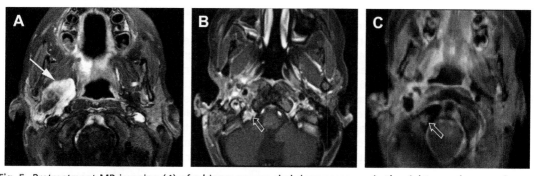

Fig. 5. Pretreatment MR imaging (*A*) of a biopsy-proven rhabdomyosarcoma in the right parapharyngeal space (*arrow*). Posttreatment MR imaging (*B*) was indeterminate for tumor recurrence at the right hypoglossal canal (*open arrow*). PET/MR imaging (*C*) demonstrated no suspicious FDG activity in the region of the right hypoglossal canal (*open arrow*), indicating posttreatment changes rather than recurrent tumor. (*A, B*) Post-gadolinium axial T1 fat-suppressed MR imaging, (*C*) axial fused FDG-PET/MR imaging. (*Courtesy of* Dr Michelle M. Miller-Thomas, Washington University in St. Louis, Mallinckrodt Institute of Radiology, St Louis, MO.)

imaging is in the evaluation of the oropharynx, which is often limited on PET/CT given streak artifact from dental hardware. This leads to more accurate T staging of the oropharyngeal SCCa and more precise evaluation of cervical level IA and IB lymph nodes.[2,29,30] Other studies examining the use of integrated PET/MR imaging for staging or restaging head and neck SCCa in the pretreatment and posttreatment setting demonstrated no significant difference between FDG-PET/CT, FDG-PET/MR imaging, and MR imaging alone.[1,31] As many patients with head and neck SCCa are treated with definitive radiation therapy, research suggests that the complementary information provided with PET/MR imaging regarding glucose metabolism and apparent diffusion coefficient may be relevant to radiotherapy planning.[12]

Some patients with SCCa of the head and neck may not experience symptoms from their primary tumor and instead will present to the clinician with a palpable abnormality in their cervical region. Often, these are enlarged lymph nodes that ultimately undergo percutaneous fine-needle aspiration or core biopsy, revealing a diagnosis of SCCa of unknown primary. These patients must then undergo both a comprehensive clinical evaluation and imaging of the head, neck, and chest to evaluate potential sites of primary malignancy. A single study has examined the potential use of PET/MR imaging in these patients and compared its accuracy with PET/CT.[32] The study demonstrated a comparable diagnostic ability between PET/MR imaging and PET/CT for detection of the primary cancer and metastases, with PET/MR imaging proving superior in the cervical region and PET/CT superior in the chest.[32] Therefore, PET/MR imaging may provide a useful imaging adjunct to the clinical examination of the head and neck when no primary malignancy can be identified on endoscopy or laryngoscopy.

A comprehensive meta-analysis of the value of PET/MR imaging for the diagnosis of head and neck cancers demonstrated high sensitivity and moderate specificity for the detection of head and neck cancer, with areas under the receiver-operator curve approaching 0.96.[33] Ultimately, PET/MR imaging may not supplant the use of PET/CT in the pretreatment or posttreatment setting of head and neck SCCa, but niche applications are being developed and further research is needed to establish its role in the management algorithm.

CANCERS OF THE SALIVARY GLANDS

Salivary gland tumors are relatively uncommon, but are most frequently present in the parotid glands (>80%) and submandibular glands (~15%) with only a minority present in the sublingual glands or minor salivary glands.[34] Unlike PET/CT, few data currently exist regarding the use of PET/MR imaging for the primary staging or restaging of salivary gland malignancies.[35,36] Because many benign or low-grade lesions within the salivary glands can be associated with significant FDG uptake, little diagnostic value is typically added by FDG-PET in the initial workup. However, MR is the imaging modality of choice in evaluating malignant salivary lesions in the head and neck.[37]

In patients undergoing PET/CT for any oncologic indication, incidental FDG uptake in the parotid gland is seen in approximately 0.4% of PET/CT scans.[38] Of these patients with incidental FDG uptake in the parotid gland, only 4% of these incidentalomas were pathologically proven as malignant.[38] Additionally, FDG-PET/CT was unable to reliably differentiate benign and malignant lesions of the parotid gland. Given the predictive ability of CT and MR imaging in salivary gland lesions, it is likely that PET/MR imaging would be superior to PET/CT; however, the utility of the FDG-PET itself is questionable. Even in cases of perineural tumor spread, MR imaging alone would be expected to have greater sensitivity than FDG-PET.[2] Currently, the role of PET/MR imaging in evaluation of salivary gland lesions is uncertain, as there is no clear evidence it offers better predictive value than MR imaging alone.

CANCERS OF THE THYROID GLAND

Cancers of the thyroid gland can generally be subdivided into 2 main classes: well-differentiated and poorly differentiated. Follicular and papillary subtypes compose the category of well-differentiated thyroid cancer, whereas anaplastic thyroid cancer is the sole poorly differentiated thyroid cancer. Medullary thyroid cancer is of intermediate aggressiveness and is often treated as a unique entity, particularly given its association with multiple endocrine neoplasia type 2. Similar to other malignancies, the more poorly differentiated the thyroid cancer, the less likely it is to behave in the same fashion as normal thyroid tissue. As a result, current clinical practice uses FDG-PET/CT for evaluation of anaplastic or poorly differentiated thyroid cancer or radioiodine refractory differentiated thyroid, whereas differentiated thyroid cancer is typically staged using radioactive iodine analogs.

In many cases, patients with differentiated thyroid cancer are not imaged before postsurgical remnant ablation with radioactive ^{131}I administration. Instead, the routine post-radioiodine therapy scan is used to evaluate the presence of metastatic disease. Some institutions choose to perform staging planar or single-photon emission CT (SPECT)/CT scans with either ^{123}I or ^{131}I before radioablation. Post-thyroidectomy ^{123}I or ^{131}I imaging, with or without SPECT/CT has been reported to yield information that could alter clinical management in 25% to 53% of patients, in single-center, retrospective studies.[39–41] Currently, FDG-PET plays little role in the initial staging of differentiated thyroid cancer. However, owing to its ability to retain iodine like normal thyroid tissue, ongoing research is being performed to evaluate the use of [124]I for staging differentiated thyroid cancer. Simultaneous PET/MR imaging is useful in staging differentiated thyroid cancer with [124]I due to fewer errors in coregistration between PET and CT scans performed at separate times or with retrospectively fused PET and MR imaging scans.[42] Particularly for cervical lymph nodes measuring less than 10 mm, PET/MR imaging offered greater reader confidence in mapping PET activity to an anatomic correlate and may allow for more precise dosimetry calculations by detecting metastases that could have been missed by conventional ^{131}I scans.[42,43]

Neck CT is most commonly used for initial staging of thyroid malignancies; however, MR imaging is used in select cases, particularly when there is suspicion of extracapsular spread. Due to the improved soft tissue contrast, MR imaging offers superior assessment for invasion of adjacent structures, such as hypopharynx extension or perineural invasion. As stated previously, for patients with known or suspected dedifferentiated thyroid cancer or patients with iodine-refractory disease, FDG-PET/CT plays a role in staging and restaging.[44] In these patients in whom distant metastatic disease occurs more commonly, FDG-PET/MR imaging has been demonstrated to be inferior to FDG-PET/CT, largely due to the decreased sensitivity of MR imaging for detection of pulmonary nodules.[45] However, because FDG-PET is more commonly performed in aggressive thyroid malignancies, PET/MR imaging may prove more beneficial than PET/CT, because the incidence of extracapsular spread may be expected to be higher. Before the availability of integrated clinical PET/MR imaging, studies demonstrated value in retrospectively fused PET and MR imaging for patients with recurrent or persistent thyroid cancer and were shown to alter treatment plans in 46% of the patients in the study cohort.[46] Additionally, recent data show that in suspected or known dedifferentiated thyroid cancer, FDG-PET/MR imaging was inferior to low-dose FDG-PET/CT for the assessment of pulmonary status.

However, for the assessment of cervical status, FDG-PET/MR imaging was equal to contrast-enhanced neck FDG-PET/CT.[45] Given that most PET/CT scans are performed as noncontrast examinations, one can speculate that the value of assessing cervical disease with PET/MR imaging is potentially superior to noncontrast PET/CT. Additionally PET/MR would also preclude radioiodinated contrast use and avoid potential delays in cases needing radioiodine therapy. Further research is needed to elucidate these differences.

Medullary thyroid cancer is a form of neuroendocrine cancer derived from the C-cells of the thyroid. These cells are responsible for the synthesis of calcitonin, which can be detected in blood samples. As a result, calcitonin can be used to monitor treatment response and as a tumor marker in medullary thyroid cancer, similar to thyroglobulin for differentiated thyroid cancer, provided the medullary thyroid cancer has not dedifferentiated. Little current published research exists regarding the use of PET/MR imaging for the detection of primary or recurrent medullary thyroid cancer, but several PET radiotracers are being studied to evaluate the diagnostic performance of PET/CT, including ^{18}F-FDG, ^{18}F-FDOPA, ^{68}Ga-somatostatin receptor imaging agents, and ^{68}Ga-gastrin analogs.[47–51] Additionally, research is being performed to examine if peptide receptor radionuclide therapy with ^{177}Lu-labeled somatostatin analogs is feasible in medullary thyroid cancer.[52]

CANCERS OF THE UPPER ESOPHAGUS

Cancers of the esophagus are often thought of as a dichotomy, with adenocarcinomas most typically arising from the lower esophagus and SCCa arising from the upper and middle esophagus. Therefore, upper or cervical esophageal cancers also should be discussed under the umbrella of head and neck cancers. SCCa of the esophagus arises in a similar patient population at risk for developing SCCa of other primary sites in the head and neck, often secondary to alcohol and tobacco use. Initial staging of esophageal cancer is performed through the use of endoscopic ultrasound (EUS) for T staging and anatomic imaging either with CT or PET/CT for detection of nodal and distant metastatic disease. A single study has examined the potential benefit of evaluating esophageal cancer with PET/MR imaging and demonstrated that PET/MR imaging had acceptable accuracy for T staging when compared with EUS, and, although not statistically significant, a higher accuracy for nodal staging.[53] The study suggested that as PET/MR imaging protocols continue to develop and become more refined,

PET/MR imaging may become the study of choice for accurate comprehensive staging of esophageal cancer in the preoperative setting.

CANCERS OF THE SKULL BASE

Cancers of the skull base can arise de novo, or be metastatic or secondary to local extension into the skull base. Because these tumors can originate in the paranasal sinuses and nasopharynx, it is important to consider skull base neoplasms as part of head and neck oncology. These patients often undergo MR imaging during the diagnostic workup and, depending on the findings, may proceed to PET/CT or directly to endoscopy and biopsy. However, there is great potential value in the pretreatment and posttreatment settings for PET/MR imaging (**Figs. 6** and **7**). Although no study has examined the role of PET/MR imaging thus far, the role of ^{18}F-NaF PET/CT and MR imaging to evaluate skull base invasion by nasopharyngeal carcinoma has been studied. The study demonstrated high sensitivity, specificity, and accuracy of both modalities, with PET/CT detecting

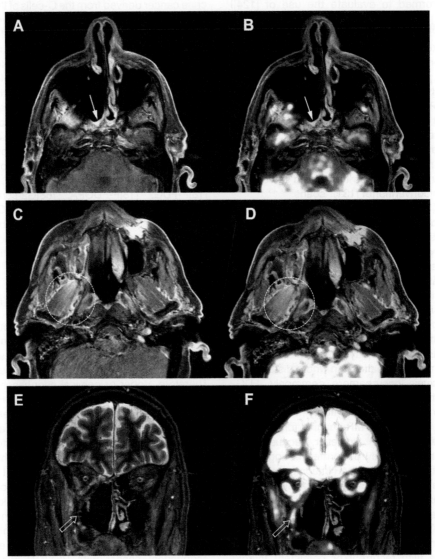

Fig. 6. Postsurgical and postradiation changes in the region of the previously treated skull base adenoid cystic carcinoma. The enhancement in the right pterygopalatine fossa (*arrows* in *A, B*) and right pterygoid musculature (*dotted circle* in *C, D*) do not demonstrate increased FDG activity, most consistent with posttreatment changes. However, abnormal linear activity along the lateral wall of the right maxillary sinus (*open arrow* in *E, F*), is suspicious for posttreatment inflammation versus perineural tumor spread. (*A, C*) Post-gadolinium axial T1 fat-suppressed MR imaging, (*B, D*) axial fused FDG-PET/MR imaging, (*E*) coronal T2 STIR MR imaging, (*F*) coronal fused FDG-PET/MR imaging.

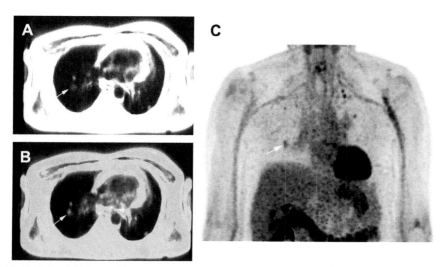

Fig. 7. Multiple FDG avid bilateral lung metastases in a patient with previously treated skull base adenoid cystic carcinoma (*arrows*). (*A*) Axial SS-FSE MR imaging, (*B*) axial fused FDG-PET/MR imaging, (*C*) partial-body maximum intensity projection image.

more lesions in the osseous skull base and MR imaging providing superior soft tissue contrast in the region.[54] The study suggests that a hybrid imaging modality, such as PET/MR imaging, may provide even higher levels of diagnostic accuracy for detecting skull base involvement; however, a clear benefit outside of workflow issues may be difficult to establish. Because CT and MR imaging are complementary in evaluating skull base lesions and frequently both are obtained, it may be difficult to justify PET/MR imaging plus CT over PET/CT plus MR imaging.

Additionally, a significant limitation to consider regarding PET/MR imaging of the skull base is the relative difficulty in attenuation correction for cortical bone during PET/MR imaging and potentially missing metastases due to alteration of standard uptake values. This is partially overcome in the skull and skull base through the use of atlas-based attenuation correction methods to account for the relative uniformity in the cranial structures between patients.[55] An additional potential role for PET/MR imaging of skull base lesions may be in the post-treatment setting, where combining the soft tissue contrast of MR imaging with the functional information provided by PET may help guide biopsies to detect recurrent or residual disease where no anatomic correlate can be found (see **Fig. 3**).

RADIATION TREATMENT PLANNING

The advantages of hybrid PET/CT in radiation treatment planning of head and neck cancer are well known and include better identification of the disease extent, biological behavior of the tumor (eg, hypoxia, proliferation), and smaller gross

tumor volumes (GTVs), clinical target volumes, and planning target volumes.[56] Integrated PET/MR imaging offers the possibility to simultaneously image anatomic, functional, and molecular characteristics of a tumor. Consequently, PET/MR imaging may be an optimal imaging modality for radiation treatment individualization.[57] A more detailed discussion on functional imaging for radiation treatment planning in head and neck cancer can be found here.[58,59] A recent study comparing integrated PET/MR imaging and CT, however, showed similar GTVs and radiation doses in a small cohort of 11 patients with head and neck cancer (10 oropharynx, 1 larynx).[60] Further studies are needed to determine the optimal use of PET/MR imaging for radiation treatment planning.

FUTURE DIRECTIONS

Although there is a relative paucity of published literature examining the use of PET/MR imaging in head and neck cancers, a great deal of research is ongoing that may potentially impact both PET/CT and PET/MR imaging utilization. As we move toward an age of personalized and molecular medicine, a major field of ongoing research involves radiotracer design. For example, research in the field of melanoma includes the development of ^{11}C tracers, tracers linked to antibodies for melanoma immunotherapy, and tracers that target melanin.[61–63] Thyroid cancer PET tracer research largely focuses on the use of [124]I and ^{68}Ga prostate-specific membrane antigen for the diagnosis and staging of differentiated thyroid cancer.[43,64,65] ^{18}F-fluorothymidine (FLT) PET has been shown to correlate with Ki-67, a proliferation index. It is therefore thought that ^{18}F-FLT may be used to monitor treatment response and therefore serve as a prognostic marker.[66] ^{18}F-Fluoromisoni-dazole, a nitriomidazole derivative can be used to image hypoxia. It is known that hypoxia indirectly correlates with structurally and functionally abnormal tumor vessels (neoangiogenesis) in the tumor bed. ^{18}F-Fluoromisonidazole can therefore be used as a biomarker for evaluating tumor progression and overall prognosis.[66] These new tracers could help identify important staging information in patients before initiation of treatment, which would provide for better targeted planning. In addition, these new biomarkers will allow better assessment of treatment response and patient management.

For justification of PET/MR imaging hybrid systems, studies will also have to focus on advances in MR imaging technology. It is possible that advances in MR imaging sequences, such as chemical exchange saturation transfer MR imaging, advanced diffusion MR imaging techniques, MR perfusion, MR spectroscopy, or hypoxia imaging (eg, blood oxygen level dependent imaging), may elicit value of PET/MR imaging over PET/CT. Because the pinnacle of hybrid PET/MR imaging likely lies in techniques in which the time-coupling of PET and MR imaging acquisition is critical, these advanced techniques are likely to yield better justification for PET/MR imaging systems than structural imaging alone.

SUMMARY

Although the current literature has relatively few publications regarding the use of PET/MR imaging in head and neck cancers, there are clear benefits for both molecular imaging with PET and anatomic imaging with MR imaging. Importantly, the research that currently exists suggests that PET/MR imaging is not inferior to PET/CT. It is therefore logical that PET/MR imaging potentially offers the simultaneous imaging benefits of both modalities while providing comprehensive diagnostic information in a single imaging session. Unfortunately, the investigation of more sophisticated functional MR imaging techniques in PET/MR imaging applications is currently lacking. It is possible that such capabilities may be the driving force for PET/MR imaging compared with PET/CT in head and neck and other cancers. More research in this realm is certainly needed, and, along with innovation in radiotracer development and molecular-targeted radiotherapy, PET/MR imaging may provide the ability for both diagnostic and therapeutic applications in head and neck cancers.

REFERENCES

1. Kubiessa K, Purz S, Gawlitza M, et al. Initial clinical results of simultaneous 18F-FDG PET/MRI in comparison to 18F-FDG PET/CT in patients with head and neck cancer. Eur J Nucl Med Mol Imaging 2014;41(4):639–48.
2. Kuhn FP, Hullner M, Mader CE, et al. Contrast-enhanced PET/MR imaging versus contrast-enhanced PET/CT in head and neck cancer: how much MR information is needed? J Nucl Med 2014;55(4):551–8.
3. Partovi S, Kohan A, Vercher-Conejero JL, et al. Qualitative and quantitative performance of (1)(8)F-FDG-PET/MRI versus (1)(8)F-FDG-PET/CT in patients with head and neck cancer. AJNR Am J Neuroradiol 2014;35(10):1970–5.
4. Queiroz MA, Hullner M, Kuhn F, et al. PET/MRI and PET/CT in follow-up of head and neck cancer patients. Eur J Nucl Med Mol Imaging 2014;41(6):1066–75.
5. Branstetter BF, Weissman JL. Role of MR and CT in the paranasal sinuses. Otolaryngol Clin North Am 2005;38(6):1279–99, x.
6. Ling FT, Kountakis SE. Advances in imaging of the paranasal sinuses. Curr Allergy Asthma Rep 2006; 6(6):502–7.
7. Zbaren P, Becker M, Lang H. Staging of laryngeal cancer: endoscopy, computed tomography and magnetic resonance versus histopathology. Eur Arch Otorhinolaryngol 1997;254(Suppl 1):S117–22.
8. Atula T, Markkola A, Leivo I, et al. Cartilage invasion of laryngeal cancer detected by magnetic resonance imaging. Eur Arch Otorhinolaryngol 2001; 258(6):272–5.
9. Boss A, Stegger L, Bisdas S, et al. Feasibility of simultaneous PET/MR imaging in the head and upper neck area. Eur Radiol 2011;21(7):1439–46.
10. Platzek I, Beuthien-Baumann B, Schneider M, et al. PET/MRI in head and neck cancer: initial experience. Eur J Nucl Med Mol Imaging 2013;40(1):6–11.
11. Covello M, Cavaliere C, Aiello M, et al. Simultaneous PET/MR head-neck cancer imaging: preliminary clinical experience and multiparametric evaluation. Eur J Radiol 2015;84(7):1269–76.
12. Rasmussen JH, Norgaard M, Hansen AE, et al. Feasibility of multiparametric imaging with PET/MR in head and neck squamous cell carcinoma. J Nucl Med 2017;58(1):69–74.
13. Martinez-Moller A, Eiber M, Nekolla SG, et al. Workflow and scan protocol considerations for integrated whole-body PET/MRI in oncology. J Nucl Med 2012; 53(9):1415–26.
14. Finck SJ, Giuliano AE, Morton DL. LDH and melanoma. Cancer 1983;51(5):840–3.
15. Jouvet JC, Thomas L, Thomson V, et al. Whole-body MRI with diffusion-weighted sequences compared

with 18 FDG PET-CT, CT and superficial lymph node ultrasonography in the staging of advanced cutaneous melanoma: a prospective study. J Eur Acad Dermatol Venereol 2014;28(2):176–85.

16. Laurent V, Trausch G, Bruot O, et al. Comparative study of two whole-body imaging techniques in the case of melanoma metastases: advantages of multi-contrast MRI examination including a diffusion-weighted sequence in comparison with PET-CT. Eur J Radiol 2010;75(3):376–83.

17. Pfannenberg C, Aschoff P, Schanz S, et al. Prospective comparison of 18F-fluorodeoxyglucose positron emission tomography/computed tomography and whole-body magnetic resonance imaging in staging of advanced malignant melanoma. Eur J Cancer 2007;43(3):557–64.

18. Burris NS, Johnson KM, Larson PE, et al. Detection of small pulmonary nodules with ultrashort echo time sequences in oncology patients by using a PET/MR system. Radiology 2016;278(1):239–46.

19. Strobel K, Dummer R, Steinert HC, et al. Chemotherapy response assessment in stage IV melanoma patients—comparison of 18F-FDG-PET/CT, CT, brain MRI, and tumormarker S-100B. Eur J Nucl Med Mol Imaging 2008;35(10):1786–95.

20. Beloueche-Babari M, Jamin Y, Arunan V, et al. Acute tumour response to the MEK1/2 inhibitor selumetinib (AZD6244, ARRY-142886) evaluated by non-invasive diffusion-weighted MRI. Br J Cancer 2013; 109(6):1562–9.

21. Liao LJ, Lo WC, Hsu WL, et al. Detection of cervical lymph node metastasis in head and neck cancer patients with clinically N0 neck—a meta-analysis comparing different imaging modalities. BMC Cancer 2012;12:236.

22. Klerkx WM, Bax L, Veldhuis WB, et al. Detection of lymph node metastases by gadolinium-enhanced magnetic resonance imaging: systematic review and meta-analysis. J Natl Cancer Inst 2010;102(4): 244–53.

23. Som PM. Detection of metastasis in cervical lymph nodes: CT and MR criteria and differential diagnosis. AJR Am J Roentgenol 1992;158(5):961–9.

24. Sakai O, Curtin HD, Romo LV, et al. Lymph node pathology. Benign proliferative, lymphoma, and metastatic disease. Radiol Clin North Am 2000;38(5): 979–98, x.

25. King AD, Tse GM, Yuen EH, et al. Comparison of CT and MR imaging for the detection of extranodal neoplastic spread in metastatic neck nodes. Eur J Radiol 2004;52(3):264–70.

26. Krabbe CA, Pruim J, Dijkstra PU, et al. 18F-FDG PET as a routine posttreatment surveillance tool in oral and oropharyngeal squamous cell carcinoma: a prospective study. J Nucl Med 2009;50(12):1940–7.

27. Hoang JK, Choudhury KR, Chang J, et al. Diffusion-weighted imaging for head and neck squamous cell

carcinoma: quantifying repeatability to understand early treatment-induced change. AJR Am J Roentgenol 2014;203(5):1104–8.

28. Abdel Razek AA, Kandeel AY, Soliman N, et al. Role of diffusion-weighted echo-planar MR imaging in differentiation of residual or recurrent head and neck tumors and posttreatment changes. AJNR Am J Neuroradiol 2007;28(6):1146–52.

29. von Schulthess GK, Kuhn FP, Kaufmann P, et al. Clinical positron emission tomography/magnetic resonance imaging applications. Semin Nucl Med 2013;43(1):3–10.

30. Huang SH, Chien CY, Lin WC, et al. A comparative study of fused FDG PET/MRI, PET/CT, MRI, and CT imaging for assessing surrounding tissue invasion of advanced buccal squamous cell carcinoma. Clin Nucl Med 2011;36(7):518–25.

31. Schaarschmidt BM, Heusch P, Buchbender C, et al. Locoregional tumour evaluation of squamous cell carcinoma in the head and neck area: a comparison between MRI, PET/CT and integrated PET/MRI. Eur J Nucl Med Mol Imaging 2016;43(1):92–102.

32. Ruhlmann V, Ruhlmann M, Bellendorf A, et al. Hybrid imaging for detection of carcinoma of unknown primary: a preliminary comparison trial of whole-body PET/MRI versus PET/CT. Eur J Radiol 2016;85(11): 1941–7.

33. Xiao Y, Chen Y, Shi Y, et al. The value of fluorine-18 fluorodeoxyglucose PET/MRI in the diagnosis of head and neck carcinoma: a meta-analysis. Nucl Med Commun 2015;36(4):312–8.

34. Pinkston JA, Cole P. Incidence rates of salivary gland tumors: results from a population-based study. Otolaryngol Head Neck Surg 1999;120(6): 834–40.

35. Razfar A, Heron DE, Branstetter BF, et al. Positron emission tomography-computed tomography adds to the management of salivary gland malignancies. Laryngoscope 2010;120(4):734–8.

36. Otsuka H, Graham MM, Kogame M, et al. The impact of FDG-PET in the management of patients with salivary gland malignancy. Ann Nucl Med 2005;19(8):691–4.

37. Lee YY, Wong KT, King AD, et al. Imaging of salivary gland tumours. Eur J Radiol 2008;66(3):419–36.

38. Makis W, Ciarallo A, Gotra A. Clinical significance of parotid gland incidentalomas on (18)F-FDG PET/CT. Clin Imaging 2015;39(4):667–71.

39. Avram AM, Fig LM, Frey KA, et al. Preablation 131-I scans with SPECT/CT in postoperative thyroid cancer patients: what is the impact on staging? J Clin Endocrinol Metab 2013;98(3):1163–71.

40. Chen MK, Yasrebi M, Samii J, et al. The utility of I-123 pretherapy scan in I-131 radioiodine therapy for thyroid cancer. Thyroid 2012;22(3):304–9.

41. Van Nostrand D, Aiken M, Atkins F, et al. The utility of radioiodine scans prior to iodine 131 ablation in

patients with well-differentiated thyroid cancer. Thyroid 2009;19(8):849–55.

42. Nagarajah J, Jentzen W, Hartung V, et al. Diagnosis and dosimetry in differentiated thyroid carcinoma using 124I PET: comparison of PET/MRI vs PET/CT of the neck. Eur J Nucl Med Mol Imaging 2011; 38(10):1862–8.

43. Santhanam P, Taieb D, Solnes L, et al. Utility of I 124 PET/CT In identifying radioiodine avid lesions in differentiated thyroid cancer; a systematic review and meta-analysis. Clin Endocrinol (Oxf) 2017; 86(5):645–51.

44. Haugen BR, Alexander EK, Bible KC, et al. 2015 American Thyroid Association management guidelines for adult patients with thyroid nodules and differentiated thyroid cancer: the American Thyroid Association guidelines task force on thyroid nodules and differentiated thyroid cancer. Thyroid 2016; 26(1):1–133.

45. Vrachimis A, Burg MC, Wenning C, et al. [(18)F]FDG PET/CT outperforms [(18)F]FDG PET/MRI in differentiated thyroid cancer. Eur J Nucl Med Mol Imaging 2016;43(2):212–20.

46. Seiboth L, Van Nostrand D, Wartofsky L, et al. Utility of PET/neck MRI digital fusion images in the management of recurrent or persistent thyroid cancer. Thyroid 2008;18(2):103–11.

47. Archier A, Heimburger C, Guerin C, et al. (18)F-DOPA PET/CT in the diagnosis and localization of persistent medullary thyroid carcinoma. Eur J Nucl Med Mol Imaging 2016;43(6):1027–33.

48. Tran K, Khan S, Taghizadehasl M, et al. Gallium-68 Dotatate PET/CT is superior to other imaging modalities in the detection of medullary carcinoma of the thyroid in the presence of high serum calcitonin. Hell J Nucl Med 2015;18(1):19–24.

49. Ozkan ZG, Kuyumcu S, Uzum AK, et al. Comparison of (6)(8)Ga-DOTATATE PET-CT, (1)(8)F-FDG PET-CT and 99mTc-(V)DMSA scintigraphy in the detection of recurrent or metastatic medullary thyroid carcinoma. Nucl Med Commun 2015;36(3): 242–50.

50. Evangelista L, Farsad M, Piotto A, et al. 18F-DOPA and 18F-FDG PET/CT, scintigraphic localization and radioguided surgery of recurrent medullary thyroid cancer: two case reports. Curr Radiopharm 2014;7(2):133–7.

51. Jiang J, Yang Z, Zhang Y, et al. Clinical value of [(18)F] FDG-PET/CT in the detection of metastatic medullary thyroid cancer. Clin Imaging 2014;38(6):797–801.

52. Salavati A, Puranik A, Kulkarni HR, et al. Peptide receptor radionuclide therapy (PRRT) of medullary and nonmedullary thyroid cancer using radiolabeled somatostatin analogues. Semin Nucl Med 2016; 46(3):215–24.

53. Lee G, I H, Kim SJ, et al. Clinical implication of PET/MR imaging in preoperative esophageal cancer staging: comparison with PET/CT, endoscopic ultrasonography, and CT. J Nucl Med 2014;55(8):1242–7.

54. Le Y, Chen Y, Zhou F, et al. Comparative diagnostic value of 18F-fluoride PET-CT versus MRI for skull-base bone invasion in nasopharyngeal carcinoma. Nucl Med Commun 2016;37(10):1062–8.

55. Yang J, Jian Y, Jenkins N, et al. Quantitative evaluation of atlas-based attenuation correction for brain PET in an integrated time-of-flight PET/MR imaging system. Radiology 2017;284(1):169–79.

56. Leclerc M, Lartigau E, Lacornerie T, et al. Primary tumor delineation based on (18)FDG PET for locally advanced head and neck cancer treated by chemoradiotherapy. Radiother Oncol 2015;116(1):87–93.

57. Leibfarth S, Monnich D, Welz S, et al. A strategy for multimodal deformable image registration to integrate PET/MR into radiotherapy treatment planning. Acta Oncol 2013;52(7):1353–9.

58. Bhatnagar P, Subesinghe M, Patel C, et al. Functional imaging for radiation treatment planning, response assessment, and adaptive therapy in head and neck cancer. Radiographics 2013;33(7):1909–29.

59. Woods C, Sohn J, Machtay M, et al. Radiation treatment planning for head and neck cancer with PET. PET Clin 2012;7(4):395–410.

60. Wang K, Mullins BT, Falchook AD, et al. Evaluation of PET/MRI for tumor volume delineation for head and neck cancer. Front Oncol 2017;7:8.

61. Garg PK, Nazih R, Wu Y, et al. 4-[11C]Methoxy N-(2-diethylaminoethyl) benzamide: a novel probe to selectively target melanoma. J Nucl Med 2017; 58(5):827–32.

62. Rizzo-Padoin N, Chaussard M, Vignal N, et al. [18F] MEL050 as a melanin-targeted PET tracer: fully automated radiosynthesis and comparison to 18F-FDG for the detection of pigmented melanoma in mice primary subcutaneous tumors and pulmonary metastases. Nucl Med Biol 2016;43(12):773–80.

63. Natarajan A, Mayer AT, Xu L, et al. Novel radiotracer for immunoPET imaging of PD-1 checkpoint expression on tumor infiltrating lymphocytes. Bioconjug Chem 2015;26(10):2062–9.

64. Kuker R, Sztejnberg M, Gulec S. I-124 imaging and dosimetry. Mol Imaging Radionucl Ther 2017; 26(Suppl 1):66–73.

65. Lutje S, Gomez B, Cohnen J, et al. Imaging of prostate-specific membrane antigen expression in metastatic differentiated thyroid cancer using 68Ga-HBED-CC-PSMA PET/CT. Clin Nucl Med 2017;42(1):20–5.

66. Lee YZ, Ramalho J, Kessler B. PET-MR imaging in head and neck. Magn Reson Imaging Clin N Am 2017;25(2):315–24.

Moving?

Make sure your subscription moves with you!

To notify us of your new address, find your **Clinics Account Number** (located on your mailing label above your name), and contact customer service at:

Email: journalscustomerservice-usa@elsevier.com

800-654-2452 (subscribers in the U.S. & Canada)
314-447-8871 (subscribers outside of the U.S. & Canada)

Fax number: 314-447-8029

Elsevier Health Sciences Division
Subscription Customer Service
3251 Riverport Lane
Maryland Heights, MO 63043

*To ensure uninterrupted delivery of your subscription, please notify us at least 4 weeks in advance of move.

Printed and bound by CPI Group (UK) Ltd, Croydon, CR0 4YY

08/05/2025

01864707-0003